Recent Results
in Cancer Research

91

Clinical Interest
of Steroid Hormone Receptors
in Breast Cancer

Edited by
G. Leclercq S. Toma R. Paridaens J. C. Heuson

With 74 Figures and 122 Tables

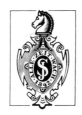

Springer-Verlag
Berlin Heidelberg New York Tokyo 1984

Professor Dr. G. Leclercq
Professor Dr. R. Paridaens
Professor Dr. J. C. Heuson
Institute Jules Bordet, Centre des Tumeurs de
l'Université Libre de Bruxelles, Service de Medicine,
Clinique et Laboratoire de Cancerologie Mammaire
Rue Héger-Bordet 1, 1000 Bruxelles, Belgium

Professor Dr. S. Toma
Istituto Nazionale per la Ricerca sul Cancro,
Istituto per lo Studio e la Cura dei Tumori,
Istituto di Oncologia Sperimentale e Clinica dell'Università,
Viale Benedetto XV n. 10, 16132 Genova, Italy

Sponsored by the Swiss League against Cancer

ISBN 3-540-13042-X Springer-Verlag Berlin Heidelberg New York Tokyo
ISBN 0-387-13042-X Springer-Verlag New York Heidelberg Berlin Tokyo

Library of Congress Cataloging in Publication Data. Main entry under title: Clinical interest of steroid hormone receptors in breast cancer. (Recent results in cancer research; 91) "Sponsored by the Swiss League against Cancer" – T.p. verso. Bibliography: p. Includes index. 1. Breast – Cancer – Endocrine aspects – Addresses, essays, lectures. 2. Steroid hormones – Receptors – Addresses, essays, lectures. I. Leclercq, G. II. Schweizerische Nationalliga für Krebsbekämpfung und Krebsforschung. III. Series: Recent results in cancer research; v. 91. [DNLM: 1. Receptors, Steroid. 2. Breast neoplasms. 3. Receptors, Estrogen. 4. Receptors, Progesterone. W1 RE106P v. 91 / WP 870 C639] RC261.R35 vol. 91 616.99'4s 83-20321 [RC280.B8] [616.99'449061].

© Springer-Verlag Berlin Heidelberg 1984
Printed in Germany.

The use of registered names, trademarks, etc. in the publication does not imply, even in the absence of a specific statement, that such names are exempt from the relevant protective laws and regulations and therefore free for general use.

Product Liability: The publisher can give no guarantee for information about drug dosage and application thereof contained in this book. In every individual case the respective user must check its accuracy by consulting other pharmaceutical literature.

Typesetting and printing: v. Starck'sche Druckereigesellschaft m.b.H., Wiesbaden
Binding: J. Schäffer OHG, Grünstadt

2125/3140—5 4 3 2 1 0

Preface

Several papers dealing with the clinical relevance of steroid hormone receptors in breast cancer have already been published. However, no publication has overviewed studies currently being conducted in Europe, nor is there a register of the european centers performing receptor assays. It has been our purpose to fill these gaps.

A large majority of authors who we contacted kindly agreed to contribute to our book. Papers were grouped into six main parts according to their contents. The abundance of clinical data relevant to receptor assays led us to add critical summaries to help the reader to form his own opinions on the subject. We would like to thank Drs. R. J. B. King, G. Contesso, L. Santi, and E. Engelsman, who helped us in this regard.

We hope that this book will enable the reader to become acquainted with the present state of European steroid hormone receptor studies devoted to breast cancer treatment. We also hope that it will promote cooperation between European oncologists involved in this field of research.

The editors

Contents

Contents

List of Contributors*

---

* The address of the principal author is given on the first page of each contribution
1 Page, on which contribution commences

Part I. Receptor Assays

Classical Methods

Sampling and Storage of Breast Cancer Tissue for Steroid Receptor Assays

G. Nicolò, A. Carbone, M. Esposito, and L. Santi

Istituto Nazionale per la Ricerca sul Caucro, Istituto Scientifico
per lo Studio e la Cura dei Tumori, Istituto di Oncologia Sperimentale e Clinica
dell' Università, Viale Benedetto XV n. 10, 16132 Genova, Italy

Introduction

Ablative or pharmacological endocrine treatment is effective in only one-third of all patients with advanced breast cancer [2, 15]. Until comparatively recently, clinical or biochemical data useful in identifying a breast cancer's hormone dependency were not available. Consequently a large number of patients needlessly underwent surgical procedures and chemotherapy was used indiscriminately, often excluding the possibility of a less damaging treatment for patients with hormone-dependent breast cancer. In the past two decades, however, basic studies on the action of steroid hormones on target tissues such as the uterus have contributed to the development of methods capable of selecting, before the start of therapy, patients who will respond to endocrine treatment.

Folca [8], in 1961, demonstrated a characteristically increased in vivo concentration of ^{3}H-hexoestrol in breast cancer metastatic tissue from patients responsive to adrenalectomy. At the same time, Jensen and Jacobson [14] suggested that target tissues such as the uterus may bind and retain estrogen steroids. In 1966, Toft and Gorsky [26], using sucrose density gradients, identified the cytoplasmic substances responsible for estrogenic retention, the so-called *estrogenic receptors* (ER).

Finally, in 1968 Koreman [17] proposed a quantitative assay of uterine ER, the dextran-coated charcoal (DCC) assay, that adsorbs the unreacted free hormone. This technique, used in conjunction with the Scatchard plot analysis, is the most commonly employed method for assaying various hormones, including 17-β-estradiol and progesterone. The DCC assay is rapid, inexpensive, and as least as sensitive as the other more complicated techniques [20].

* The authors would like to thank the following colleagues who kindly cooperated in filling out the questionnaire: Dr. H. Braunsberg, Department of Clinical Pathology, St. Mary's Hospital Medical School, London, England; Dr. G. Contesso, Institut Gustave Roussy, Villejuif, France; Dr. M. F. Duffy, Nuclear Medicine Laboratory, St. Vincent's Hospital, Dublin, Ireland; Dr. R. A. Hawkins, Department of Clinical Surgery, University Medical School, Edinburgh, Scotland; Dr. R. Leake, Department of Biochemistry, University of Glasgow, Scotland; Dr. G. Leclercq, Istitut Jules Bordet, Bruxelles, Belgium; Dr. H. Magdalenat, Institut Curie, Paris, France; Dr. A. Piffanelli, Instituto di Radiologia, Università di Ferrara, Italy; Dr. S. Saez, Centre Leon Berard, Lyon, France

Recent studies involving the application of this quantitative assay of steroid receptors in primitive and advanced breast cancer have provided the following clinical results:

1. The percentage of primitive breast cancers with ER positivity ranges from 63% in patients under 50 years old to 76% in patients over 50 years old [19], and from 67% in premenopausal patients to 78% in postmenopausal patients [16]. The absolute receptor content also varies with age [18].

2. For metastatic breast cancer tissue, the percentage of ER positivity ranges from 48% in patients under 50 years old to 69% in patients over 50 years old [19]. A recent review of the literature shows that the worldwide ER+ percentages range from 67% in 2,250 cases of primitive breast carcinoma to 57% in 775 cases in which metastatic breast cancer tissue was analyzed.

3. ER determinations from different tumor sites in a patient with multiple metastases coincide in 85% of simultaneously performed biopsies [1]. Assay values agree in 91% of two or more biopsy samples (primitive tumor and metastasis) obtained at separate times from the same patients [16], while the percentage of agreement decreases to 82% when the ER determination has been carried out on samples of metastatic tissue obtained at different times in a patient who has undergone various types of therapy [16]. Moreover, the absolute ER content may decrease after endocrine treatment [1]. These results demonstrate that the determination of hormone dependency in the majority of primitive tumors is of value in planning therapeutic strategy. This is true even several years after the initial diagnosis, when metastases occur. The progression of disease and endocrine treatment can, however, modify the hormone dependency of the tumor.

4. For advanced carcinoma of the breast the average rate of response to different types of endocrine therapy is 54% [12] and seems to be strictly correlated with the absolute content of receptors [2].

5. The percentage of response to endocrine therapy increases to 77% in the ER+ PgR+ (progesterone receptor) groups [23] and may increase to 90% in the ER+ PgR+ subgroup with positive nuclear receptor values [4].

6. A response rate of less than 10% occurs in those patients whose tumors are lacking ER [18]. A response rate of about 30% may be encountered in the ER+ PgR− group [19], while the rate of response has not been evaluated in the ER− PgR+ group because of its low frequency [19]. Finally, the response rate to endocrine therapy is 0% in the ER− PgR− subgroup with nuclear receptor negativity [4].

7. In a study based on 281 patients with primitive breast cancer, Knight et al. [15] demonstrated that during a 24-month follow-up the risk of recurrence was significantly higher in ER− than in ER+ groups.

8. Independently, Hähnel [10] and Furmansky et al. [9] reported a statistically significant difference of survival between ER+ and ER− groups, irrespective of lymph node status. Their studies were based on 335 and 422 primitive breast carcinoma patients respectively, and the follow-up periods were 58 and 40 months.

Even though many observations still need further confirmation, global clinical results appear to be very important and in some ways conclusive in breast cancer management. For this reason it is mandatory that the quantitative determination of steroid receptor levels is reliable and reproducible. It is consequently of major interest to handle with a precise and possibly standardized procedure all tumor tissues which have to be sampled and stored for the hormone dependency biochemical assay.

Some Guidelines for a Standardized Sampling and Storage Procedure

A good working relationship between the surgical pathologist and the biochemist is extremely important for the correct *sampling* and *storage* of specimens for the receptor assay.

If one reviews the steps occurring between the operating room and the biochemical laboratory, the following points must be emphasized:

1. Each tissue sample should be sent to the laboratory with a special form containing the recommended guidelines for collecting and delivering specimens for steroid receptor analyses. This form should stress that the receptors (ER, PgR) are particularly thermolabile proteins. It should be clearly stated that the specimens must be cooled immediately after excision. To this end it may be useful to place the sample in a clean dry plastic bag sealed by squeezing out excess air, packed with ice on all sides.
2. The following information must be listed by the clinician on the above-mentioned form: (a) type and source of tissue, (b) time of excision and/or loss of blood supply to the nearest minute, (c) time of placing on ice, and (d) time of freezing.
3. The following pertinent clinical data should be reported: (a) endocrine status of premenopausal patients (date of commencement of the most recent menstrual bleeding), (b) postmenopausal status (early or late), (c) previous castration, (d) prior radiotherapy, (e) types of gonadal steroid therapy performed during the past 6 months, and (f) smoker or nonsmoker (preliminary results of Daniell's [7] study suggested that breast tumors are more frequently ER+ in nonsmokers [68%] than in smokers [39%] patients).

Sampling

The surgical pathologist, if not part of the surgical team, must be located as close as possible to the operating room. He/she has the responsibility of grossly analyzing the surgical specimen, detecting the lesion, and taking the samples for frozen section examination and the steroid receptor assay.

It is our experience, and that of others [3], that tissue sampling by someone other than a pathologist may lead to an incorrect microscopic diagnosis or false-negative receptor assay due to incorrect gross examination of the excised tissue, particularly when the tumor is very small.

A correct plan of tissue sampling for steroid receptors is based on some well-established concepts. A wide range of cytoplasmic receptor concentrations, varying from two- to sevenfold, have been observed in different zones of control endocrine-dependent organs such as the uterus and in breast tumors [11, 24, 25]. Therefore the pathologist should follow a standardized tissue sampling procedure similar to the one elaborated by Silfverswärd et al. [25] in their study on a sample mapping of the cytoplasmic and nuclear ER concentrations. They examined 0.5 cm thick slices obtained by two parallel cuts close to the "equator" of the tumor. The slices were further subdivided into four quadrants or into concentric rings. Quadrants taken from a single slice of the same tumor showed approximately two fold differences in receptor levels. Furthermore, in postmenopausal women cytoplasmic ER concentrations were lower in the central zones while the intranuclear receptor levels were lower at the periphery of the disc. In premenopausal women, higher levels of intranuclear receptors were observed in the central areas of the tumor, while the total amount of receptors in the cytoplasm was much lower than that in

Table 1. ER values and neoplastic cellularity in breast carcinoma tissue and lymph node metastases

Case no.	Age (years)	pTNM classification[a]	Grading (G) (WHO)	ER value[b] (fmol/mg prot. cyt.)	Cellularity[c]	Fibrosis[c]	Necrosis[c]
1	78	pT4b pN1biii	G2	T 39.77	++++	+/−	−
2	63	pT2a pN0	G1	T 22.00	++++	+/−	−
3	63	pT4b pN0	G3	T 43.50	++	++	−
4	66	pT2a pN0	G2	T 56.00	++++	+/−	−
5	58	pT4b pN2	G3	T 79.60	++++	+/−	+/−
6	47	pT2a pN0	G2	T 13.72	++	++	−
7	57	pT1a pN1biii	G2	T 40.00	++	++	−
8	53	pT1a pN0	G1	T 15.00	++	++	−
9	38	pT1a pN1a	G1	T 21.80	+++	+	−
10	41	pT3b pN1biii	G2	T −	++	++	−
				L 15.10	++++	−	−
11	48	pT4b pN1biii	G2	T −	++	++	−
				L −	+++	+	−
12	45	pT4b pNIbiii	G2	T 9.50	++	++	−
				L 16.20	++++	− −	−
13	57	pT4b pN1biii	G3	T −	++	+/++	+/−
				L −	+/−	++	+++
14	51	pT4b pN1biii	G3	T −	++	+	−
				L −	++	++	+
15	38	pT3a pN1biv	G1	T 0.90	++	++	−
				L 8.00	+++	+/−	−

[a] Classification according to the guidelines of the International Union Against Cancer
[b] T, primary tumor; L, lymph node metastasis
[c] The degree of cellularity was evaluated on histological specimens. −, absent; +/−, 0−25%; +, 25%

the nucleus, possibly reflecting an effective in vivo translocation of receptor to the nucleus.

In conclusion, sampling must include the center and periphery of a complete equatorial slice of the tumor. Particular attention should be paid to eliminating non-neoplastic tissue, such as fatty and necrotic tissue, which may interfere with the assay.

The pathologist should also perform a parallel tissue section for microscopic evaluation on frozen sections and for investigation of other morphological parameters (degree of cellularity, fibrosis, elastosis, necrosis, lymphocyte infiltration).

Furthermore receptor levels in recurrent carcinomas should be tested, even when primary values are available, and involved lymph nodes, which due to their high neoplastic cellularity often reflect the true receptor status of the tumor, should be routinely assayed. Lymph node assays showing an increased level of steroid receptors can better predict a positive response to hormone therapy, without being subject to the intratumoral variations [13] seen in the primitive tumor. Table 1 shows a series of consecutive ER assays in primitive breast cancer and lymph node metastasis. One can see a good correlation between neoplastic cellularity and ER positivity. In five of nine cases (numbered 1−9) the neoplastic cellularity of the primary tumor was very high and in none of the remaining cases was it less than 50% of total cellularity. In three of six cases with additional metastatic tissue analysis (numbered 10−15), ER value positivity was correlated with neoplastic cellularity. In two of these three cases only the ER assay on metastatic lymph nodes was positive.

Usually, the amount of material required for a reliable assay with the DCC method and Scatchard plot analysis of at least six points ranges from 200 to 500 mg for each type of steroid receptor. However, in some instances so much material is not available, e.g., when a patient is not operable owing to an advanced cancer or when there are small cutaneous recurrences or visceral or skeletal metastases. In these cases the receptor content can be assayed on as little as 25−30 mg of tissue using the single saturating concentration method.

In our laboratory, correlation of results obtained with (a) the DCC method in conjunction with the Scatchard plot and (b) a single saturating concentration method was very good in 36 consecutive assays, with $r = 0.99$ and $P < 0.001$ (Fig. 1).

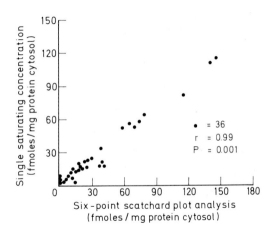

Fig. 1. Comparison between results obtained with a single saturating concentration method and the six-point Scatchard plot

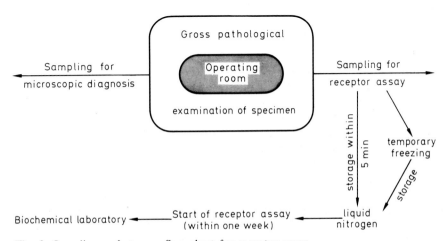

Fig. 2. Sampling and storage flow chart for receptor assay

Table 2. Handling of breast cancer tissue for steroid hormone receptors assay

Questionnaire	Ferrara	Brussels	Paris	Lyon
1. Who selects the specimens	A nuclear physician	A pathologist	A pathologist	A pathologist and a biochemist
2. Plan of sampling and type of material	On "growing head" of primary tumor and lymph nodes	On primary tumor at random	On primary tumor; at random on drill biopsy	Several pieces on primary tumor, nodes and any kind of metastases
3. Amount of tissue sampled lacking necrotic and fatty areas	–	–	25 mg	250 mg (DCC) 160 mg (hydroxyl-apatite)
4. Freezing method	Liquid nitrogen	Liquid nitrogen	At −30° C (large surgical samples); liquid nitrogen (small or drill biopsy)	Liquid nitrogen
5. Time of storage in liquid nitrogen	10−20 days	7−14 days	8 days at −30° C	2−14 days
6. Histological checking of tumor tissue	Routinely performed (including tumor grading)	Routinely performed	Routinely performed	Routinely performed
7. Method of checking cellularity	None	None	Fluorimetric DNA determination	Histologically

Two other kinds of specimens can be utilized for the steroid receptor assay: (a) a frozen section fluorescently stained by immunological and/or cytochemical means and (b) material obtained by fine-needle aspiration which may be analyzed with polyacrylamide isoelectrofocusing. A major advantage of the cytochemical technique is its ability to identify those breast carcinomas having a heterogeneous cellular population with only a small number of ER+ cells. These carcinomas, though often giving a positive biochemical result, fail to respond to endocrine therapy.

These procedures are relatively new methods of steroid receptor assays whose sensitivity has yet to be evaluated.

Villejuif	Glasgow	London	Dublin	Edinburgh	Genova
A pathologist	A surgeon or a pathologist	A surgeon	A pathologist	A pathologist or a biochemist	A pathologist
On primary tumor and metastatic nodes	On many parts of primary tumor and other localizations	–	On the section opposite that used for histology	On the centre of the primary tumor and lymph node/s	On a central disc of the primary tumor nodes and recurrences
100–200 mg (DCC) 20 mg (microtechnique)	–	25–50 mg	–	160–250 mg	250 mg
Liquid nitrogen	At −20° C in 50% glycerol; in liquid nitrogen	–	Liquid nitrogen	Usually tumor is analyzed fresh by homogenization at 0° C	Liquid nitrogen
2–3 days	Within 30 days	–	Not longer than 30 days	1–7 days	7–30 days
Routinely performed	Routinely performed	Routinely performed	Routinely performed	Routinely performed	Routinely performed
Histologically	DNA assay	DNA assay	None	None	Histologically

Freezing and Storage

Rapid cooling of the sample to below 0° C and its storage at a very low temperature are important steps in reducing the number of borderline and false-negative results.

To minimize the amount of ER protein denaturation, a tumor slice of 0.5–1 g obtained by the aforementioned procedures should be trimmed, dry bottled, and quick frozen directly in liquid nitrogen ($-321°$ F, $-196°$ C), 5 or 10 min after surgical excision. Steroid binding activity seems to be stable for up to 3 or 4 months in liquid nitrogen.

Hawkins [11] has demonstrated that repeated control assays of amounts of rabbit uterus cytosol from samples stored at −196° C showed 16.6% variation over a 4-month period. Greater variation was seen beyond this time. Muschenheim [21] reported that shipment of a sample from a peripheral hospital to the central biochemical laboratory in liquid nitrogen seems to increase the incidence of positive ER tests (69.3% > 3 fmol/mg protein cytosol) when compared with shipment in dry ice or by other means (56%).

If immediate freezing in liquid nitrogen is not possible, fairly quick and effective preliminary freezing can be performed using a dry ice system or by the cryostat technique at −20° C. Organic solvent must be avoided. The related risk of denaturing with these methods may be eliminated by wrapping the tissue samples in tin foil.

Brown [6] reported that results analogous to those obtained with liquid nitrogen were obtained by a fast-freezing technique employing a fluorinate hydrocarbon spray, Criokwik (commonly used in several pathology laboratories), and further storage at −70° C for up to 1 week. The storage of samples at −70° C for more than 4 weeks should be avoided due to the enormous amount (80%) of receptor lost [22].

It seems that reliable results are closely related to the time interval between surgical excision and the beginning of the freezing procedure. This interval must not be greater than the time needed for the pathologist to perform a gross examination of the specimen (Fig. 2). The procedure of sample and storage depicted in Fig. 2 has led to an increase in the number of positives from 53.8% to 70% in Bordin's laboratory [5].

However, it seems worth emphasizing that the sampling and consequent storage for the steroid receptor assay should be avoided in the following instances:

1. *When a diagnostic doubt exists about the nature of the lesion.* Histological interpretation of the specimens is more difficult on sections obtained from paraffin-embedded tissues which have been frozen.
2. *When a tumor consists of multiple small foci* (of 2−3 mm in diameter) *with intraductal carcinoma or in situ lobular carcinoma.* In these instances a cytochemical analysis of steroid receptors should be considered.

In conclusion, Table 2 lists some important points in the handling and storage of breast cancer tissue for the steroid receptor assay as performed by 10 european laboratories, according to the answers to a questionnaire recently circulated by us.

References

1. Allegra JC, Barlock A, Huff K, Lippman ME (1980) Changes in multiple or sequential estrogen receptor determinations in breast cancer. Cancer 45: 792−794
2. Allegra JC, Lippman ME, Thompson EB, Simon R, Barlock A, Green L, Huff KK, Do HMT, Aitken SC, Warren R (1980) Estrogen receptor status: an important variable in predicting response to endocrine therapy in metastatic breast cancer. Eur J Cancer 16: 323−331
3. Assor D, Meyer DL (1979) Estrogen receptor assay. Letter to the editor. Am J Clin Pathol 72: 130
4. Barnes DM, Skinner LG, Ribeiro GG (1979) Triple hormone receptor-assay: a more accurate predictive-tool for the treatment of advanced breast cancer? Br J Cancer 40: 862−865
5. Bordin GM (1979) Estrogen-receptor assay. Letter to the editor. Am J Clin Pathol 72: 129
6. Brown PW, Witorsch J, Banks WL, Lawrence W (1977) Freezing and storage of breast cancer tissue for estrogen receptor protein assay. Arch Surg 112: 183−185
7. Daniell HW (1980) Estrogen receptors, breast cancer, and smoking. N Engl J Med 302: 1478
8. Folca PJ, Glascock RF, Irvine WT (1961) Studies with tritium-labelled hexoestrol in advanced breast cancer: comparison of tissue accumulation of hexoestrol with response to bilateral adrenalectomy and oophorectomy. Lancet 2: 796−798

9. Furmanski P, Saunders DE, Samuel BS, Brooks C, Marvin AR, The Breast Cancer Prognostic Study Clinical and Pathology Associates (1980) The prognostic value of estrogen receptor determinations in patients with primary breast cancer. Cancer 46: 2794—2796

10. Hähnel R, Woodgings T, Vivian AB (1979) Prognostic value of estrogen receptors in primary breast cancer. Cancer 44: 671—675

11. Hawkins RA, Hill A, Freedman B, Gore SM, Roberts MMO, Forrest APM (1977) Reproducibility of measurements of oestrogen receptor concentration in breast cancer. Br J Cancer 36: 355—361

12. Hawkins RA, Roberts MM, Forrest APM (1980) Oestrogen receptors and breast cancer: current status. Br J Surg 67: 153—169

13. Hoen JL, Plotka ED, Dickson KB (1978) Comparison of estrogen receptor levels in primary and regional metastatic carcinoma of the breast. Ann Surg 100: 69—71

14. Jensen EV, Jacobson HI (1962) Basic guides to the mechanism of estrogen action. Recent Prog Horm Res 18: 387

15. Knight WA III, Osborne CK, Yochmowitz MG, McGuire LW (1980) Steroid hormone receptors in the management of human breast cancer. Ann Clin Res 12: 202—207

16. Koenders A, Beex L, Smals A, Kloppenborg P, Benraad TH (1980) Oestradiol and progesterone receptors in multiple tumors specimens from patients with breast cancer. Neth J Med 23: 62—67

17. Korenman SG (1968) Radioligand binding assay of specific estrogen using a soluble uterine macromolecule. J Clin Endocrinol Metab 28: 127—130

18. Lippman ME, Allegra JC (1978) Receptors in breast cancer. N Engl J Med 299: 930—933

19. McGuire WL (1980) Steroid receptors and clinical breast cancer. In: Bresciani F (ed) Perspective in steroid receptor research. Raven, New York, p 239

20. McGuire WL, Carbone PP, Sears ME, Escher GC (1975) Estrogen receptors in human breast cancer: an overview. In: McGuire WL, Carbone PP, Vollmer EP (eds) Estrogen receptors in human breast cancer. Raven, New York, p 1

21. Muschenheim F, Furst J, Bates HA (1978) Increased incidence of positive tests for estrogen binding in mammary carcinoma specimens transported in liquid nitrogen. Am J Clin Pathol 70: 780—782

22. Namkung PC, Moe RE, Petra PM (1979) Stability of estrogen receptor assay in frozen human breast tumor tissue. Cancer Res 39: 1124—1125

23. Osborne KC, McGuire WL (1979) The use of steroid hormone receptors in the treatment of human breast cancer: a review. Bull Cancer 66: 203—210

24. Romano M, Cerra M, Cecco L, Panza N (1979) DNA and oestradiol receptor distribution in human breast cancer. Tumori 65: 687—694

25. Silfverswärd G, Skoog L, Humla S, Gustafsson SA, Nordenskföld D (1980) Intratumoral variation of cytoplasmatic and nuclear estrogen receptor concentrations in human mammary carcinoma. Eur J Cancer 16: 59—65

26. Toft D, Gorski J (1966) A receptor molecule for estrogens: isolation from the rat uterus and preliminary characterization. Proc Natl Acad Sci USA 55: 1574

Routine Assays for Steroid Hormone Receptors*

G. Leclercq

Institut Jules Bordet, Centre des Tumeurs de l'Université Libre de Bruxelles,
Service de Médicine, Clinique et Laboratoire de Cancérologie Mammaire,
Rue Héger-Bordet 1, 1000 Bruxelles, Belgium

Introduction

Breast cancers contain specific receptors for estrogens, progestins, androgens, and corticoids. Numerous biochemical methods have been developed for their detection. All are based on the demonstration of a saturable binding capacity for a given radiolabeled steroid. Up to now, almost all assays have been restricted to cytoplasmic receptors. Recently, however, some laboratories have introduced tests for nuclear receptors. One may speculate that this new trend will gather momentum in the near future (see chapter by S. Cowan et al.).

It is not the purpose of the present chapter to review all methods; only routine assays will be described. For additional information, I refer the reader to an extensive review [1].

Main Steps in the Receptor Assays

The homogenization of the tumor sample is the first step in the assay. The homogenate is then centrifuged at 100,000 g to obtain the cytosol fraction. In the next step, the cytosol is incubated with appropriate ^{3}H-labeled steroids and competitors (see below). Thereafter, most unbound and nonspecifically bound steroids are removed by a dextran-coated charcoal (DCC) treatment. The remaining radioactivity is finally measured by scintillation counting in order to evaluate the concentration of labeled complexes.

Specific labeled complexes may be distinguished from the nonspecific binding by one of the following two methods.

1. In the incubation step, two cytosol fractions are incubated with a saturating concentration of ^{3}H-steroid. A large excess of an unlabeled steroid or specific competitor is added to one of the fractions in order to distinguish specific from nonspecific binding. The difference in bound radioactivity between the two fractions gives the receptor concentration.

2. Aliquots of cytosol are incubated with increasing amounts of ^{3}H-steroid (an excess of unlabeled competitor is often used in a parallel incubation to measure the nonspecific

* This work was supported by a grant from the Fonds Cancérologique de la Caisse Générale d'Epargne et de Retraite de Belgique

binding). The specificity of the binding reaction is determined by the graphical method of Scatchard [2]. A sloping straight line pattern indicates the presence of only one binder. The dissociation constant of the binding reaction (K_d) is measured by the magnitude of the reverse of the slope of the line. K_d values of the order of $10^{-10}-10^{-9} M$ are indicative of a specific receptor. The binding capacity of the cytosol (i.e. the receptor concentration) is measured at the intersection of the line with the abscissa. Nonlinear patterns are usually obtained when the cytosol is contaminated by large amounts of plasma binding proteins (SHBG, CBG, etc.). In such cases, an extrapolating procedure is required for evaluating the binding parameters of the specific reaction (see chapter by H. Braunsberg).

Several studies have shown that these techniques are equivalent for evaluating receptor concentration. The area of uncertainty is only in the low range which is at the limit of sensitivity of both assays [3−5]. Nevertheless, in practice the measurement of an appropriate K_d value always adds confidence to the specificity of the binding reaction. The "single-point assay" should therefore be recommended only when multiple steroid receptor analyses are required in small biopsy specimens.

Additional information about the specificity of the binding reaction can be obtained from agar gel electrophoresis, which clearly distinguishes receptors from contaminating serum proteins [6]. This technique, requiring expensive equipment, has been introduced in only a limited number of laboratories, most of which are located in the Federal Republic of Germany or the Netherlands. On the other hand, the molecular size of the binding proteins may be obtained from sucrose density gradient sedimentation. The receptors usually migrate as aggregates of which the sedimentation coefficients are close to 4 and 8 S. The therapeutic relevance of the evaluation of these coefficients is still a matter of controversy [7, 8].

Appropriate ³H-Labeled Steroids for Receptor Assays

Accurate measurement of steroid hormone receptors requires the use of specific ligands with low binding affinity for plasma contaminants.

Estrogen Receptors

³H-estradiol is widely used for the measurement of the estrogen receptor. The use of another potent estrogen, *moxestrol* (R-2858; 11β-methoxy-17-ethynyl estratriene-3,17β-diol), has been proposed in order to improve the accuracy of the assay. Unlike estradiol, this steroid does not bind with high affinity to plasma SHBG. In a correlation study with ³H-moxestrol and ³H-estradiol, Raynaud et al. [9] reported that determination with ³H-estradiol usually overestimated the binding reaction at low binding site concentration. A similar study from our laboratory partially confirmed this observation (Fig. 1). Thus in most cases bound ³H-estradiol was higher than bound ³H-moxestrol at low binding site concentration (≤ 40 fmol/mg tissue protein). However, almost all cytosols devoid of ³H-moxestrol binding sites were also devoid of ³H-estradiol binding sites (34/40), indicating that the latter ligand rarely produced false-positive results. At high binding site concentration, determinations with both ligands correlated extremely well (only 2 discrepancies out of 39 assays). Methodological differences in receptor assay might be

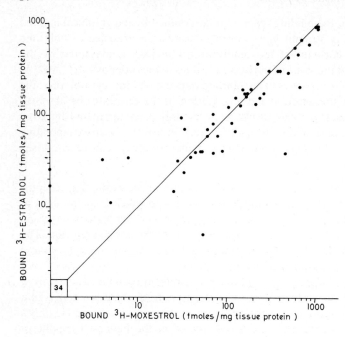

Fig. 1. Correlation between estrogen binding sites assayed with ^{3}H-estradiol and ^{3}H-moxestrol. The assays were conducted according to the EORTC recommendations [21]

responsible for the partial discrepancy between Raynaud's study and ours. In the former, determinations were carried out with a single-point assay. We used a Scatchard plot analysis, which is more accurate than the single-point assay at low binding site concentrations. Therefore it is our impression that the use of ^{3}H-moxestrol instead of ^{3}H-estradiol would not markedly improve the accuracy of the assay in a Scatchard plot analysis. In single-point assays, ^{3}H-moxestrol might be recommended.

Progesterone Receptors

Progesterone binds with high binding affinity to plasma CBG. In the progesterone receptor assay this problem has been solved by replacing ^{3}H-progesterone with one of two ^{3}H-progestins: *promegestone* (R-5020; 17,21-dimethyl-19-nor-4,9-pregnadiene-3,20-dione) [10] or *ORG-2058* (16α-ethyl-21-hydroxy-19-nor-4-pregnene-3,20-dione) [12]. These two steroids appear equally effective [12].

Androgen Receptors

Dihydrotestosterone binds with high affinity to plasma SHBG. ^{3}H-Dihydrotestosterone cannot be used for measuring the androgen receptor since this ligand cannot be removed from SHBG by a DCC treatment (*note:* ^{3}H-DHT can be used with agar gel electrophoresis [6]). In contrast, another ^{3}H-androgen, *methyltrienolone* (R-1881; 17β-hydroxy-17α-methylestra 4,9,11-trien-3-one) has proved powerful in the detection of the androgen receptor [13, 14]. However, this compound also binds to the progesterone receptor, and an excess of triamcinolone acetonide is required to suppress this undesirable reaction [14].

Corticoid Receptors

Corticoid receptor assays using ³H-dexamethasone as radioligand and unlabeled dexamethasone as competitor do not discriminate between glucocorticoid and mineralocorticoid receptors which could be present either alone or together in the cytosols [15]. Each receptor may be assayed according to the following protocol: (a) glucocorticoid: ³H-dexamethasone in the presence of aldosterone; (b) mineralocorticoid: ³H-aldosterone alone.

The Need for Quantitative Assessment

Several investigators have classified mammary cancers into two distinct populations on the basis of the presence or absence of steroid receptors. For this purpose, they usually used the lower limit of accuracy of their assay as a cut-off point. However, no evidence was offered on the existence of two such populations. With regard to estrogen and progesterone receptors (those which were mainly studied), binding sites range from very low to very high values. These values appear to fall in a log normal distribution. Finally, some benign mammary lesions also contain small amounts of receptors, and consequently cannot be distinguished from neoplastic lesions on a qualitative basis.

These considerations led to the suggestion that quantitative rather than qualitative assessment is required for characterization of the tumors. This is supported by the fact that the receptor concentration is influenced by endogenous hormonal levels (i.e., estrogen receptor levels are usually lower in pre- than in postmenopausal women; see chapter by S. Saez and C. Chouvet). Moreover, in advanced disease the probability of obtaining a remission with endocrine therapy is directly related to the estrogen receptor concentration [16].

Various reference parameters have been used to define the receptor concentration [17]. In most recent studies, the binding capacity is expressed in femtomoles (10^{-15} mol) per milligram of total cytosol protein. In some laboratories, including ours, it is expressed in femtomoles per milligram of tissue protein after correction for contaminating serum proteins. For assessing tissue protein, serum albumin is measured by radialimmunodiffusion and the following formula applied [6]:

tissue protein = total protein − serum albumin × 100/60.

Limitations of the DCC Assay

In the DCC assay, underestimation of the receptor concentration occurs if the protein concentration is below a critical level (~ 1 mg/ml) [3, 18, 19]. This leads to inaccurate measurement in cytosols from very small tumor specimens and considerably limits the usefulness of the technique. However, for estrogen receptors this underestimation can be minimized if 1 mg/ml of bovine serum albumin is added to the DCC solution [19].

Suggestion for Future Development of Routine Assays

During the past 5 years particular emphasis has been placed on the measurement of estrogen and progesterone receptors. In contrast, only a few investigations have been devoted to androgen and corticoid receptors. Therefore in future studies it would be of interest to evaluate whether assaying all steroid receptors will increase the therapeutic value of the test. However, the difficulty of obtaining large amounts of tissue is a considerable drawback with this approach.

The development of routine assays requiring less tissue is another topic of interest for clinical laboratories (see chapters by H. Magdelenat and C. Silfverswärd et al.). In this regard, a single test using a mixture of ^{125}I-estradiol and ^{3}H-R-5020 for the simultaneous measurement of estrogen and progesterone receptors [20] might be extremely helpful. Finally, efforts should be made to standardize assays [21, 22] in order to limit the source of errors in cooperative trials.

References

1. Chamnes GC, McGuire WL (1979) Steroid receptor assay methods in human breast cancer. In: Thompson EB, Lippman ME (eds) Steroid receptors and the management ov cancer. CRC, Boca Raton, pp 3−30
2. Scatchard G (1949) The attraction of proteins for small molecules and ions. Ann NY Acad Sci 51: 660−672
3. Leclercq G, Heuson JC, Schoenfeld R, Mattheiem WH, Tagnon HJ (1973) Estrogen receptors in human breast cancer. Eur J Cancer 9: 665−673
4. McGuire WL, de la Garza M, Chamness GC (1977) Evaluation of estrogen assays in human breast cancer tissue. Cancer Res 37: 637−639
5. Mulder J, Verhaar MAT (1979) A comparative study on estradiol receptor assays in human breast tissue. Clin Chim Acta 99: 129−134
6. Wagner RK (1972) Characterization and assay of steroid hormone receptors and steroid-binding proteins by agar-gel electrophoresis at low temperature. Hoppe Seylers Z Physiol Chem 353: 1235−1245
7. Wittliff JL, Lewko WM, Park D, Kute TE, Baker DT, Kane LN (1978) Steroid binding proteins of mammary tissues and their clinical significance in breast cancer. In: McGuire WL (ed) Hormones, receptors and breast cancer. Raven, New York, pp 325−359
8. Freedman B, Hawkins RA (1980) Sedimentation profiles of the oestrogen receptor from breast tumours of man and rat using vertical-tube rotor centrifugation. J Endocrinol 86: 431−442
9. Raynaud JP, Martin PM, Bouton MM, Ojasoo T (1978) 11β Methoxy-17-ethynyl-1,3,5(10)-estratiene-3,17β-diol (Moxestrol), a tag for estrogen receptor binding site in human tissues. Cancer Res 38: 3044−3050
10. McGuire WL, Raynaud JP, Baulieu EE (1977) Progesterone receptors in normal and neoplastic tissues. Raven, New York
11. Keightley DD (1979) The binding of progesterone, R-5020 and ORG-2058 to progesterone receptor. Eur J Cancer 15: 785−790
12. Duffy MJ, Duffy GJ (1979) Studies on progesterone receptors in human breast carcinomas: use of natural and synthetic ligands. Eur J Cancer 15: 1181−1184
13. Bonne C, Raynaud JP (1975) Methyltrienolone, a specific ligand for androgen receptors. Steroids 26: 227−232
14. Zava DT, Landrum B, Horwitz KB, McGuire WL (1979) Androgen receptor assay with [^{3}H]methyltrienolone (R 1881) in the presence of progesterone receptors. Endocrinology 104: 1007−1012
15. Martin PM, Rolland MP, Raynaud JP (1981) Macromolecular binding of dexamethasone as evidence for the presence of mineralo-corticoids in human breast cancer. Cancer Res 41: 1222−1226
16. Paridaens R, Sylvester RJ, Ferrazzi E, Legros N, Leclercq G, Heuson JC (1980) Clinical significance of the quantitative assessment of estrogen receptors in advanced breast cancer. Cancer 46: 2889−2895

17. Hähnel R, Twadde E (1978) Estradiol binding by human breast carcinoma cytosols: the influence of commonly used reference parameters on the results. Eur J Cancer 14: 125–131
18. Poulsen HS (1981) Oestrogen receptor assay. Limitation of the assay. Eur J Cancer 17: 495–501
19. Powel BL, de la Graza M, Clark GM, McGuire WL (1981) Estrogen receptor measurement in low protein breast cancer cytosols. Breast Cancer Res Treat 1: 33–35
20. Thibodeau SN, Freeman L, Jiang NS (1981) Simultaneous measurement of estrogen and progesterone receptors in tumor cytosols with use of ^{125}I-labeled estradiol and ^{3}H-R 5020. Clin Chem 27: 687–691
21. EORTC Breast Cancer Cooperative Group (1973) Standard for the assessment of estrogen receptors in human breast cancer. Eur J Cancer 9: 379–381
22. EORTC Breast Cancer Cooperative Group (1980) Revision of the standards for the assessment of hormone receptors in human breast cancer. Eur J Cancer 16: 1513–1515

Mathematical Analysis of Data from Receptor Assays

H. Braunsberg

Department of Chemical Pathology, St. Mary's Hospital Medical School,
London W2 1PG, United Kingdom

Introduction

Work on the receptor status of human malignant breast tumours has passed from an initial qualitative stage to the realization that quantitative aspects may be of clinical importance [12, 15]. Estimates of receptor site concentrations depend not only on the chemical analytical technique used but also on the method of calculation [4, 5, 13, 17]. Several approaches to the mathematical analysis of receptor data can be considered and recent work has shown that accuracy may be improved by the use of techniques not previously applied to receptor assays [4, 5, 13].

In their target tissues, steroids may be bound by (a) intracellular hormone receptors, (b) other intracellular binding sites and (c) components thought to be derived from plasma constituents, such as albumin, sex hormone binding globulin (SHBG) and corticosteroid binding globulin (CBG). The hormone receptors display high affinities for their natural hormones. Oestradiol receptors (ER) of human tissues have dissociation constants (K_d) in the range $10^{-11}-10^{-10}$ M, while those for complexes of progesterone receptors (PgR) with progesterone are of the order of 10^{-9} M. The receptor binding sites are present at relatively low concentrations and receptors are characterized as high affinity-low capacity components. Binding sites other than those of receptors generally have lower affinities and greater capacities for steroid hormones. In this class, intracellular components which bind to oestradiol with K_d 40 times greater than those for receptors have been described [6]. It has been suggested that these may play a role in hormone action [6]. Even lower affinities and very large capacities generally characterize other binding sites, including those believed to be of extracellular origin, but the CBG-like material may have an affinity for progesterone which is of the same order as that of PgR.

The estimation of specific receptor parameters involves the resolution of binding data into high affinity-low capacity (receptor) and low affinity-high capacity (non-receptor) components as well as the estimation of receptor site concentrations, $[R]_T$, and the association or dissociation constants, K_a or K_d, as measures of affinity. Calculations can be effected by estimating total and non-receptor ("non-specific") binding and subtracting the latter before use of equations based on a single type of binding component (Receptor Model). This approach is used widely at present. Alternatively, curves representing total binding and covering four to five orders of magnitude of ligand concentrations can be resolved mathematically into several distinguishable binding sites (Multicomponent Model). There is no fundamental difference between these two approaches, and as computers and programmable calculators are now available for use in this work, it is possible that the Multicomponent Model, mathematical analysis of which is more complex, will be explored and used more widely.

Receptor Model

The interaction between a hormone and its receptor can be described by the equilibrium

$$R + H \rightleftharpoons RH$$

In the absence of any other binding components, an expression for the concentration of steroid bound to the receptor can be derived from the mass action equation:

$$[R][H]/[RH] = K_d \qquad (1)$$

where $[R]$ and $[H]$ are the concentrations of unbound receptor and hormone, respectively, and $[RH]$ is the concentration of receptor-bound hormone. The total receptor concentration is given by:

$$[R]_T = [R] + [RH] \qquad (2)$$

and writing B and F for concentrations of bound and unbound steroid one obtains

$$K_d = ([R]_T - B)F/B \qquad (3)$$
$$B = F[R]_T/(F + K_d) \qquad (4)$$

It should be noted that B is the concentration of steroid bound to a class of receptor molecules, not necessarily to a single compound only. The estimation of $[R]_T$ and K_d (or $K_a = 1/K_d$) is facilitated by the rearrangement of Eq. (3) and various forms of linear plots have been derived [8, 13, 14, 19]. However, all tissues contain steroid binding components other than receptors and these equations can only be applied after correction for non-receptor binding.

Correction for "Non-specific" Binding Components

Binding to non-receptor sites can be estimated or eliminated by making use of their greater capacity [cf. 6], lower affinity [9] or greater heat stability [11, 20] as compared with receptors. The use of hormone analogues which bind to receptors but not to components related to steroid binding globulins may reduce non-specific binding [16] but these steroids bind to other sites present, including albumin, and their use still requires correction of binding data.

Provided that the concentration of steroid bound to non-specific sites and in equilibrium with a given concentration of unbound hormone can be estimated with some accuracy, the receptor-bound moiety in a mixture can be determined. A survey of methods of calculation used in 19 specialist laboratories [3] revealed that such corrections were made by four different methods, only one of which [18] was theoretically sound. In practice, the use of such erroneous methods of calculation led to relatively small discrepancies for estimates of $[R]_T$, though larger errors in estimates of K_d were encountered [4]. With the use of a programmable calculator the correct method [18] of subtracting non-specific components presents no problem, and it has the advantage of simultaneously correcting for reagent blanks and for any dissociation of ligand from low affinity components during analysis [4]. The relationship between estimates of non-specifically bound and unbound steroid can be determined in the absence of receptor binding [11, 20] or at high ligand concentrations at which receptor binding is negligible as compared with non-specific binding. If $[P]$, the total concentration of non-specific sites, and K_{NS}, their dissociation constant, are very large compared with $[R]_T$ and K_d, then at ligand concentrations not exceeding $10^{-6} M$

$$B_{NS}/F_{NS} \sim [P]/K_{NS}$$

where B_{NS} and F_{NS} are non-specifically bound and unbound ligand moieties in the absence of significant receptor binding. If B_N/F_{NS} can be shown to be constant in the range of ligand concentrations used in the receptor assay, then a straight line

$$B_{NS} = k\ F_{NS}$$

can be fitted to non-specific binding data, where k is a constant. For any concentration of unbound ligand in equilibrium with receptor, a value of B_{NS} can be subtracted from the total ligand bound in the presence of receptor.

If several distinguishable classes of non-receptor sites are present, or if $[P]$ or K_{NS} are relatively low, B_{NS}/F_{NS} may not be constant in the relevant range of ligand concentrations. In addition, methodological factors may cause changes in this ratio [4]. In this situation, curve fitting presents a more complex problem. In practice, however, approximations based on pairs of estimates of B_{NS} and F_{NS} permit sufficiently accurate estimates of non-specifically bound ligand to be deducted [4].

A linear relationship between B_{NS} and F_{NS} cannot be assumed and should be established in each receptor assay. This is best done by examining the B_{NS}/F_{NS} ratios over a wide range of ligand concentrations.

Linear Plots

Several equations derived from the Mass Action equation can be used to obtain linear plots [cf. 4, 7, 13]. It should be noted that all these expressions relate to equilibrium between receptor and hormone and are not strictly applicable in non-equilibrium situations. The Scatchard plot [19] has been used most widely in one of its forms:

$$B/F = [R]_T/K_d - B/K_d \tag{5}$$

Both B and F depend on the total ligand concentration, T, and neither B/F nor B is an independent variable. The data should, therefore, also be plotted according to the equation

$$B = [R]_T - (B/F)K_d \tag{6}$$

For perfect data these equations give identical estimates of $[R]_T$ and K_d. Analytical results are rarely perfect and the arithmetic or geometric means of estimates of each parameter obtained by means of both equations may give more reliable results [17]. This applies to other linear plots.

Use of the Lineweaver-Burk plot [14] has been examined recently [4, 13]. The equations can be written

$$1/B = (K_d/[R]_T)(1/F) + 1/[R]_T \tag{7}$$
$$1/F = ([R]_T/K_d)(1/B) - 1/K_d \tag{8}$$

Table 1. Data from Colquhoun [cf. 13] recalculated by least squares (L.S.) and unweighted robust (U.R.) regression fitting using Eqs. (5) (Scatchard) and (9) (Woolf). The theoretical values for $[R]_T$ and K_d were 30.0 and 0.150 respectively

	Scatchard		Woolf	
	$[R]_T$	K_d	$[R]_T$	K_d
L.S.	28.29	0.121	30.64	0.145
U.R.	27.99	0.120	28.20	0.123

When this method is employed, accuracy is improved by inclusion of more low ligand concentrations than are usually used for Scatchard plots. With an experimental design more suitable for Scatchard plots, Eq. (7) performed poorly in the presence of outliers [13]. However, this method might offer some advantages for analytical methods with higher precision at low than at high ligand concentrations. This may apply, for example, to dextran-coated charcoal methods for the separation of bound from unbound steroids, since very large amounts of unbound hormone (at high concentrations) may be adsorbed incompletely and cause variable contamination of the bound moiety.

$$F/B = (1/[R]_T)F + K_d/[R]_T \tag{9}$$
$$F = ([R]_T F/B) - K_d \tag{10}$$

Equation (9) has been claimed to give more accurate results than the Scatchard and Lineweaver-Burk plots when "outliers" are present [13]. However, this conclusion is hardly justified. The results calculated by Keightley and Cressie [13] from data of Colquhoun contained an error, and there was, in fact, little difference between results calculated from Scatchard and Woolf plots, as shown in Table 1.

Keightley and Cressie reported values of 30.64 and 30.87 for $[R]_T$ and 0.145 and 0.147 for K_d for the Woolf plot and concluded that this method was independent of the line fitting technique. The correct values, however, show more variation than the Scatchard results, which are also close to the theoretical values.

The direct linear plot [8] is obtained by expressing the Mass Action equation as

$$([R]_T/B) - (K_d/F) = 1 \tag{11}$$

and its use has been explained in detail [4]. The best estimates of K_d and $[R]_T$ are obtained by finding the median values of

$$X_{i,j} \ (i \neq j) = (B_j - B_i)/(B_i/F_i - B_j/F_j) \tag{12}$$
$$Y_{i,j} \ (i \neq j) = (B_i/F_i)X_{i,j} + B_i \tag{13}$$

This method of calculation may give more accurate results than the Scatchard plot fitted by least squares regression [5, 7].

Non-linear Plots

The Proportion Graph [1] consists of plotting log B/T and log F/T against log T, where $T = B + F$. This yields two curves from which $[R]_T$ and K_a can be estimated. The authors point out its relative complexity and suggest that its use may not be justified when only a single binding system is present. The method requires ligands with high specific activity since very low concentrations are required for accurate estimation of K_a, while $[R]_T$ is estimated from higher ligand concentrations.

Non-logarithmic curves of B and F against T can be fitted to avoid certain statistical disadvantages of the linear plots [17]. With a single class of binding site the equations are:

$$B^2 - (R + T + 1/K_a)B + RT = 0 \qquad\qquad (14)$$
$$F^2 + (R - T + 1/K_a)F - 1/K_a = 0 \qquad\qquad (15)$$

T can be considered the independent variable with relatively small errors (1%−2%), and the variances of B and F are likely to be more uniform than those of B/F or F/B used in Scatchard or Woolf plots [1, 17].

The calculation of receptor parameters from both types of non-linear plot is more complex than that using linear plots. It can, however, be carried out on computers or programmable calculators and several programs have been developed [1, 17].

Applicability of the Receptor Model

The Receptor Model is almost invariably used after correction for non-specific binding in assays applied to breast cancer tissues. However, it is by no means certain that it is always appropriate. Non-receptor species whose dissociation constants or capacities or both do not exceed those of receptors by more than one or two orders of magnitude cannot be estimated by means of the higher ligand concentrations frequently used for estimating non-specific sites. Examples are the CBG-like binding sites for progesterone and the "type II" intracellular binding sites for oestradiol [6]. When such components present a problem, methods employing heat denaturation [11] or the exploitation of differences in affinity [6] can lead to accurate receptor assays. These approaches have not been used widely. Another situation in which the Receptor Model cannot be applied arises from incomplete dissociation of ligand bound to low affinity sites as reported [2] when the method of Feherty et al. [9] was used.

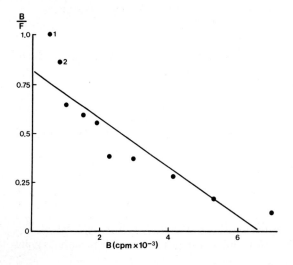

Fig. 1. Scatchard plot with two possible outliers

Detection of deviations must take experimental errors into account and would require 10 or more ligand concentrations ranging over two or three orders of magnitude. Even then it is often difficult to decide whether an apparent divergence is real or due to outliers. The Scatchard plot shown in Fig. 1 shows an example. Point 1 could be considered an outlier and the line refitted after rejecting it. As shown in Fig. 2, this leads to point 2 appearing as an unacceptable outlier. Recalculation after rejection of both points 1 and 2 produces a reasonable linear plot with some scatter of points (Fig. 3). However, a hand-drawn curve (which may or may not accurately represent a multicomponent system) would appear to give a better fit (Fig. 4). In such a case a full analysis requires goodness of fit data for several possible models rather than arbitrary rejection of data. In assays on breast tumours, the receptor binding sites, after correction for non-specific binding, generally appear to represent a single class of high affinity-low capacity components. However, many laboratories employ only four or five ligand concentrations with a limited range. Thus multiple classes of binding sites may not be detected and high-affinity components may be overestimated more often than is realized [6]. The detection of multiple binding sites may

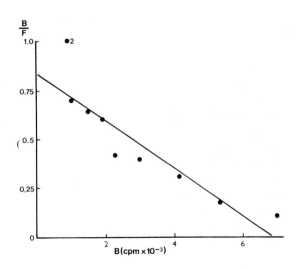

Fig. 2. Line fitted to data of Fig. 1 after rejection of one outlier

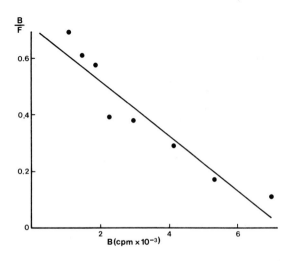

Fig. 3. Line fitted to data of Fig. 2 after rejection of a further point

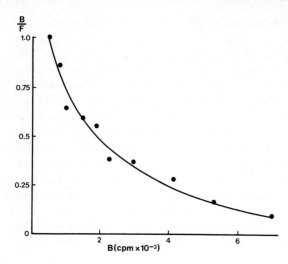

Fig. 4. Data shown in Fig. 1 showing curvature

require a study of the affinity distributions of tissue preparations [17]. Relatively large amounts of tissue with an adequate number of ligand concentrations (20 or more) are required for such studies, and suitable large tumours are often available. So far, this aspect has not been examined adequately.

Multicomponent Model

When no correction is made for non-receptor binding or when such corrections are inadequate, the "linear" equations yield curved plots which must be resolved into their components. Alternatively, the Proportion Graph [1] or the plots suggested by Rodbard et al. [17] can be used.

The resolution of the Scatchard plot into two or more components has received considerable attention [6, 17, 18]. The graphical curve peeling of Rosenthal [18] has been criticised as being tedious and subjective while failing to produce estimates of precision of the fitted parameters [17]. An improved iterative technique has been proposed [17] but no comparisons of the use of these methods for experimental data are available.

The Proportion Graph has been used to resolve oestradiol receptor and non-specific binding as well as testosterone binding to both SHBG and CBG, for which association constants appeared to differ by a factor of 5. The number and range of ligand concentrations needed in these experiments were not stated. No comparisons of this method with that of Rosenthal have been published.

Plots of B or B/T against T [17] can be resolved into two or three classes of binding sites given sufficient data points. The appropriate equations are given by Rodbard et al. [17], and computer programs are available for their solution. Applications of this method to experimental data and comparisons with other techniques remain to be examined.

The Effects of Outliers

Receptor assays are subject to considerable errors. Apart from pipetting and other analytical errors, cumulative counting errors may increase the variance of B or F at high or low ligand concentrations [4]. Attention has also been drawn to the non-uniformity of variance of B/F (used in the Scatchard plot), which may be subject to very large errors at high ligand concentrations [17]. Most workers use a least squares (L.S.) method of regression analysis for Scatchard plots. It has been suggested that a "weighted" method should be used and that outliers must be rejected using reliable and objective rules [17]. However, the estimation of appropriate weights presents some problems, as does the definition of criteria for rejecting outliers. A recent survey of methods of calculation used in 19 specialist laboratories indicated that arbitrary rejection of data was the major cause of variation between estimates of receptor parameters [3]. Often, the rejection of one point leads to a further apparent outlier (Figs. 1, 2).

Methods other than L.S. linear regression analysis have recently been tried [13]. An unweighted robust (U.R.) regression analysis appeared to give more reliable estimates of receptor parameters when outliers were present. As in the direct linear plot, all possible pairs of values for B and F are used to calculate medians of estimates of the slope, β, and of the intercept, α, on the ordinate axis:

$$\beta = \operatorname*{med}_{i \neq j} (B_i/F_i - B_j/F_j)/(B_i - B_j) \tag{16}$$

$$\alpha = \operatorname*{med}_{i \neq j} \{ {}^1\!/_2 (B_i/F_i + B_j/F_j - {}^1\!/_2\beta(B_i + B_j)) \} \tag{17}$$

Comparisons of the Scatchard, Lineweaver-Burk and Woolf plots indicated that the latter was least affected by outliers when the U.R. regression analysis was used [13]. However, the examination of the effect of outliers was based on a five-point assay (in duplicate) over a 25-fold range of concentrations with three of the duplicates at relatively high concentrations and none near the ordinate axis of the Scatchard plot. This may have created unfavourable conditions for the Scatchard plot in comparison with the Woolf plot. When these data are recalculated using five single points only (Table 2), there is little to choose between the Scatchard and Woolf plots (Table 3). As shown by Keightley and Cressie [13], the effect of outliers is reduced considerably when the U.R. rather than L.S. regression analysis is used. The direct linear plot performed well in the presence of an

Table 2. Data for a five-point assay adapted from Keightley and Cressie [13] without (B) and with (B′) outliers. Total = bound plus unbound ligand present

Total	B	B′	Code
53.4	16.1	8.0	1A
		24.6	1B
102.7	26.2	–	–
361.8	43.4	22.2	3A
		65.1	3B
653.5	45.9	–	–
1,320.1	49.6	24.9	5A
		74.4	5B

Table 3. Effect of outliers in a five-point assay on estimates of $[R]_T$ obtained by three linear plot methods. Data and codes as shown in Table 2. Least squares (L.S.) and unweighted robust (U.R.) regression analysis. Figures in parentheses represent values expressed as per cent of results without outliers

Outlier	Scatchard		Woolf		Direct linear
	L.S.	U.R.	L.S.	U.R.	
None	53.3	53.4	52.5	52.6	54.9
1A	71.9 (135)	53.0 (99)	56.3 (107)	54.0 (103)	89.0 (162)
1B	49.4 (93)	50.5 (95)	51.4 (98)	51.0 (97)	47.0 (86)
3A	53.7 (101)	53.0 (99)	55.2 (105)	52.6 (100)	52.2 (95)
3B	76.5 (144)	61.9 (116)	51.5 (98)	52.6 (100)	60.3 (110)
5A	54.6 (102)	53.9 (101)	25.4 (48)	50.1 (95)	53.4 (97)
5B	72.2 (135)	60.0 (112)	81.3 (155)	60.1 (114)	57.7 (105)

Table 4. Effect of outliers in a five-point assay on estimates of K_d obtained by three linear plot methods. The results without outliers are expressed in arbitrary units and those with outliers are shown as per cent of result without an outlier in each case. Data and codes as shown in Table 2; r, correlation coefficient for least squares (L.S.) regression analysis

Outlier	Scatchard			Woolf			Direct linear
	r	L.S.	U.R.	r	L.S.	U.R.	
None	− 0.996	8.35	8.34	1.000	7.85	8.09	8.34
1A	− 0.606	290	109	0.989	196	70	96
1B	− 0.866	48	59	0.999	73	67	62
3A	− 0.714	136	110	0.943	243	106	96
3B	− 0.712	195	127	0.993	56	100	101
5A	− 0.620	139	105	0.970	Negative	86	68
5B	− 0.892	178	122	0.960	300	126	123

underestimate of B at a relatively low concentration. Estimates of K_d were more seriously affected by outliers even when the U.R. regression was used (Table 4). The direct linear and Woolf plots tended to give low and the Scatchard plot high estimates of K_d. The three linear plots were further compared for results with 10 single points more evenly spread over a 30-fold range of ligand concentrations (Table 5). Outliers were calculated by reducing or increasing the total bound ligand of tubes 1, 5, 7, and 10 by 25% without altering the non-specific binding (Fig. 5). The correction for non-specific binding was made by a Rosenthal-type calculation from a L.S. regression line for bound versus unbound ligand [4]. The results shown in Table 6 and Fig. 6 indicate that when the U.R. regression analysis was used, estimates of $[R]_T$ by Scatchard plots were marginally better than those by Woolf plots. The direct linear plot performed poorly with outliers at very low ligand concentration but seemed satisfactory in all other cases. Results for K_d are shown in Table 7 and Fig. 7. The direct linear plot gave consistent estimates for K_d while those from Scatchard plots were slightly better than those from Woolf plots.

Table 5. Data for ten-point receptor assay

Tube	Total ligand (cpm)	Total bound (cpm)	Non-specifically bound (cpm)
1	214	88	20
2	275	104	36
3	452	167	54
4	651	222	65
5	984	329	104
6	1,289	364	214
7	2,046	581	221
8	2,885	736	300
9	4,362	905	466
10	6,334	1,167	709

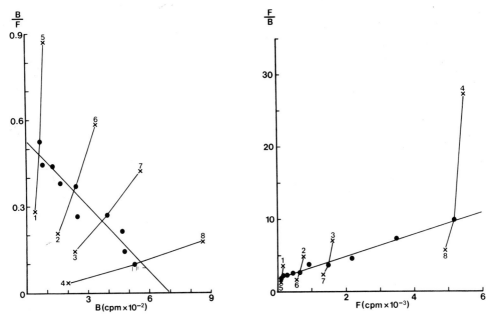

Fig. 5. Data of Table 5 shown as *(left)* Scatchard and *(right)* Woolf plots. Outliers were calculated by reducing (points 1−4) or increasing (points 5−8) the values of total ligand bound for samples 1, 5, 7, and 10 by 25%

Thus, the claim that the Woolf plot performs better in the presence of outliers than the Scatchard plot [13] is not supported by these results, while the improved performance obtained by U.R. regression analysis is confirmed. It would be of interest to compare results obtained with these calculations and those proposed by Rodbard et al. [17]. The effect of outliers on the resolution of multicomponent models has not been evaluated. It would be of interest to examine the performance of different methods of mathematical analysis with a view to choosing one least affected by outliers.

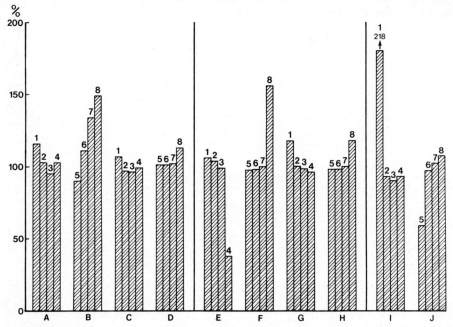

Fig. 6. Effect of single outliers on estimates of receptor site concentration calculated from Scatchard (A−D) and Woolf (E−H) plots using L.S. (A, B, E, F) and U.R. (C, D, G, H) regression and from direct linear plot (I, J). The numbers of columns correspond to those of outliers in Fig. 5. Results expressed as per cent of value obtained in the absence of an outlier

Table 6. Effect of outliers on estimates of $[R]_T$ using a ten-point assay. Results expressed as pmol per gram tissue. Regression coefficients (r) for L.S.

Outlier	Scatchard			Woolf			Direct linear
	r	L.S.	U.R.	r	L.S.	U.R.	
None	− 0.957	4.72	4.70	0.994	4.48	4.52	4.16
1A	− 0.827	5.49	5.05	0.975	4.77	5.36	9.06
1B	− 0.803	4.25	4.75	0.989	4.37	4.45	2.47
5A	− 0.851	4.86	4.57	0.964	4.67	4.51	3.86
5B	− 0.758	5.22	4.77	0.987	4.39	4.45	4.04
7A	− 0.868	4.49	4.54	0.947	4.45	4.43	3.74
7B	− 0.715	6.31	4.80	0.978	4.46	4.51	4.24
10A	− 0.661	4.87	4.64	0.902	1.71	4.33	3.86
10B	− 0.850	7.03	5.31	0.898	6.99	5.36	4.45

Conclusions

National and international analytical quality control schemes have revealed considerable variations in the quantitative results returned by different laboratories. Discrepancies may arise from differences in methods and equipment for the disintegration of tissues, in analytical techniques, in random rejection of data and in methods of calculation of receptor

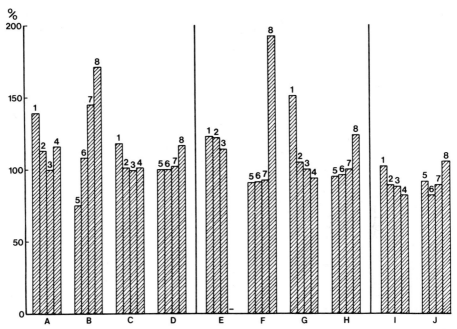

Fig. 7. Effect of single outliers on estimates of dissociation constant. For explanation see legend to Fig. 6. Outlier 4 caused a negative estimate when the Woolf plot was fitted by L.S. regression

Table 7. Effect of outliners on estimates of K_d (pM) using a ten-point assay

Outlier	Scatchard		Woolf		Direct linear
	L.S.	U.R.	L.S.	U.R.	
None	41.0	40.5	37.7	38.4	40.5
1A	56.8	47.9	46.5	57.9	41.1
1B	30.7	40.5	34.1	36.4	37.1
5A	46.4	40.9	45.9	40.2	36.0
5B	43.4	40.5	34.6	36.7	33.2
7A	41.1	40.3	43.2	38.6	35.7
7B	59.6	41.1	35.0	38.3	36.0
10A	47.5	36.1	Negative	36.1	33.2
10B	69.9	47.5	72.4	47.5	42.5

parameters. If results of receptor assays carried out in different laboratories are to be compared, attention must be paid to details of all these aspects of methodology.

The calculations used routinely in clinical studies on breast cancer are seriously affected by variations resulting from experimental error. Furthermore, the model based on a single class of binding sites may not be applicable in all cases, and the imposition of such an assumption on data obtained with too few, or too narrow a range of, ligand concentrations may lead to considerable errors in estimates of receptor site concentrations. The use of assays with 10 or more ligand concentrations and additional estimates of non-specific binding may not be feasible in busy laboratories or when amounts of tissue are limited. Several methods of detecting multiple classes of binding sites have been proposed recently [17] and more thorough studies of the binding components of breast tumours are still needed. If the Receptor Model is found to be valid, then U.R. regression analysis of Scatchard plots would seem to be the method of choice and apparent outliers should not be rejected. If, however, convincing evidence were obtained of frequent interference by non-receptor components, the reliability of different multicomponent curve fitting procedures should be investigated.

The accuracy of receptor assays depends as much on the choice of a reliable method of calculation as on good analytical techniques. Improved mathematical treatments and computer programs for their use are becoming available and should help to improve the reliability of quantitative receptor data.

References

1. Baulieu EE, Raynaud JP (1970) A "proportion graph" method for measuring binding systems. Eur J Biochem 13: 293–304
2. Braunsberg H (1975) The determination of high-affinity oestrogen receptors in human breast tumours. Eur J Cancer 11: 101–103
3. Braunsberg H, Hammond KD (1979) Methods of steroid receptor calculation: an interlaboratory study. J Steroid Biochem 11: 1561–1565
4. Braunsberg H, Hammond KD (1980) Practical and theoretical aspects in the analysis of steroid receptors. J Steroid Biochem 13: 1133–1145
5. Braunsberg H, Hammond KD (1981) The calculation of receptor parameters. In: Safarty GA, Nash AR, Keightley DD (eds) Quality assurance in estrogen receptor assays. Masson, New York
6. Clark JH, Peck EJ (1979) Female sex steroids. Receptors and function. Springer, Berlin Heidelberg New York
7. Cressie NAC, Keightley DD (1979) The underlying structure of the direct linear plot with application to the analysis of hormone-receptor interactions. J Steroid Biochem 11: 1173–1180
8. Eisenthal R, Cornish-Bowden A (1974) The direct linear plot: a new graphical procedure for estimating enzyme kinetic parameters. Biochem J 139: 715–720
9. Feherty P, Farrer-Brown G, Kellie AE (1971) Oestradiol receptors in carcinoma and benign disease of the breast: an in vitro assay. Br J Cancer 25: 697–710
10. Haldane JB (1957) Graphical methods in enzyme chemistry. Nature 179: 832
11. Hammond KD, Braunsberg H (1979) Assay of human endometrial progesterone receptors using the natural hormone and a polyethylene glycol precipitation technique. J Steroid Biochem 13: 1147–1156
12. Heuson JC, Longeval E, Mattheiem WH, Deboel MC, Sylvester RJ, Leclercq G (1977) Significance of quantitative assessment of estrogen receptors for endocrine therapy in advanced breast cancer. Cancer 39: 1971–1977
13. Keightley DD, Cressie NAC (1980) The Woolf plot is more reliable than the Scatchard plot in analysing data from hormone receptor assays. J Steroid Biochem 13: 1317–1323
14. Lineweaver H, Burk D (1934) The determination of enzyme dissociation constants. J Am Chem Soc 56: 658–666
15. McGuire WL, Zava DT, Horwitz KB, Garola RE, Chamness GC (1978) Receptors and breast cancer: do we know it all? J Steroid Biochem 9: 461–466
16. Ojasoo T, Raynaud JP (1978) Unique steroid cogeners for receptor studies. Cancer Res 38: 4186–4198

17. Rodbard D, Munson PJ, Thakur AK (1980) Quantitative characterization of hormone receptors. Cancer 46: 2907–2918
18. Rosenthal HE (1967) A graphic method for the determination and presentation of binding parameters in a complex system. Anal Biochem 20: 525–532
19. Scatchard G (1949) The attractions of proteins for small molecules and ions. Ann NY Acad Sci 51: 660–672
20. Wagner RK (1972) Characterization and assay of steroid hormone receptors and steroid binding serum proteins by agargel electrophoresis at low temperature. Hoppe Seylers Z Physiol Chem 353: 1235–1245

New Methods

Estrogen and Progestin Receptor Analysis in Human Breast Cancer by Isoelectric Focusing in Slabs of Polyacrylamide Gel

Ö. Wrange, S. Humla, I. Ramberg, B. Nordenskjöld, and J.-Å. Gustafsson

Department of Medical Nutrition, Department of Tumor Pathology and Oncology, Karolinska Institutet, Huddinge University Hospital F 69, 141 86 Huddinge, Sweden

Introduction

The use of estrogen- and progestin receptor-quantitation as prognostic indicators and for predicting response to endocrine treatment in individual cases of human breast cancer has created a need for convenient methods of receptor analysis. In our experience isoelectric focusing is an efficient method for routine analysis of estrogen receptors [8, 9] and progestin receptors [7] in surgical biopsies of human breast cancer.

Materials and Methods

Reagents

[2,4,6,7-³H]Estradiol (specific radioactivity 85 Ci/mmol) and [17α-methyl-³H]promegestrone, R-5020 (specific radioactivity 78 Ci/mmol), were purchased from the New England Nuclear Co. Ferritin (horse spleen), lyophilized hemoglobin (beef), activated charcoal and 2-hydroxyethylmercaptan were obtained from Sigma Chemical Co., St. Louis, Mo. Dextran T-500 was purchased from Pharmacia Fine Chemicals, Uppsala, Sweden. Trypsin, crystallized twice, dialyzed, and lyophilized ($\sim$ 211 µg/mg), was obtained from Worthington, Freehold, N.J. Glycerol, acrylamide, N_1N'-methylenebisacrylamide and riboflavin were purchased from Merck, Darmstadt, West Germany. Ampholine and ready-made polyacrylamide gel for isoelectric focusing (pH 3.5−9.5) were purchased from LKB-produkter, Bromma, Sweden. Ready-made gels containing 20% (w/v) glycerol were kindly provided by LKB-produkter AB.

Tissue Material

Pieces of human mammary carcinoma were excised immediately after surgery and kept on ice in isotonic saline. Within 1−2 h they were frozen without buffer at −70° C.

Sample Preparation

Tumor tissue was thawed, minced, and suspended in approximately 3 ml buffer A [5 mM potassium phosphate pH 7.4; 2 mM 2-hydroxyethylmercaptan; 10% (w/v) glycerol] per gram tissue and homogenized with a Polytrone (Kinematica, Lucerne, Switzerland). The homogenate was centrifuged at 100,000 g for 45 min and the floating lipid layer removed. The pellet was taken for DNA determination [1] to measure receptor amounts in femtomoles per microgram of DNA. The supernatant (cytosol) was incubated with 7.5 nM [³H]estradiol (estrogen receptor assay) or 20 nM [³H]R-5020 (progestin receptor assay). For control of nonspecific (nonsaturable) binding one may use a parallel incubation (containing the same concentration of tritium labeled ligand and also a 100-fold excess concentration of unlabeled diethylstilbestrol (for the estrogen receptor assay) or R-5020 (for the progestin receptor assay). It is not, however, necessary to have any control incubation for nonspecific binding when using isoelectric focusing in routine receptor analysis (see below).

Estrogen Receptor

For estrogen receptor assay [³H]estradiol was incubated with cytosol for 1.5 h at 0° C. An aliquot of the cytosol was also taken for spectrophotometric analysis. The absorbance at 280 nm and 310 nm was measured and the difference used as a rough estimate of the protein concentration in the cytosol, being expressed as absorbance units (A 280−310 nm). After the 1.5-h incubation, trypsin was taken from a freshly prepared solution and added to give a final trypsin amount of 5 µg/A 280−310 nm of cytosol protein; in addition, one-ninth volume of 20 mM $CaCl_2$ was added to give a final Ca^{2+} concentration of 2 mM. The incubation was kept at 10° C for 30 min followed by cooling on ice. It was then mixed with one-third volume of a dextran-coated charcoal suspension (final concentrations of charcoal and dextran were 1% w/v and 0.1% w/v respectively) and kept on ice for 5 min, followed by centrifugation at 3,000 × g for 5 min. An aliquot of the supernatant was taken for isoelectric focusing.

Progestin Receptor

For progestin receptor assay the cytosol was incubated with [³H]R-5020 for 2 h at 0° C followed by dextran-coated charcoal treatment (as above) and the supernatant was taken for isoelectric focusing analysis. No trypsin digestion was performed (see below).

Gel Preparation

Preparation of the gel for isoelectroc focusing was essentially as described by Winter and Andersson [6]. The "self-made" gel was 245 × 110 × 2 mm and contained Ampholine of pH ranges 3.5−10 and 5−8 at concentrations of 0.6% (w/v) and 0.4% (w/v) respectively. The polyacrylamide gel had a value of T = 5% (w/v) and C = 3% (w/v) [2], and glycerol was added to a concentration of 20% (w/v). Riboflavin 1 µg/ml was added and the gel allowed to polymerize in light [6] for 2 h.
Ready-made gels (LKB-produkter AB) containing 2.4% (w/v) Ampholine, pH 3.5−9.5, were also used for routine receptor measurements (see below).

Isoelectric Focusing

Isoelectric focusing was performed with an LKB Multiphor connected to a constant power supply and a cooling system (LKB-multitemp). Double layers of electrode strips soaked in

1 *M* sodium hydroxide (cathode) or 1 *M* sulphuric acid (anode) were used. The gel was prefocused for 30 min at 30 mA and 30 W (ready-made gel) or 30 min at 20 mA and 20 W (self-made gel).

Sample frames of acrylic plastic were used in order to apply up to 0.3 ml of sample solution to the gel. Inner diameter was about 7 × 10 mm, and height, 3 mm. After prefocusing the gel, the sample frames were placed on the gel surface 0.9–1 cm from the cathode electrode strip, where the final pH was about 8–8.5. (The hormone-receptor complex is dissociated or destroyed in the acid pH near the anode.) Ferritin and hemoglobin dissolved in water were placed between the sample frames as small drops directly on the gel surface (they may also be added to the sample solution as an internal marker). Ferritin was focused as a yellow band around pH 4.5 and hemoglobin as a brown band around pH 7.6.

Each sample was pipetted into a sample frame. Usually eight samples were analyzed simultaneously. If enough tumor material was available, it was convenient to place a sample volume containing 0.5–1 A 280–310 units of tumor cytosol in each frame. This amount of cytosol protein was sufficient to detect low amounts of receptor (0.01 fmol/µg DNA). In some experiments, more than 4 A 280–310 units of tumor cytosol was applied without affecting the analysis of the receptors, which demonstrates that the risk of overloading the gel is small. The power unit was set at 20 mA, 20 W and 1,200 V and focusing was carried out for another 1.5 h. When the ferritin standard was focused near the anode and the hemoglobin standard in front of the sample frame (after about 1 h), the liquid inside the sample frames was aspirated with a Pasteur pipette and the sample frames removed. Any remaining sample solution on the gel surface was removed with a filter paper to minimize the risk of radioactive contamination.

The isoelectric focusing was continued until the current ceased to diminish. The total focusing time from the application of sample was about 1.5 h. Effective cooling is of utmost importance because of the rapid dissociation of the hormone-receptor complex when exposed to heat. Insufficient cooling is easily detected, since in this case condensation occurs on the inside of the inner lid above the gel. If condensation is noticed, the power should be decreased. pH was measured at 2°–4° C using a surface pH electrode (type 403-30, Ingold, Zurich, Switzerland).

Fractionation of the Gel

The 2-mm-thick home-made gel was cut into strips, one for each sample track, and each strip was transferred to a slicing frame made of razor blades. A sheet of Parafilm (American Can Co., Greenwich, Conn.) was placed on the gel, which was then pressed down between the razor blades with the help of a cork ring. The Parafilm was removed and each 3.3-mm-broad gel slice transferred to a plastic vial uwing a pair of forceps. Five milliliters of Instagel (Packard Instrument Co., Inc., Warrenville, Downess Grove, Ill.) was added to each vial. The vials were shaken vigorously and kept at 50° for 1 h and then shaken again and assayed for radioactivity in a liquid scintillation spectrometer. The incubation at 50° C was sufficient to allow the tritium-labeled steroid to diffuse out of the gel (data not shown). The 1-mm-thick ready-made gels (LKB 1804 Ampholine PAG plate) had a cellophane support sheet. A strip of gel containing one sample track and still on its support sheet was out of the PAG plate, and a similarly sized strip of millimeter graph paper was placed upside down on the gel surface. The gel strip could then be conveniently handled, with the cellophane sheet on one side and the paper on the other. Gel slices were easily obtained with a sharp pair of surgical scissors; the graph paper used as a template could be clearly seen through the gel. The gel was routinely cut into 4-mm slices. Each gel slice was placed in a plastic vial and 5 ml Instagel added; the vials were then handled as described above.

Receptor Quantitation

The radioactivity in the vials was measured and the efficiency calculated according to the external standard technique. For the [³H]estradiol-labeled sample a peak of radioactivity with a maximum at pH 6.5−6.7 represented estrogen receptor-bound ligand. For the [³H]R-5020-labeled cytosol a peak of radioactivity with a maximum at pH 6.1−6.3 represented progestin receptor bound ligand. Routinely only a 5-cm-long gel strip between pH 8 and pH 4.7 was fractionated and assayed for radioactivity.

Results and Discussion

The preparation of cytosol can be carried out in many other ways than those described above; however, to avoid disturbance of the isoelectric focusing procedure it is important to use a buffer with low ionic strength and low buffering capacity.
It is not necessary to remove the unbound hormone with dextran-coated charcoal, since free hormone will not move from the sample application point. This simple step is recommended, however, to minimize the risk of radioactive contamination.

Estrogen Receptor

As illustrated in Fig. 1, the nontrypsinized tumor cytosol is usually focused as a double peak with maxima at pH 5.9−6.1 and 6.5−6.7; both these peaks disappear when a 100-fold excess of unlabeled diethylstilbestrol is present in the incubation medium. After trypsin digestion (Fig. 1B), only one sharp peak, with a maximum at pH 6.5−6.7, is seen; this radioactivity peak also disappears when a 100-fold excess of unlabeled diethylstilbestrol is present in the incubation medium, which demonstrates that it represents receptor-bound estradiol. It has previously been shown [8] that limited trypsin digestion results in the formation of a hormone-binding fragment of the estrogen receptor with a sedimentation coefficient of 4 S in low ionic strength solutions and a pI of 6.5−6.7. The nontrypsinized (native) estrogen-receptor complex has a sedimentation coefficient of 8 S in low ionic strength solutions and a pI of 5.9−6.1. Cytosol preparations from breast cancer tissue usually contain a mixture of the 8 S and the 4 S estrogen receptor complexes and such samples are thus focused as a double peak (see Fig. 1A). This may be due to endogenous protease activity in the cytosol during sample preparation. In the experiment illustrated (Fig. 1), more receptor (11%) was recovered in the trypsinized sample than in the nontrypsinized sample, as is usually the case [1]; this may be due to a greater tendency for the native receptor to aggregate and stay at the application point as compared with the trypsin-induced receptor fragment. Human serum labeled with [³H]estradiol also gives rise to a peak of radioactivity focusing at pH 5.5 (not shown). This peak of radioactivity represents sex hormone-binding globulin (SHBG). Extensive mix experiments with cytosol and human serum have shown that SHBG does not interfere with estrogen receptor quantitation in surgical biopsies of human breast cancer by isoelectric focusing [3]. The pH

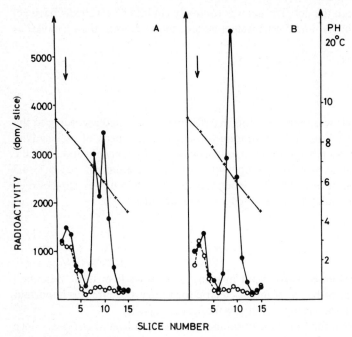

Fig. 1A, B. Isoelectric focusing of [³H]estradiol-labeled cytosol from human breast cancer tissue with (O———O) or without (●———●) a 100-fold excess of diethylstilbestrol. **A** was not trypsinized and **B** was trypsinized as described in methods. The *arrow* marks the sample application point and (×———×) signifies the pH gradient

of SHBG does not change as a result of trypsin digestion (data not shown). Limited trypsin digestion of the tumor cytosol prior to isoelectric focusing is thus recommended for the following reasons:

1. Increased specificity of the assay, due to increased separation of the trypsin-induced receptor fragment focusing at pH 6.5−6.7 from SHBG focusing at pH 5.5 as compared with the native receptor (focusing at pH 5.9−6.1).
2. Increased sensitivity of the assay, due to sharper peaks and minimized risk of losses due to receptor aggregation.

As reported elsewhere [8], the loss of estrogen receptor due to proteolytic degradation during digestion with trypsin is insignificant with the recommended dose of trypsin, and the loss is 8% and 25% respectively when 4 or 8 times the recommended amount of trypsin is used.

Recovery of the estrogen-receptor complex after limited trypsin digestion and isoelectric focusing is about 85% when compared with the amount of specifically bound [³H]estradiol determined by dextran-coated charcoal treatment in the presence and absence of a 100-fold excess of unlabeled diethylstilbestrol.

The peak focused at pH 6.6 has been found by repeated experiments to represent receptor-bound estradiol and is always absent in a control incubation containing an excess of unlabeled estradiol or diethylstilbestrol. These and other data [8] have shown that no estradiol-binding protein other than the proteolytically induced estradiol receptor fragment is focused at or near pH 6.6, and thus we have found that a control incubation with an excess of unlabeled competitor is unnecessary in the routine assay.

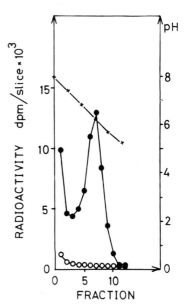

Fig. 2. Isoelectric focusing of [³H]R-5020-labeled cytosol from human breast cancer in the presence (O−−−−O) or absence (●———●) of a 100-fold excess of unlabeled R-5020

Progestin Receptor

The progestin receptor should not be exposed to proteolysis by trypsin prior to analysis by isoelectric focusing since the so obtained smaller receptor fragment will not move in the gel. This may be due to a too alkaline pI of the trypsin-induced receptor fragment or to a too low charge or insufficient stability [7]. The [³H]R-5020-labeled progestin receptor is focused as a somewhat broader peak than the estrogen receptor. The progestin receptor forms a maximum at pH 6.4−6.0 (Fig. 2), which is always saturable with an excess of unlabeled R-5020. That this peak represents the progestin receptor has been shown by its high affinity and specificity for progestins [7]. Human serum contains components that interact with [³H]R-5020 and forms a peak at pH 5.0−5.4 when analyzed by isoelectric focusing. This peak is not saturable with a 100-fold excess of unlabeled R-5020 [7]. Heavily blood-contaminated tumor biopsies will increase the background radioactivity in the gel, but the receptor peak is separated from the nonspecific peak by isoelectric focusing. The stability of the progestin receptor-ligand complex is improved by the presence of glycerol in the buffer [4]. We found it advantageous to have glycerol present in the gel: its stabilizing effect is easily seen in the form of sharper peaks and reduced tailing radioactivity between the receptor peak and the point of sample application (Wrange and Humla, unpublished data). We have previously compared progestin receptor assay by isoelectric focusing and sucrose gradient centrifugation [7]. The amount of progestin receptor detected by isoelectric focusing and the specific 8 S and 4 S binding in the gradients showed a correlation ($r = 0.76$). This study has been repeated using sucrose gradient centrifugation in vertical rotor since Powell et al. [5] demonstrated in 1979 that this technique of sucrose gradient centrifugation is superior to conventional horizontal gradients when analyzing progestin receptors because only ca. 2 h of centrifugation is needed. Powell et al. [5] showed that the [³H]R-5020 binding in the 8 S peak after vertical gradient centrifugation correlates well with other methods of progesterone receptor quantitation (batch techniques based on hydroxyapatite or dextran-coated charcoal) but that the saturable binding in the 4 S peak does not. We have therefore correlated the amount of saturable [³H]R-5050

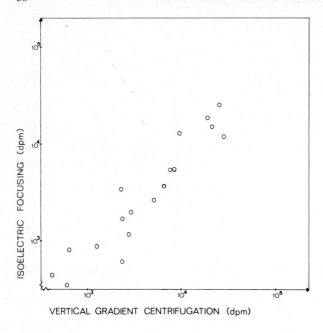

Fig. 3. A comparison of progestin receptor assay by vertical sucrose gradient centrifugation and isoelectric focusing on "home-made" gels. 10%−30% (w/v) sucrose gradients were prepared manually in homogenization buffer. 200 µl of [^{3}H]R-5020-labeled sample after dextran-coated charcoal treatment was taken for each experiment and analysed concomitantly. Gradients were centrifuged for 2 h at 64,000 rpm in a Beckman VT:65 rotor. A parallel sample also containing a 100-fold excess of unlabeled R-5020 was analyzed in each case to control nonspecific binding

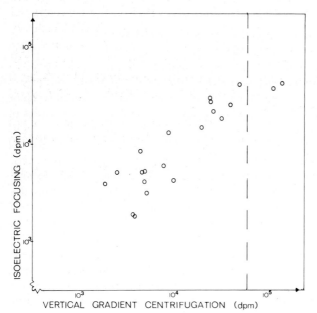

Fig. 4. A comparison of progestin receptor assay by vertical sucrose gradient centrifugation and isoelectric focusing on ready-made gels containing 20% glycerol

binding in the 8 *S* peak by vertical sucrose gradient analysis with the amount of hormone focused as a pH 6.4−6.0 peak. Gels with and without glycerol were also tested in this way (Wrange and Humla, unpublished data). Eighteen progestin receptor-positive tumors analyzed with self-made gels (see methods) showed a good quantitative correlation with 8 *S* receptor analyzed by vertical rotor (Fig. 3) [slope (calculated by least square linear regression) 0.93; $r^* = 0.96$]. A similar comparison with 15 tumors analyzed on ready-made gels without glycerol showed a decreased recovery and also broader peaks and increased tailing of radioactivity from the application point (slope 0.33; $r = 0.82$; not shown); when such ready-made gels were synthesized in the presence of 20% glycerol, the correlation (analyzing 21 tumors) with the amount of 8 S progestin receptor detected by vertical rotor sucrose gradients was slope 0.30, $r = 0.82$. In this case, however, there was a tendency for deviation to occur at high absolute progestin receptor volumes, indicating lower recovery on isoelectric focusing at high protein concentrations. This is demonstrated by the great effect on the slope calculated by linear regression when the two highest absolute receptor values detected by vertical centrifugation are excluded (cf. dotted line in Fig. 4) ($\mu = 19$; slope 0.74; $r = 0.92$). The radioactivity peaks were more narrow and there was less tailing of radioactivity from the sample application point when ready-made gels containing 20% glycerol were used instead of gels lacking glycerol.

Conclusion

We advise the use of 20% glycerol in the polyacrylamide gel when measuring progestin receptors, the positive effect of glycerol probably being due to a decreased dissociation of the hormone-receptor complex [4]. The estrogen receptor may be analyzed concomitantly in parallel incubations on the same gel.

There was a tendency toward a decrease in progestin receptor recovery at high absolute values, probably reflecting increased aggregation at high cytosol protein concentration. Control experiments have shown that recovery of progestin receptor is not affected by applying up to 1 mg of protein to the gel (sample volume 200 µl) (7 and unpublished observations). It is thus recommended that about $0.5-1$ A $280-310$ units of cytosol protein is applied to the gel for analysis of the progestin receptor. The estrogen receptor analysis is not affected by high cytosolic protein concentrations owing to the trypsin digestion, which effectively prevents receptor aggregation.

Only one incubation is needed for each routine receptor analysis since no non-receptor hormone binders are focused at the same pH as the receptor and thus the pI may be used as an internal control of what is actually being measured.

The small amount of tissue needed for analysis makes it possible to assay receptors in fine needle aspirates from human breast cancer (see pp. 41−44).

References

1. Burton K (1968) Determination of DNA concentration with diphenylamide. In: Grossman L, Moldave K (eds) Methods in enzymology, vol 12, part B. Academic, New York, p 163
2. Hjertén S (1962) Molecular sieve chromatography on polyacrylamide gels, prepared according to a simplified method. Arch Biochem Biophys (Suppl) 1: 147−151
3. Okret S, Wrange Ö, Nordenskjöld B, Silfverswärd C, Gustafsson JÅ (1978) Estrogen receptor: assay in human mammary carcinoma with the synthetic estrogen II β-methoxy-17α-ethinyl-1,3,5(10) estratriene-3,17β-diol (R2858). Cancer Res 38: 3904−3909
4. Pichon MF, Milgrom E (1977) Characterization and assay of progesterone receptor in human mammary carcinoma. Cancer Res 37: 464−471
5. Powell B, Garola RE, Chamness GC, McGuire WL (1979) Measurement of progesterone receptor in human breast cancer biopsies. Cancer Res 39: 1678−1682
6. Winter A, Ek K, Andersson UB (1977) Analytical electrofocusing in thin layers of polyacrylamide gels. LKB application note 250

7. Wrange Ö, Humla S, Ramberg I, Gustafsson S, Skoog L, Nordenskjöld B, Gustafsson JÅ (1981) Progestin-receptor analysis in human breast cancer cytosol by isoelectric focusing in slabs of polyacrylamide gel. J Steroid Biochem 14: 141–148
8. Wrange Ö, Nordenskjöld B, Gustafsson JÅ (1978) Cytosol estradiol receptor in human mammary carcinoma: An assay based on isoelectric focusing in polyacrylamide gel. Anal Biochem 85: 461–475
9. Wrange Ö, Ramberg I, Gustafsson JÅ, Nordenskjöld B (1978) Estradiol receptor analysis in human breast cancer tissue by isoelectric focusing in polyacrylamide gel. LKB application note No 313

Estrogen Receptor Analysis on Fine Needle Aspirates from Human Breast Carcinoma

C. Silfverswärd, A. Wallgren, B. Nordenskjöld, and S. Humla

Departments of Tumor Pathology and Oncology, Karolinska Hospital, Stockholm, and Department of Oncology, Regionssjukhuset, Linköping, Sweden

Introduction

The concentration of estrogen receptor protein (ER) in breast carcinoma is a useful indicator of the likelihood of response to endocrine therapy [3]. A correlation between low receptor values and early recurrence of the carcinoma has also been shown [7]. In most centers the ER analysis is performed on surgically removed tumor specimens. However, in many patients with inoperable or recurrent carcinoma, surgical specimens for ER determinations are not readily available, and after preoperative irradiation ER determination is unreliable as the primary tumor often undergoes advanced degenerative changes or totally disappears [6]. In such cases ER determination on fine needle aspirates could be a method of choice. Two earlier reports based on a small number of patients [4, 5] indicated that reproducible ER levels may be obtained from analysis of fine needle aspirates from breast carcinoma. The present study of 168 patients examines the results of ER analysis on fine needle aspirates collected from patients with primary or recurrent breast carcinoma prior to surgery. For comparison, analysis was also performed on histologic tissue material after surgical biopsy or mastectomy.

Material and Methods

Collection of Material

In 158 cases of cytologically diagnosed primary breast carcinoma and in 10 cases of chest wall or lymph node recurrences, a percutaneous needle aspirate was taken from the tumor using the technique described by Franzén and Zajicek [2]. The same needle (outer diameter 0.7 mm) was used as that usually used to obtain material for cytological diagnosis. Double aspirations were performed and the material was ejected into a solution of ^{3}H-estradiol. The needles were also rinsed with the same solution in order to remove the tumor material otherwise retained in the needle. The presence of tumor cells was verified in all cases by microscopic analysis of a drop of the diluted aspirate smeared onto a slide, which was stained according to the May-Grünwald-Giemsa method. All cases were also histologically verified and a piece of tumor was taken for conventional ER analysis at the time of surgery.

Recent Results in Cancer Research. Vol. 91
© Springer-Verlag Berlin · Heidelberg 1984

Biochemical Methods

Thin needle aspirates were injected into 0.5 ml of 5 nM ^{3}H-estradiol (New England Nuclear, 141 Ci per mmol) in 0.01 M Tris-HCl, 0.001 M EDTA (ET buffer) and frozen within 15 min. The material was then kept at $-70°$ C for a few weeks. After thawing, the aspirates were homogenized in an all-glass homogenizer and further incubated at $0°$ C for 45 min. The aspirates were then centrifuged at 15,000 g for 20 min. The supernatants were trypsinized, treated with dextran-coated charcoal for 10 min, centrifuged at 800 g for 10 min, and subjected to polyacrylamide electrofocusing as previously described [8]. Sediments after centrifugation of tumor homogenate contained the cell nuclei and were taken for measurement of DNA according to Burton [1] as a reference for quantitation of specific binding.

The ER content in the histologic tissue specimens was measured as previously described [8]. Three specimens were analysed from each tumor and the mean value was calculated by dividing the total amount of ER by the total amount of DNA.

Results

The Amount of DNA in Aspirates

In Table 1 the aspirates were divided according to the amount of cellular material, expressed as micrograms of DNA. Approximately 60% of the aspirates contained more than 10 µg DNA, corresponding to 10^6 cells.

Correlation Between Estrogen Receptor Contents in Aspirates and in Tissue Samples

There was a significant correlation ($r = 0.63$, $P < 0.001$) between the ER contents in aspirates and those in tissue samples (Fig. 1). However, in a number of cases which contained ER according to the analysis of tissue samples, the analysis of aspirated material failed to show any receptor. As shown in Figs. 2 and 3, which depict the same correlations for cases containing 10 µg DNA or less per aspirate and for cases containing more than 15 µg DNA per aspirate, almost all of these "false-negative" cases were found among those with sparse tumor material. In aspirates containing more than 15 µg DNA there were even

Table 1. Amount of cellular material in aspirates

DNA in aspirate (µg)	No. of cases	%
5	30	17.9
6−10	35	20.8
11−15	35	20.8
16−30	30	19.9
30	38	22.6
Total	168	100.0

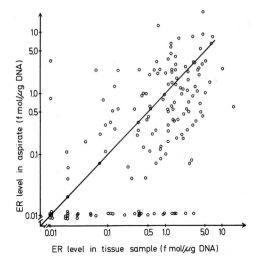

Fig. 1. Correlation between ER determination on surgical tissue samples and on aspirated material. All 168 cases

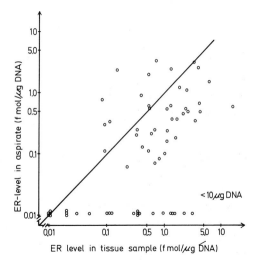

Fig. 2. Correlation between ER determination on surgical tissue samples and on aspirated material. Cases with up to 10 µg DNA in aspirates

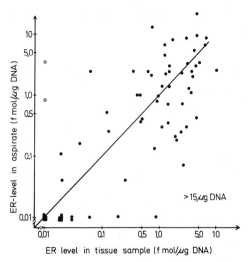

Fig. 3. Correlation between ER determination on surgical tissue samples and on aspirated material. Cases with more than 15 µg DNA in aspirates

a few cases which contained ER according to the analysis of aspirated material, but where the analysis of tissue material failed to show any receptor.

Discussion

This study verifies our earlier findings [4, 5] that it is possible to assess ER contents in breast tumors reliably through analysis of fine needle aspirates using the same aspiration technique as for diagnostic needle biopsy, provided that aspiration has yielded a sufficient amount of tumor material (measured as the amount of DNA). If the amount of DNA in the aspirate is lower than $10-15 \mu g$, the analysis is of limited practical value since false-negative results are frequent. In inoperable or recurrent breast carcinoma the fine needle aspiration technique is an easy and rapid method both for morphological verification of the tumor and for obtaining material for ER analysis. As has been shown earlier [5], aspirates from inoperable breast carcinomas usually contain abundant and sufficient cellular material for a reliable determination of the ER content. Receptor analysis of aspirated material from such tumors and from recurrences is done routinely at the Department of Oncology (Radiumhemmet) in Karolinska Hospital in Stockholm. We are presently investigating whether our method of ER determination is applicable to patients with distant metastases (skeletal, lung, liver).

References

1. Burton K (1968) Determination of DNA concentration with diphenylamine. In: Grossman L, koldave K (eds) Methods in enzymology, vol 12, part B. Academic Press, New York, p 163
2. Franzén S, Zajicek J (1968) Aspiration biopsy in diagnosis of palpable lesions of the breast. Acta Radiol 7: 241−262
3. McGuire WL, Carbone PP, Vollmer EP (1975) Estrogen receptors in human breast cancer. Raven, New York
4. Silfverswärd C, Humla S (1980) Estrogen receptor analysis on needle aspirates from human mammary carcinoma. Acta Cytol 24: 54−57
5. Silfverswärd C, Gustafsson JÅ, Gustafsson SA, Nordenskjöld B, Wallgren A, Wrange Ö (1980) Estrogen receptor analysis on fine needle aspirates and on histologic biopsies from human breast cancer. Eur J Cancer 16: 1351−1357
6. Wallgren A, Arner O, Bergström J, Blomstedt B, Granberg PO, Karnström L, Räf L, Silfverswärd C (1978) Preoperative radiotherapy in operable breast cancer. Cancer 42: 1120−1125
7. Westerberg H, Gustafsson SA, Nordenskjöld B, Silfverswärd C, Wallgren A (1980) Estrogen receptor levels and other factors in early recurrence in breast cancer. Int J Cancer 26: 429−433
8. Wrange Ö, Nordenskjöld B, Gustafsson JÅ (1978) Cytosol estradiol receptor in human mammary carcinoma: an assay based on isoelectric focusing in polyacrylamide gel. Anal Biochem 85: 461−475

Estrogen and Progestin Receptors on Drill Biopsy Samples of Human Mammary Tumors

H. Magdelénat

Section Médicale et Hospitalière, Institut Curie, 26 Rue d'Ulm, 75231 Paris Cedex 5, France

Introduction

In recent years, a major contribution to the strategy of breast cancer therapy has been provided by the determination of steroid receptors. The presence of estrogen and progesterone receptors in such tumors is not only predictive of the response to hormonetherapy (which itself has been greatly improved by antiestrogens) but is also a powerful independent prognostic factor [4, 11].

It is now generally agreed that estrogen and/or progestin receptors should tentatively be assayed in every case of breast carcinoma. As conservative treatments, e.g., radiotherapy, have proved to be as efficient as surgery at certain stages of the disease [3] and are applied to a great number of patients, tissue sampling is the limiting problem for systematic receptor assay. Drill biopsy and fine needle aspiration are two means of obtaining representative samples of tumor tissue and are currently practiced to establish diagnosis. Histological sampling (drill biopsy) is sometimes preferred to cytological sampling (fine needle aspirate) since it yields a more complete description of the tumor, including histological grading [14].

In this chapter a method for assaying estrogen (ER) and progestin (PgR) receptors in tissue samples obtained by drill biopsy is presented.

Materials and Methods

Drill Biopsy

The method has been described by Rousseau [12]. After alcoholic disinfection of the skin, light local anesthesia is induced with 1% lidocaine. This anesthesia is generally limited to the skin since drill biopsy is usually painless. After anesthesia, it is essential to make a 3−5 mm incision throughout the entire width of the skin with a surgical blade so that drilling will not be done through fibrous material, which may cause local heating and introduce epidermal debris into the tumor. A rotating bore (diameter, 2 mm; length, 10 mm) actuated by a motor-driven flexible is progressively introduced through the tumor and, after disconnecting the flexible, the tissue sample located in the bore is aspirated into a syringe and *immediately* frozen in liquid nitrogen. A second sample is obtained by drill biopsy and fixed in Bouin solution for histological examination.

Receptor Assay

Chemicals. [^{3}H]-R-2858 (moxestrol or 11β-methoxy-17α-ethynyl, 17β-estradiol), 80–90 Ci/mmol, and R-2858 (NEN, Germany); [^{3}H]-R-5020 (promegestone or 17,21-dimethyl-19-nor-pregna-4,9-diene-3,20-dione, 80–90 Ci/mmol, and R-5020 (NEN, Germany). Tritiated hormone stock solutions are changed or purified every month.
TRIS [tris(hydroxypropyl)aminomethane], HCl, NH$_4$OH, glycerol, sucrose, KCl (Merck). Dithiothreitol (DTT), Norit A, 3.5 p-diaminobenzoic acid (DABA) (Sigma), Dextran 70 (Pharmacia). Coomassie G 250 (Biorad Protein Assay Reagent), Triton X-100, scintillation grade (Nuclear Enterprise). Aqualuma Plus liquid scintillator (Lumac).

Material. Ninety-six well microtiter plates (Nunc), waterproof tape (Cook), Polytron homogenizer with the smallest, 7 mm axis (Kinematika). Beckmann L 5-75 ultracentrifuge, Beckmann 40.2 or 40.3 rotor with thick wall polycarbonate tubes (Beckmann). Giratory shaker (Brunswick). Centrifuge with buckets for microtiter plates (Heraus), SL 4000 liquid scintillation counter (Intertechniques), Uvicon 810 spectrophotometer (Kontron). JY 3D spectrofluorometer (Jobin Yvan). Desk computer (Tektronix 4051).

Buffers. Estrogen receptor assay: Tris-HCl 10 mM, 0.25 M sucrose, 0.4 M KCl, pH 7.4 at 20° C.
Progestin receptor assay: phosphate 5 mM, glycerol 10%, DTT 1 mM, pH 7.4 at 20° C.

Tissue Homogenization. Samples weighing less than 20 mg are considered improper for receptor assay. Samples weighing between 20 and 60 mg are homogenized in 0.5 ml of buffer (1 : 26 to 1 : 11 dilution). Samples weighing more than 60 mg are homogenized in 9 volumes/weight of buffer. Homogenization is carried out directly in the polycarbonate ultracentrifuge tubes with 5-s runs of the Polytron at half maximum speed (5–6 setting), with 15-s cooling periods when more than one run is necessary. Homogenates are centrifuged for 1 h at 105,000 g at 0° C. Supernatants (cytosols) are collected for steroid (450 µl) and protein (10 µl) assays. Pellets are stored at −30° C for DNA assay.

Receptor Assay. One hundred microliter cytosol aliquots and 10 µl of the tritiated hormone (1 nM and 2 nM final concentrations for ER and PgR respectively) are incubated in duplicate in microtiter plates in the absence (total binding) or presence (nonspecific binding) of a 100-fold excess of unlabeled steroid (10 µl).
Incubation is for 3 h at 25° C for ER determination and 4 h at 0° C for PgR determination. Incubation is terminated by the addition of 120 µl of a dextran-coated charcoal suspension in buffer (Norit A: 0.5%; Dextran 70: 0.05%). Microtiter plates are covered with waterproof tape, vigorously shaken on a giratory shaker for 10 min at 0° C, and centrifuged at 1,500 g for 10 min at 0° C. The radioactivity of 120-µl supernatant aliquots is measured in the presence of 3.5 ml liquid scintillator, and converted to dpm after quenching corrections (mean cpm : dpm ratio = 0.42).
Specific binding sites are derived, with computer assistance, from the radioactivity which is displaced by the 100-fold excess of unlabeled steroid.
Results are expressed as femtomoles per gram of fresh tissue (fmol/gT).

Protein Assay. The Bradford protein assay [2] is applied to 10 µl of cytosol diluted in 2 ml water, using Biorad reagent and microprocedure, and BSA as the standard.

DNA Assay. The DNA assay is adapted from the fluorometric method of Fiszer-Szafarz [5]. The 105,000 g pellet is suspended in 2 ml NH_4OH 1 N containing 0.2% Triton X-100 and hydrolyzed for 1 h in a boiling water-bath. The hydrolyzate is cleared by centrifugation for 5 min at 1,000 g. 60 μl of a charcoal-cleared 2 M solution of DABA in 4 N HCl is added to 50-μl aliquots of hydrolyzate.
Reaction is allowed for 30 min at 60° C and is terminated by the addition of 2.9 ml HCl 1 N.
Fluorescence intensity is measured with a spectrofluorometer (excitation 410 nm, emission 515 nm) and compared with a standard curve from calf thymus DNA.

Quality Control. Systematically, a cytosol reconstituted from a lyophilized rabbit uterus primed with estradiol before killing is introduced in the assay.

Results

Sample Characteristics

Size and Weight. Tissue samples obtained by drill biopsy consist of fragments 3−25 mm long and 1.5−2 mm in diameter. Several small fragments are obtained in soft tumors. Samples containing well-defined fragments generally weigh more than 20 mg. Such samples are obtained in 90% of cases. When the tumor is particularly soft, debris can be obtained; this pertains to 9% of cases. Complete failure to obtain a tissue sample is generally due to technical problems and is very rare (1% of cases).
The mean weight observed with 184 samples (including 15 benign tumors) was 40 mg (extremes 10 and 75 mg). Twelve samples (6.5%) weighed less than 20 mg (see below), six of them being characterized later as benign tumors.

Biochemical Parameters. Negative results for ER and PgR are only valid when cellularity of the sample is sufficient [10]. DNA assay of the 105,000 g gives the best estimation of this cellularity and is highly correlated with the cellularity estimated at histological examination. Values of less than 500 μg DNA per gram tissue are representative of poorly cellular samples which should therefore be rejected. In the 184 cases studied, 21 samples (11.4%) weighing more than 20 mg were rejected owing to insufficient cellularity. Six of these samples were benign tumors, as confirmed at histological examination.
Protein concentration of cytosol should not be too low [6], the limit being 1.5 mg/ml during incubation. One sample out of the 184 studied, weighing more than 20 mg and with more than 500 μg DNA/gT, had a cytosol protein concentration of less than 1.5 mg/ml and was rejected. Protein concentration was always low in samples weighing less than 20 mg.
Finally, even if the above objective criteria are fulfilled, some samples are macroscopically "bad looking" (debris, blood, fat, jelly), and negative ER and PgR results which are obtained should be considered as suspicious. Such a situation was found in 13 out of the 184 cases studied, three of them being benign tumors, as proved afterward at histological examination.
Causes of sample rejection are summarized in Table 1.

Positivity Rates Observed in Clinical Practice

A previous study [7, 8] comparing drill biopsy with corresponding surgical samples showed for both ER and PgR a correspondence close to 90% in terms of positivity when drill

Table 1. Causes of sample rejection in a series of 184 drill biopsies samples (169 adenocarcinomas and 15 benign tumors)

	All cases (184)	Adenocarcinoma (169)
Weight < 20 mg	12 (6.5%)	6 (3.5%)
DNA < 500 µg/gT (weight > 20 mg)	21 (11.4%)	15 (9.0%)
Other (DNA > 500 µg/gT, weight > 20 mg)	14 (7.6%)	11 (6.5%)
Total	47 (25.5%)	32 (19%)

Table 2. Positivity rates (threshold: 250 fmol/gT) in 114 drill biopsies of primary breast adenocarcinoma

ER$^+$	54/91	(59%)
PgR$^+$	48/99	(48%)
ER$^+$PgR$^+$	39/76	(51%)
ER$^+$PgR$^-$	9/76	(12%)
ER$^-$PgR$^+$	1/76	(1%)
ER$^-$PgR$^-$	27/76	(36%)

samples weighed more than 20 mg. From this study it appeared that the practical threshold of positivity for drill biopsy specimens was 250 fmol/gT (about 6 fmol/mg protein) for ER and PgR. Positivity rates were then established in a series of 114 drill biopsies on primary breast adenocarcinomas of common histological type. Both ER and PgR were assayed in 76 of these 114 cases. Results are shown in Table 2.

These positivity rates are comparable to those generally reported for large surgical samples in the literature [1].

Discussion

The results presented here, together with previous results already published, show that drill biopsy samples can be used for estrogen and/or progestin assays, provided that accurate quality controls are carried out.

Owing to the small mass of tissue obtained, only one receptor can be reliably assayed. We currently give priority to assaying progestin receptor since it gives more reliable clinical information [11, 13]. The use of an homogenizing buffer containing 0.4 M KCl allows the extraction of all present receptors, cytosolic and nuclear, avoiding the false-negative levels of purely cytosolic receptors when levels of endogenous circulating hormones are elevated (premenopausal women). In the presence of KCl, the progestin tag R-5020 does not bind to glucocorticoid receptors which may be present in the tumor, so that no addition of unlabeled cortisol is required. The choice of a rather low concentration of labeled hormone (1 nM for ER and 2 nM for PgR) allows only high affinity receptors to be detected and leads to greater accuracy of moderate receptor levels by minimizing nonspecific binding. Quality control of the tissue sample must be done in every case. Tissue DNA must be systematically assayed since control of cellularity by histological techniques is not possible on the assayed sample. Protein assay is also recommended in order to control the dilution of the cytosol.

The following rules should be observed to ascertain the validity of receptor levels determined on drill biopsies:
1. Samples should weigh more than 20 mg,
2. Tissue DNA should be above 500 µg/gT,
3. Cytosol protein concentration should be above 1.5 mg/ml.

In our experience, these conditions are met in about 80% of samples from adenocarcinoma.

In our institute, drill biopsy sampling has been routinely practiced for 30 years for histological diagnosis and for the past 3 years for steroid hormone receptors. Progestin receptor determination is therefore extended to nearly all patients with breast tumor and can be proposed prior to any treatment other than surgery. The technique has proved of great clinical value in predicting hormonosensitivity and in prognosis: correlations of ER and PgR values obtained from drill biopsy specimen with prognostic factors and the course of the disease have already been published: (i.e., correlations with histological grading [8], disease-free interval [13] and survival rates [9]).

References

1. Allegra JC, Lippman ME, Thompson EB, Simon R, Barlock A, Green L, Huff KK, Do HMT, Aitken SC (1979) Distribution, frequency and quantitative analysis of estrogen, progesterone, androgen and glucocorticoid receptors in human breast cancer. Cancer Res 39: 1447–1454
2. Bradford MM (1976) A rapid and sensitive method for the quantitation of microgram quantities of protein utilizing the principle of protein-dye binding. Anal Biochem 72: 248–254
3. Calle R, Pilleron JP, Schlienger P, Vilcoq JR (1978) Conservative management of operable breast cancer. Ten year experience at the Fondation Curie. Cancer 42: 2045–2053
4. Cooke T, George D, Shields R, Maynard P, Griffiths K (1979) Estrogen receptors and prognosis in early breast cancer. Lancet 1: 995–997
5. Fiszer-Szafarz B, Szafarz D, Guevara de Murillo A (1981) A general, fast and sensitive micromethod for DNA determination: application to rat and mouse liver, rat hepatoma, human leukocytes, chicken fibroblasts and yeast cells. Anal Biochem 110: 165–170
6. Garola RE, McGuire WL (1978) A hydroxyapatite micromethod for measuring estrogen receptor in human breast cancer. Cancer Res 38: 2216–2218
7. Magdelénat H, Durand JC, Calle R (1977) Dosage des récepteurs d'oestrogènes et de progestogènes sur forage-biopsies de tumeurs mammaires humaines. In: Bohuon C, Jardillier JC (eds) 2nd Symposium de biochimie clinique carcinologique, Institut Jean Godinot, Reims, 2–3 Dec.
8. Magdelénat H, Toubeau M, Picco C, Bidron C (1980) Détermination des récepteurs d'oestrogènes et de progestérone sur forages-biopsies des tumeurs mammaires. In: Martin PM (ed) Récepteurs hormonaux et pathologie mammaire. MEDSI, Paris
9. Magdelénat H, Pouillart P, Iouve M (1982) Progesterone receptor as a more reliable pronostic parameter than estrogen receptor in patients with advanced breast cancer. Breast Cancer Res. Treat. 2: 195–196
10. Martin PM, Rolland PH, Jacquemier J, Rolland AM, Toga M (1979) Multiple steroid receptors in human breast cancer. II. Estrogen and progestin receptors in 672 primary tumors. Cancer Chemother Pharmacol 2: 107–113
11. Pichon MF, Pallud C, Brunet M, Milgrom E (1980) Relationship of presence of progesterone receptors to prognosis in early breast cancer. Cancer Res 40: 3357–3360
12. Rousseau J (1955) La biopsie par forage. Bull Cancer 42: 398–418
13. Toubeau M (1981) Intérêt clinique du dosage des récepteurs d'hormones stéroides dans les cancers du sein. Expérience de l'Institut Curie. Medical dissertation, Paris
14. Veith F, Picco C (1977) Cancer du sein: pronostic histologique sur matériel biopsique. Bull Cancer 64: 537–556

The Value of Determination of Nuclear Oestrogen Receptors in Breast Cancer Biopsies*

S. Cowan, C. Love, and R. E. Leake

Department of Biochemistry, University of Glasgow, Glasgow G12 8QQ, United Kingdom

Introduction

The oestrogen receptor status of the soluble fraction of a tumour biopsy is now accepted as a valuable tool in the management of advanced breast cancer [11]. Soluble receptor status of primary disease may also be of value as a prognostic index [3, 20], although this value might be limited to patients with intermediate nodal involvement [19]. However, the presence of soluble receptors alone is not an absolute index of hormonal dependence [22]. Hormone-receptor complex might fail to undergo translocation/activation [37] or to bind to the correct acceptor sites on the DNA [33]. Loss of hormonal dependence through a breakdown at the post-transcriptional level is also a possibility. For these reasons several parameters of oestrogen response have been studied in breast tumour biopsies. Measurement of the presence of progesterone receptor (a product of oestrogen action) has proved productive [11]. The suggestion that a useful index of hormonal dependence might simply be the presence of nuclear-bound oestrogen receptor [21] has been followed up by several groups [2, 15, 29, 38].

This chapter describes the methods currently in use for determining nuclear oestrogen receptor concentration and suggests a method that might be useful for routine laboratory assay. The relevant properties of the nuclear receptor in breast tumour biopsies are considered. The potential value of nuclear oestrogen receptor status both in prognosis and in selection of therapy is reviewed.

Nuclear Exchange Assay

Early work with rat uterus [1] suggested that at a low temperature the rate of exchange of labelled steroid for endogenously bound oestrogen was too slow for a successful exchange assay. However, incubation of nuclear preparations at 37° C in the absence of protease inhibitors leads to rapid degradation of receptor. This objection may have been overcome by the recent demonstration [34] that the addition of 5 mM Ca^{2+} permits rapid exchange of

* Work from our own laboratory was supported, in part, by the Cancer Research Campaign, to whom we are very grateful. C. L. is pleased to acknowledge receipt of a Medical Research Council studentship. We are much indebted to our various surgical colleagues and, in particular, to David Smith and Ken Calman

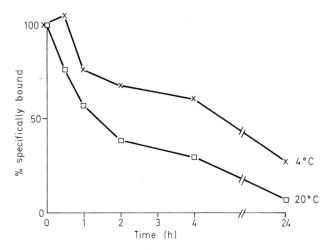

Fig. 1. Rate of dissociation of specifically bound oestradiol from nuclear receptor at 4° C and 20° C. Nuclei were pre-labelled at 37° C for 30 min in 2×10^{-9} M ^{3}H-oestradiol. Incubation medium contained 0.25 M sucrose, 1.5 mM MgCl$_2$, 10 mM Hepes, pH 7.4, plus 2×10^{-7} M unlabelled oestradiol

Table 1. Re-labelling of nuclear pellet after 24 h to show relative stability of receptor at 4° C and 20° C[a]

Temperature (° C)	Time of incubation		
	0 h	24 h	26 h
4	29.4 ± 15.5 (32)	12.9 ± 6.7 (25)	23.7 ± 14.0 (25)
20	29.4 ± 15.5 (32)	2.7 ± 2.4 (7)	18.8 ± 13.0 (7)

[a] Figures represent specifically bound ^{3}H-oestradiol expressed as cpm/μg DNA − mean ± standard deviation (no. of experiments). Nuclei were incubated as described in the legend to Fig. 1. After 24 h an aliquot was re-incubated with ^{3}H-oestradiol for 2 h and specifically bound steroid again determined

filled rat nuclear receptor at 37° C without significant degradation. In the case of human tumour receptor, oestradiol comes off its receptor and may be exchanged with tritiated steroid even at lower temperatures (Fig. 1), so that exchange assays can be conducted with minimal interference from either protease or nuclease attack. A second exchange (at 20° C) after incubation at 4° C for 24 h shows that little receptor is lost during this period (Table 1). Not surprisingly, whilst the exchange of unlabelled oestradiol for labelled hormone appears to be more complete at 20° C over 24 h, the loss of receptor, shown by the failure to re-label the sites at 26 h, is much greater.

Alternative nuclear exchange procedures have been proposed by Garola and McGuire [14] using high salt extraction of the nuclear pellet and absorption of receptor on to hydroxyapatite and by Hospelhorn and Jensen (personal communication) using glass beads and displacement by silver. The procedure using high salt concentration assumes that all nuclear receptor is extracted under these conditions, although this has been disputed by Clark and Peck [8]. Both the Ca^{2+} and glass bead/silver methods have considerable potential, and comparison of results obtained by these methods with those from current techniques is urgently needed.

It should be noted that although exchange of free for bound oestrogen can be achieved at 4° C with intact nuclei, the hormone-receptor complex, as extracted with high salt, seems stable at such low temperatures. Taking the mean of three experiments using receptor extracted with high salt, specific receptor content at 4° C was initially 43.2 cpm/µg DNA (100%), after 24 h 38.8 cpm/µg DNA (90%) and after 48 h 32.4 cpm/µg DNA (75%). Similar stability of high salt-extracted nuclear receptor has been found by others [14, 41].

All procedures used in our laboratory have been described in detail [23, 25].

Handling and fractionation of tissue and the nuclear assay were carried out as follows: Tissue was collected fresh and transported from the operating theatre to the laboratory on ice. Wherever possible, oestrogen-receptor assay was performed the same day; when this was not possible, storage was at −20° C in sucrose buffer: 0.25 M sucrose, 1.5 mM MgCl$_2$, 10 mM Hepes, pH 7.4, 50% glycerol (v/v). Soluble and nuclear fractions were then prepared by excising approximately 150 mg tissue from the area adjacent to that removed for pathological examination. Homogenisation was carried out at 50 mg/ml in HED buffer [20 mM Hepes, 1.5 mM EDTA, 0.25 mM dithiothreitol (DTT), pH 7.4] for two 10-s bursts at a setting of 150 on an Ultra-Turrax, model TP 18/2, followed by further homogenisation with a glass tissue grinder (Kontes Duall). The homogenate was centrifuged at 5,000 g for

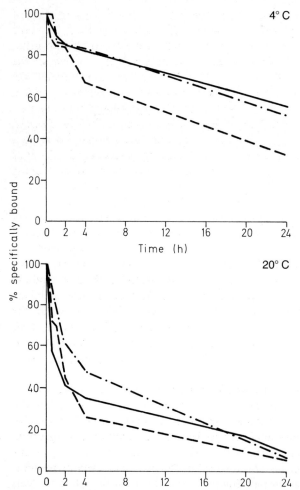

Fig. 2. Effect of protease inhibitors on the off-rate of ^{3}H-oestradiol from nuclear receptor. Nuclei were labelled and incubated as described in the legend to Fig. 1. Results represent the percentage of specifically bound counts retained at the time indicated. Incubation medium contained no additions (———), 2 mM PMSF (− · −) or 2,000 U/ml Trasylol (−−−)

5 min at 4° C to yield a 'cytosol' supernatant and a crude nuclear pellet. The pellet was washed three times in 0.15 M NaCl, 20 mM Hepes (pH 7.4), and finally resuspended, using the Kontes grinder, to the original volume in buffered saline. A wash with 0.1% Triton X-100 was sometimes incorporated at this stage to further purify the nuclear material, but this did not appreciably alter the level of nuclear binding. Further purification of the pellet fraction by differential centrifugation through sucrose (finally 2.4 M sucrose, 1.5 mM MgCl$_2$) was carried out for the initial experiments on characterization of the exchange process. The integrity of the nuclei was checked by phase-contrast microscopy.

To determine the concentration of receptors present in the nuclear suspension, 150-µl aliquots were added to 50-µl aliquots of ^{3}H-oestradiol-17β to give final concentrations of steroid of 1, 1.5, 2, 4, 6, 8, and 10 × 10^{-10} M. A parallel set of tubes were also set up containing ^{3}H-oestradiol with a 100-fold concentration of unlabelled diethylstilboestrol (DES) to determine the specificity of binding. All tubes were then incubated at 4° C for 18 h or 20° C for 2 h − results obtained at the two temperatures were not found to be significantly different. The inclusion of protease inhibitors, aprotinin (Trasylol) and/or PMSF (phenylmethylsulphonyl fluoride), in the incubation medium did not appear to enhance receptor measurement or modify the off-rate of bound ligand (Fig. 2). After incubation the amount of steroid bound was determined as follows: 100-µl aliquots from each tube were placed into 5 ml 0.9% saline. The mixture was poured down the chimney of a Millipore filter apparatus on to a pre-wetted Whatman GF/C glass-fibre filter. The tube was washed out with 5 ml saline, the washing poured on to the filter and the filter further washed, under suction, three times, each time with 4 ml saline. After removal of the chimney, the edge of the filter was washed and the filter removed into a scintillation vial prior to drying overnight at 60° C. Ten millilitres toluene/PPO (5 g/l) scintillant was added, and the samples counted at 35% efficiency in a Searle Mark III liquid scintillation counter. More recently the washing procedure has been semi-automated (see this chapter, "Discussion"). The Scatchard plot of specific bound material was constructed using a computer program. An unambiguous Scatchard plot yielding a K_d of less than 5 × 10^{-10} M reflected positive nuclear receptor status. The assay was sensitive down to 25 fmol/mg DNA.

Reproducibility

Nuclear oestrogen receptor in intact tumour biopsies appears to be stable under the storage conditions for at least 2 months. Some samples have been stored for much longer without apparent loss of receptor concentration although there is a gradual change in shape of the sucrose density gradient peak of receptor (data not shown). However, given the intratumoral variation of both soluble and nuclear receptor content (Table 2) [see also Refs 35, 39], it is not possible to give an exact figure for stability in intact biopsies. Nuclear receptor content of lyophilised tumour has, in the three cases tested, been unchanged over a period of 1 year.

Six independent assays were carried out simultaneously on aliquots of the nuclear pellet from a large breast tumour and the variation was found to be less than 20%. When different sections of tumour were excised from a single large biopsy and assayed for nuclear receptor content, a three- to fourfold variation was observed (Table 2). Further studies suggest [6] that the variation in nuclear receptor concentration across large tumours can occasionally be much larger than this and that central (non-necrotic) portions may even be receptor negative whilst the periphery is receptor positive.

Table 2. Variation in nuclear and soluble oestrogen receptor concentration in six parallel sections from a single tumour biopsy

Section	Soluble fraction		Nuclear fraction	
	Receptor content (fmol/mg protein)	Dissociation constant (mol)	Receptor content (fmol/mg DNA)	Dissociation constant (mol)
A	124	0.9×10^{-10}	1,933	3.8×10^{-10}
B	171	1.05×10^{-10}	1,395	2.0×10^{-10}
C	484	1.02×10^{-10}	658	2.5×10^{-10}
D	146	1.6×10^{-10}	658	2.9×10^{-10}
E	423	1.02×10^{-10}	1,778	2.6×10^{-10}
F	526	1.2×10^{-10}	753	2.7×10^{-10}

Response to Hormone Therapy

Response to hormone therapy was assessed in patients with secondary disease for whom the receptor status had been determined prior to initiation of any therapy. Hormone therapy alone was applied as primary treatment during the period of assessment. The criteria for response were those suggested by the British Breast Group [5] and reinforced by the UICC (Union International Contre le Cancer) [17]. In brief, these involve at least 50% regression of existing lesions, and no appearance of new lesions within a 6-month period. Only patients who satisfied these criteria for at least 6 months were recorded as having responded.

Using the assay procedure described and adopting the above criteria, the response of patients to hormone therapy was recorded relative to the particular receptor category of the biopsy (Table 3). Four categories of receptor status were found. Biopsies containing receptor in both soluble and pellet fraction (+/+) are referred to as containing functional receptor. Two categories, those with receptor in the soluble fraction alone (+/zero) or the nuclear fraction alone (zero/+) are said to contain abnormal receptor (not necessarily implying physical abnormality). The final category is that in which there was no detectable receptor in either fraction (zero/zero).

Patients whose biopsies showed an intact receptor system (+/+) had a very good chance of responding to some type of endocrine therapy (most commonly tamoxifen treatment) (Table 3). Only five patients (9%) in the truly receptor-negative class showed complete response. In each case, these patients had received tamoxifen and may have responded to one of the actions of this drug which is not receptor mediated [40]. It is striking that the patients whose biopsies contained receptor in only one fraction, irrespective of which one, behaved in a manner similar to the receptor-negative group. Such an observation suggests that these receptors are non-functional, although it gives no indication as to whether the fault lies in the receptor itself or in some cellular recognition site. Preliminary evidence from our laboratory suggests that in the case of biopsies containing soluble receptor alone (+/zero), a fault in transformation can be detected in some but not all samples. Failure of such receptors to bind to DNA has also been reported [33]. This could be due either to loss of a transformation/activation factor or to the loss of the appropriate recognition signal from the chromatin.

Table 3. Response of breast tumour patients to hormone therapy in relation to the oestrogen receptor status of the biopsy

Receptor status (R_c/R_n)	Total number of patients	Patients with complete response	
		No.	%
+/+	45	32	71
Zero/zero	63	5	8
+/zero	17	4	24
Zero/+	9	1	11

Table 4. Stage of disease of patients who did not have a complete response to hormone therapy, in relation to the oestrogen receptor status of the biopsy

Receptor (R_c/R_n)	Total number of patients	Partial response	Static disease	Progressive disease
+/+	13	4	1	8
Zero/zero	58	2	5	51
+/zero	13	2	1	10
Zero/+	8	–	–	8

Of the 134 patients considered (Table 3), only 27 were premenopausal and 10 were menopausal. The response rates quoted (42 out of 134 = 31%), therefore, apply principally to postmenopausal disease. Of the 42 patients experiencing complete response, 18 had had local recurrence, 10 recurrence in gland and/or skin, seven in bone and the remainder at one or more distant sites. Of the 77 patients with progressive disease, 13 had local recurrence, 21 skin and/or gland, 21 bone, seven pleura, seven liver and the remainder at one or more distant sites.

The patients who did not experience a complete response for 6 months were divided into three groups: partial response, static and progressive disease (Table 4).

From the data presented in Tables 3 and 4, it may be concluded that over 80% of patients (51 out of 63) with receptor-negative tumours will experience progressive disease whilst on hormone therapy. Progressive disease seems equally inevitable for patients whose biopsies have nuclear receptor alone (8 out of 9). Determination of both nuclear and soluble receptor status clearly allows this group to be identified and treated as very unlikely to benefit from endocrine therapy. Patients who have soluble receptor alone fare slightly better (only 10 out of 17 with progressive disease). However, they are at a much higher risk of progressive disease (when on endocrine therapy, at least) than are the fully receptor positive group (8 out of 45). The use of both soluble and nuclear receptor status again allows them to be identified as a separate group for treatment and follow-up.

Nuclear Receptor Status and Prognosis

Since determination of both soluble and nuclear receptor status enabled us to identify subgroups of patients with advanced disease whom we should not have detected on the

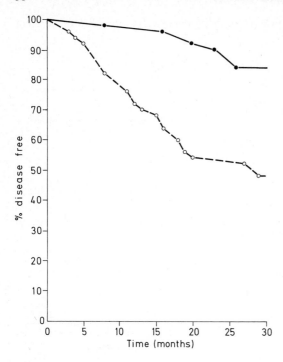

Fig. 3. Oestrogen receptor status in relation to disease-free interval of breast cancer patients. The probability of surviving for 30 months was significantly greater for patients whose biopsies contained functional receptor (●———●) than for those who had receptor negative biopsies (○− − −○). $P \ll 0.01$

basis of soluble receptor alone, we examined receptor status of primary disease in relation to nodal involvement and disease-free interval. Soluble oestrogen receptor status has already been reported to be a useful prognostic index [3, 20], although its value may be confined to patients with intermediate nodal involvement [19]. Our results are based on patients who presented with operable breast cancer at least 36 months prior to the time of writing. The majority of patients with primary disease were treated by simple mastectomy and axillary clearance to the level of the axillary vein. Depending on their age and the presence or absence of axillary lymph node metastases, some patients were entered into trials of adjuvant chemotherapy (RT vs RT + CMF vs CMF) or adjuvant endocrine therapy (tamoxifen vs nil). All patients were followed up at regular intervals at hospital clinics; information on a few was obtained from the appropriate family doctor. The date and site of recurrence was recorded in relation to the nodal status and oestrogen receptor status of the primary disease.

Disease-free interval recorded for each patient is the time which elapsed between initial diagnosis of primary breast cancer and detection of recurrent disease.

Oestrogen receptor status was determined on a biopsy of the primary disease prior to initiation of any adjuvant therapy. In most cases, nodal status was determined by routine pathological dissection of the axillary tissue and histological examination of all identified nodes. If disease recurred simultaneously at both local (e.g., wound flap) and distant sites, it was recorded as distant recurrence. As stated above, all patients in the study were diagnosed as having primary breast cancer at least 36 months prior to the time of writing, and all those reported as still well have been checked at least 30 months after initial diagnosis.

The study involved 50 patients with functional oestrogen receptor (+/+) and, for direct comparison, 50 patients selected at random from those with no detectable receptor in either fraction (zero/zero). Our results (shown in Fig. 3) and those of others [3, 16] are

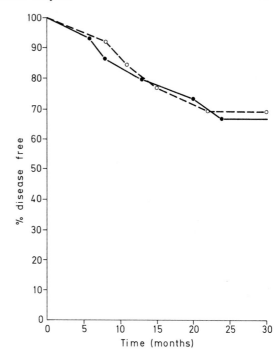

Fig. 4. Disease-free interval of breast cancer patients whose primary biopsies contained abnormal receptors. Data are plotted for 15 patients whose biopsies contained only soluble receptor (●────●) and for 13 patients whose biopsies contained only nuclear receptor (○−−−○)

compatible with the idea that a subgroup of patients with receptor-negative disease progress very rapidly. Thereafter, the remaining receptor-negative patients relapse at about the same rate as the receptor-positive group. However, the study will have to be extended over at least 5 years before this can be confirmed.

The two groups of patients whose biopsies yielded abnormal receptor status (i.e., those with receptor in one fraction only; see Ref [26]) were indistinguishable with respect to disease-free interval (Fig. 4), and both lay between the patterns for the (+/+) and (zero/zero) groups. It is significant that the group with soluble receptor alone (which would have been included in the receptor-positive group had not the nuclear assay been performed) behaved so differently from the group with functional receptors. There is no evidence, as yet, that the abnormal receptor status is more common in one nodal group than another [26]. Our study showed a significant difference in disease-free interval between receptor-positive and receptor-negative patients even in the node-negative subgroup (the difference in probability of surviving > 30 months using Fisher's Exact Test for a 2 × 2 table (because of the 100% survival for node negative/(+/+) patients at 30 months) gave $P = 0.095$). This observation differs from those of others [3, 19], possibly because they would include the (+/zero) patients in their receptor-positive groups.

Discussion

Measurement of nuclear oestrogen receptor status in breast cancer biopsies was originally proposed [21] to overcome possible "false-positives" due to either breakdown in the translocation/transformation process [37] or the loss of appropriate chromosomal recognition site(s) [33, 36]. Use of a nuclear exchange assay which eliminated protease degradation would also ensure that women with high levels of circulating oestrogens (such that most oestrogen receptor was in the nucleus) would not automatically be classified as receptor poor [38]. Subsequently several groups have studied nuclear oestrogen receptor content in relation to both patient management and prognosis [3, 13, 15, 21, 25−27].

In selecting an assay method, a compromise has to be made between protease degradation and loss of nuclear receptor through processing at 37° C [11, 18], and exchange rate at low temperatures. Salt-extracted nuclear receptor does not appear to undergo significant exchange at 4° C [7]. In our experience, exchange of nuclear-bound oestrogen occurs gradually at 4° C in intact nuclei (Fig. 1, Table 1), although more rapid exchange rates have been observed by others [4]. A variable proportion of empty nuclear receptors have been reported in breast cancer biopsies [29, 34]. Edwards et al. [12] claim that in the case of MCF-7 cells these empty sites can be extracted into the soluble fraction during purification of the nuclei. However, our results suggest that for breast cancer biopsies the total number of nuclear receptors detected is similar whether assayed at 4° C or 20° C and that purification of nuclei makes minimal difference to receptor concentration on a DNA basis. In conclusion, the functional role, if any, of unfilled nuclear receptors in breast tumours is undecided. For this reason, an exchange assay procedure which measures most, if not all, nuclear receptors, both filled and unfilled, should be adopted for clinical purposes. Alternative nuclear exchange assays to the one described here measure salt-extracted nuclear receptors. Protease activity must be inhibited in such high temperature assays and they are still open to the criticism that the biologically active hormone-receptor complex might be that which is not extracted by high salt [8, 31]. No information on the application of the theoretically promising glass bead/silver nitrate exchange assay to human breast cancer nuclei is yet available.

Selection of breast cancer patients to receive endocrine therapy on the basis that they have soluble oestrogen receptor-positive tumours, although an improvement on previous discriminants, still only achieves a 54% (range 39%−62%) response rate [16]. Selection of patients on the basis of tumours with functional receptor (i.e., those that have both soluble and pellet receptor) raises the response rate to 71% [25]. Measurement of one of the parameters reflecting later events in oestrogen-induced growth [9, 10] has only been related to clinical response for a significant number of patients in the case of progesterone receptor synthesis [11, 28]. In this case the response rate of patients with both soluble oestrogen receptor and soluble progesterone receptor was 74%. In a small study [2] measurement of both soluble and nuclear oestrogen receptor together with soluble progesterone receptor suggested that response rate might be slightly higher, but a much greater number of patients would have to be studied for this result to become significant.

Several groups have shown that the higher the concentration of soluble receptor, the better the chance of response to therapy [11, 30]. Presumably, if total functional (soluble and nuclear) receptor were used, the response rate would be even better because cases of abnormal receptor would at least in part be eliminated.

The presence of soluble oestrogen receptor in the breast tumour biopsy has been related to increased disease-free interval and total survival time [16, 20, 32] although this may only apply to patients with one to three nodes involved [3, 19]. However, incorporation of nuclear receptor data, and so elimination of patients whose biopsy specimens contain soluble receptor alone, may indicate that node-negative patients whose tumours contain functional receptor may also have a better prognosis [26].

Given that a nuclear assay of the type described is needed for routine testing of both primary and advanced breast cancer biopsies, a more rapid, semi-automated procedure would be desirable. Initial attempts to use a 12-channel cell harvester (Ilacon) to facilitate throughout appear very encouraging.

At the present time it is clear that measurement of either nuclear oestrogen receptor or of soluble progesterone receptor in breast tumour biopsies gives a better indication of oestrogen dependence than does measurement of soluble receptor alone. At least one and preferably both additional measurements should, therefore, be included in routine assays for either prognosis or therapy selection.

References

1. Anderson JN, Clark JH, Peck EJ Jr (1972) Oestrogen and nuclear binding sites: determination of specific sites by [^{3}H] oestradiol exchange. Biochem J 126: 561−567
2. Barnes DM, Skinner LG, Ribeiro GG (1979) Triple hormone-receptor assay: a more accurate predictive tool for the treatment of advanced breast cancer? Br J Cancer 40: 862−865
3. Bishop HM, Blamey RW, Elston CW, Haybittle JL, Nicholson RI, Griffiths K (1979) Relationship of oestrogen-receptor status to survival in breast cancer. Lancet 2: 283−284
4. Blankenstein MA, Peters-Mechielsen MJ, Mulder E, Van Der Molen HJ (1980) Estimation of total oestrogen receptors in DMBA-induced rat mammary tumors by exchange of nuclear bound ligand at low temperature; a comparison with rat uterus. J Steroid Biochem 13: 557−564
5. British Breast Group (1974) Assessment of response to treatment in advanced breast cancer. Lancet 2: 38−39
6. Castagnetta L, Lo Casto M, Mercadante T, Polito L, Cowan S, Leake RE (1983) Intratumoural variation of oestrogen receptor status in endometrial cancer. Br J Cancer 47: 261−267
7. Chamness GC, McGuire WL (1980) Methods for analyzing steroid receptors in human breast cancer. In: McGuire WL (ed) Breast cancer, vol 3. Plenum Medical, New York, p 149
8. Clark JH, Peck EJ Jr (1976) Nuclear retention of receptor-oestrogen complex and nuclear acceptor sites. Nature 260: 635−637
9. Delarue JC, Bohoun C (1980) Utilization of the measurement of hormone receptors in the treatment of breast cancer in women. Ann Biol Clin (Paris) 38: 293−296
10. Duffy MJ, O'Connell M (1981) Estrogens, estradiol receptors and peroxidase activity in human mammary carcinomas. Eur J Cancer 17: 711−716
11. Edwards DP, Chamness GC, McGuire WL (1979) Estrogen and progesterone receptor proteins in breast cancer. Biochim Biophys Acta 560: 457−486
12. Edwards DP, Martin PM, Horwitz KB, Chamness GC, McGuire WL (1980) Subcellular compartmentalization of estrogen receptors in human breast cancer cells. Exp Cell Res 127: 197−213
13. Fazekas AG, MacFarlane JK (1980) Studies on cytosol and nuclear binding of estradiol in human breast cancer. J Steroid Biochem 13: 613−622
14. Garola RE, McGuire WL (1977) An improved assay for nuclear oestrogen receptor in experimental and human breast cancer. Cancer Res 37: 3333−3337
15. Hahnel R, Partridge RK, Gavet L, Twaddle E, Ratajczak T (1980) Nuclear and cytoplasmic estrogen receptors and progesterone receptors in breast cancer. Eur J Cancer 16: 1027−1033
16. Hawkins RA, Roberts MM, Forrest APM (1980) Oestrogen receptors and breast cancer: current status. Br J Surg 67: 152−169
17. Hayward JL, Carbonne PP, Heuson JC, Kumaoka S, Segaloff A, Rubens RD (1977) Assessment of response to therapy in advanced breast cancer. Eur J Cancer 13: 89−94
18. Horwitz KB, McGuire WL (1980) Nuclear estrogen receptors: effect of inhibitors on processing and steady state levels. J Biol Chem 255: 9699−9705
19. Howat JMT, Barnes DM (1981) Oestrogen receptor status and management of breast cancer. Lancet 1: 1317

20. Knight WA, Livingston RB, Gregory EJ, McGuire WL (1977) Estrogen receptor as an independent prognostic factor for early recurrence in breast cancer. Cancer Res 37: 4669–4671

21. Laing L, Smith MG, Calman KC, Smith DC, Leake RE (1977) Nuclear oestrogen receptors and treatment of breast cancer. Lancet 2: 168–169

22. Leake RE (1976) Current views on oestrogen receptors. Trends Biochem Sci 1: 137–139

23. Leake RE, Laing L, Smith DC (1979) A role for nuclear oestrogen receptors in prediction of therapy regime for breast cancer patients. In: King RJB (ed) Steroid receptor assays in human breast tumours. Alpha Omega, Cardiff, p 73

24. Leake RE (1980) Methodology of steroid hormone receptor determination in breast cancer. In: Taylor RW (ed) Progestogens in the management of hormonal responsive carcinomas. Medicine Publishing Foundation, Oxford, p 3

25. Leake RE, Laing L, Calman KC, Macbeth FR, Crawford D, Smith DC (1981) Oestrogen-receptor status and endocrine therapy of breast cancer: response rates and status stability. Br J Cancer 43: 59–66

26. Leake RE, Laing L, McArdle C, Smith DC (1981) Soluble and nuclear oestrogen receptor status in human breast cancer in relation to prognosis. Br J Cancer 43: 67–71

27. MacFarlane JK, Fleiszer D, Fazekas AG (1980) Studies on estrogen receptors and regression in human breast cancer. Cancer 45: 2998–3003

28. Osborne CK, Yochmowitz MG, Knight WA, McGuire WL (1980) The value of estrogen and progesterone receptors in the treatment of breast cancer. Cancer 46: 2884–2888

29. Panko WB, MacLeod RM (1978) Uncharged nuclear receptors for estrogen in breast cancers. Cancer Res 38: 1948–1951

30. Paridaens R, Sylvester RJ, Ferrazzi E, Legros N, Leclercq G, Heuson JC (1980) Clinical significance of the quantitative assessment of estrogen receptors in advanced breast cancer. Cancer 46: 2889–2895

31. Ruh TS, Baudendistel LJ (1977) Different nuclear binding sites for antiestrogen and estrogen receptor complexes. Endocrinology 100: 420–426

32. Samaan NA, Buzdar AU, Aldinger KA, Schultz PN, Yang KP, Romsdahl MM, Martin R (1981) Estrogen receptor: a prognostic factor in breast cancer. Cancer 47: 554–560

33. Sato B, Nomura Y, Nakao K, Ochi H, Matsumoto K (1981) DNA binding ability of estrogen receptor from human breast cancer. J Steroid Biochem 14: 295–303

34. Schoenberg DR, Clark JK (1980) A simple modification of the estrogen receptor exchange assay: validation in nuclei from the rat uterus and a mouse mammary tumor. Endocrinology 106: 56–60

35. Silfverswärd C, Skoog L, Humla S, Gustafsson SA, Nordenskjöld B (1980) Intratumoral variation of cytoplasmic and nuclear estrogen receptor concentrations in human mammary carcinoma. Eur J Cancer 16: 59–63

36. Taylor RN, Swaneck GE, Smith RG (1980) Correlation of nuclear acceptor sites for oestrogen receptors with gene transcription in vitro. Biochem J 192: 385–393

37. Thorsen T, Stoa KF (1979) Nuclear uptake of oestradiol-17β in human mammary tumour tissue. J Steroid Biochem 10: 595–599

38. Thorsen T (1980) Occupied and unoccupied oestradiol receptor in human breast tumour cytosol. J Steroid Biochem 13: 405–408

39. Tilley WD, Keightley DD, Cant ELM (1978) Inter-site variation of oestrogen receptors in human breast cancers. Br J Cancer 38: 544–546

40. Tisdale MJ (1977) Inhibition of prostaglandin synthetase by anti-tumour agents. Chem Biol Interact 18: 91–102

41. Zava DT, Harrington NY, McGuire WL (1976) Nuclear estradiol receptor in the adult rat uterus: a new exchange assay. Biochemistry 15: 4292–4297

Histochemical Methods

Immunocytochemical Demonstration of Steroid Receptors*

E. Marchetti and I. Nenci

Istituto di Anatomia e Istologia Patologica, Università di Ferrara,
Via Fossato di Mortara 66, 44100 Ferrara, Italy

Introduction

Immunocytochemistry as an investigative method is now as sensitive as radiometric, cell-free methods, and thus provides the opportunity of detecting hormones at their sites of action [28]. Immunocytochemical demonstration of steroid receptors on cells and tissues is based on the detection of the steroid hormone bound to its own receptor by specific antibodies. The aim of this contribution is first to report the authors' and other workers' experience and then to provide a critical evaluation of the advantages and limitations of immunocytochemistry of steroid receptors when applied to the problem of breast cancer.

Methodology

Immunocytochemistry was originally applied to the demonstration of estrogen receptors in vital cells from human breast cancer [14] and then extended to tissue slices and to other steroid hormones.

Cell Suspensions

Isolated cell suspensions were obtained from specimens of human breast cancer immediately after surgical removal by gently mincing tissue fragments in cold phosphate-buffered saline (pH 7.2) (PBS) without any enzymatic treatment. Incubation of cells in estradiol 2×10^{-8} M then followed. The incubation step was generally carried out at 4° C for 1 h, sometimes followed by postincubation in PBS at 37° C for various lengths of time. On occasions the incubation step was carried out at 18° C or 37° C from the beginning.
After incubation, cells were thoroughly washed in cold PBS, cytocentrifuged, or placed on slides and left to dry at a cold temperature without any fixation step.

* This experimental work was supported in part by grant No. 80.01568.96 from the Progetto Finalizzato CNR "Controllo della crescita neoplastica"

For the visualization of the bound estradiol a double immunocytochemical technique was applied: In the first step slides were treated with specific anti-17β-estradiol antibody raised by immunization of rabbits with 17β-estradiol-6-carboxymethyloxime-bovine serum albumin (dilution of serum = 1 : 100 in PBS). After several washes in cold PBS, cells were covered with a fluorescein-labeled goat anti-rabbit Ig antiserum. Both the immune reactions were performed in a moist chamber at 4° C. After the final washes in cold PBS, cell preparations were mounted in buffered glycerol in PBS (1 : 1) and immediately inspected by means of ultraviolet microscopy.

Tissue Sections

Immunocytochemical techniques have also been applied to demonstrate estrogen receptors on frozen sections from estrogen target tissues.

One approach is based on the immune tracing of estradiol on frozen tissue sections. Several technical variations have been devised independently by different workers.

To enhance the visualization of specific receptors, 17β-estradiol has been substituted by the polymeric derivative polyestradiol phosphate (PEP), which acts as a large antigen for the antibody [24, 25]. After incubation with PEP, frozen sections were treated with a double antibody method using fluorescein as a tracer. Alternatively, estradiol has been detected by immunofluorescence [29] and by the peroxidase-antiperoxidase method [30] on frozen sections; the latter appears to be a more sensitive technique than the usual double antibody method. Both of the aforementioned methods have the advantage of tracing not only the hormone bound in vitro but also the hormone prebound in vivo.

In another approach frozen sections are exposed to a soluble immunocomplex comprising PEP and anti-17β-estradiol antibody, which is then displayed by a second fluorescein- or peroxidase-labeled antibody [19]. The availability of estradiol reactive groups to estradiol antibody of the immunocomplexed polyestradiol has been tested by the double immunodiffusion technique [18].

A double labeling immunofluorescence assay using fluorescein and rhodamine as tracers has been proposed to simultaneously detect estradiol and progesterone in individual target cells [10].

Frozen sections have been used not only to detect estradiol given in vitro but also to localize the specific binding of the hormone administered in vivo, the chosen display system being immunofluorescence [21] or immunoperoxidase [8]. In this respect the combined use of immunocytochemistry and cryoultramicrotomy seems to be a valuable technique for detecting specific steroid binding at the ultrastructural level [3, 11].

In contrast to the above techniques, which involve frozen tissue sections, an immunocytochemical estrogen receptor assay in paraffin sections has been proposed. This assay is compatible with routine histologic preparations [9]. In order to protect receptor sites against conformational changes resulting from fixation and embedding, estradiol was added before and during the fixation steps.

The most recently devised immunocytochemical approach makes use of specific receptor antibodies. Such a technique has been applied to the dynamic tracing of the intracellular compartmentalization of glucocorticoid receptor in vital target cells [7, 22]. Preliminary results have also been reported with estrogen receptor [26]. It is worthy of note that the pattern of positivity mirrors the features obtained by steroid antibodies in analogous experimental conditions.

Validation

To establish the specificity of the immune tracing of estradiol, the following control tests must be performed [28]:

1. In the first step of the immune reaction the specific anti-17β-estradiol antibody is substituted either by a nonimmune rabbit serum or by the specific anti-17β-estradiol antiserum saturated with 17β-estradiol in excess.

2. In the second step either an unlabeled goat antirabbit antiserum is applied before the fluoresceinated one or only the fluorescein-conjugated antibody is applied without previous exposure to specific anti-17β-estradiol antiserum.

The question of the availability to the antibody of estradiol bound to the receptor has been raised. On the basis of the immobilized antibody [1, 5], it has been shown that estradiol antibody cannot react with estradiol already bound to its receptor. Nevertheless, the consistency of the immunocytochemical approach has been validated by other analogous techniques involving steroid antibodies. The kinetics of binding reactions in the experimental conditions of immunocytochemistry are also different from those of biochemical methods and probably account for this apparent discrepancy.

The main question in the immunocytochemical demonstration of steroid receptors is whether immune-traced steroid-binding sites can be confidently assumed to be true receptors. According to the current concept of "receptor", the demonstrated binding must exhibit the following characteristics [2]:

1. *Finite binding capacity:* Pre-coincubation of cells and tissues with a series of estrogenic or antiestrogenic substances which are known to compete with estrogen for specific receptors is performed to assess the finite binding capacity. In this way cells and tissues which are shown to be positive by the standard techniques appear completely negative.

2. *Steroid specificity:* This is demonstrated by the lack of inhibition by nonestrogenic steroids, i.e., the binding of estrogen to its receptor is unaffected by unrelated steroids. Steroid specificity can be tested by pre-coincubating tissues and cells with nonestrogenic steroids such as progesterone and testosterone and their synthetic analogs in a high molar excess.

3. *High affinity:* Demonstration of the high affinity of binding cannot be undertaken readily using immunocytochemical techniques; however, if the binding withstands prolonged cold washing steps this may be taken as acceptable proof, since low affinity binding would undergo dissociation.

4. *Tissue specificity:* Immunocytochemical techniques give a positive staining in known target tissues such as human breast and rat uterus, while no positivity is apparent in several known estrogen nontarget tissues and tumours when they are processed in the same way.

In conclusion, the available evidence supports the contention that the binding sites displayed by immunocytochemical techniques represent specific recognition sites for estrogen. The question arises as to what kind of binding sites are demonstrated in this way. Since the binding appears to fulfill the accepted criteria for estrogen receptors [13], the receptor nature of the immunocytochemical estrogen-binding sites may be inferred and, in the absence of other explanations for the observed results, this represents a tenable proposal.

Some Clues to Cell Biology

Different experimental conditions during the incubation step were chosen to monitor the uptake and intracellular compartmentalization of the hormone. The pattern of fluorescent staining of the cells varied according to the temperature and time of incubation with the hormone: at 4° C estradiol-binding sites were traced diffusely in the cytoplasm while at 37° C nuclear staining was appreciable [14]. Moreover, by prolonging the postincubation step at 37° C it was possible to follow the nuclear retention time course [15]. After the leakage of the hormone a finite number of long-lived retention sites were traced on the chromatin network, probably corresponding to nuclear acceptor sites.

The double antibody method has also been applied to the dynamic monitoring of estradiol uptake, retention and distribution in isolated breast cancer cells at the electron microscopic level [20]. The experimental methodology was identical to that employed for immuno-fluorescence, except that horseradish peroxidase was used as a tracer.

The pattern of immunoperoxidase positivity upon electron microscopy varied according to the temperature and time of the incubation step and agreed strictly with the localizations of receptor-bound steroid as traced by immunofluorescence. While at 4° C estradiol-binding sites were traced as diffuse cytoplasmic constituents and mainly as polyribosomes, at 37° C the nuclear binding sites, identified as nuclear bodies, were stained. Moreover it has been possible to study the structural counterpart of the transportation process by modulating the temperature-dependent transport rates of the protein-bound estrogen into the nucleus [17]. During the transportation process cytoplasmic estradiol-bearing particles were traced which interacted with the nuclear membrane, seemingly inducing the formation of nuclear pore complexes. These transient intracellular organelles mediating the transport of steroids into the nucleus, at first named "transferosomes", were afterwards identified as coated vesicles. In this respect it seems worth noting the analogy of this shuttle system with the more recently identified "receptosomes" involved in another reported intracellular delivery system of receptor-ligand complexes [31].

Some Clues to Cancer Biology

The immunocytochemical tracing of steroid receptors has been particularly useful when applied to the study of estrogen receptors in human breast cancer [12, 13, 19].

Among all the examined tumours (several hundreds up to now), very few were composed of homogeneous cell populations with respect to cell hormone receptivity — more often receptor-positive and receptor-negative cells were displayed in the same tumour. In addition, a variable degree of staining intensity among positive cells was apparent, this being indicative of a continuous gradient of cytoplasmic receptor endowment among individual cells of the same tumour. This cell heterogeneity in cytoplasmic estrogen binding appears to occur at the very beginning of tumour development, as is apparent in both ductal and lobular carcinoma in situ.

By monitoring the intracellular distribution of the bound hormone it was possible to demonstrate a defective nuclear translocation of estrogen receptors in cells with a normal cytoplasmic uptake. Such a failure of the intranuclear translocation bears a strong analogy to a physiological behavior observed in target tissues of very young rats. In fact, at a time when the nuclear accumulation was accomplished in older animals, a perinuclear concentration of the bound hormone was evident in 5-day-old animals, with no appreciable nuclear positivity [21]. These observations, which have been confirmed by biochemical studies [4, 23], and later investigation at the ultrastructural level [17], support the hypothesis that a regulatory role is played by the nuclear membrane in the steroid action mechanism.

Although no relationship could be established between receptor endowment and peculiar morphological characteristics, cells with differentiated features displayed evident cytoplasmic uptake and nuclear translocation of the bound hormone more often than did the undifferentiated cell population [13, 19].

Conclusions

Immunocytochemistry has been instrumental in increasing our understanding of the physiology and pathophysiology of steroid hormone action. By combining the visual approach with the sensitivity of specific antibodies it has been possible not only to confirm the results yielded by biochemical approaches but also to acquire a deeper insight into some biological aspects of hormone responsiveness relevant to the problem of breast cancer. The observation of heterogeneity of cell hormone receptivity of breast cancer has also affected deeply the theoretical approach to tumour therapy. Evidence that each tumour is a pool of receptor-positive and receptor-negative cells has prompted the search for new treatment schedules which, taking this constant heterogeneity into account, involve combined cytotoxic and endocrine therapy.

Immunocytochemical methods have been extremely valuable in the investigation of the mechanism of hormone action and are the methods of choice for study at the ultrastructural level. Nevertheless, the fairly long technical procedures as well as the numerous and complex control tests have favored the replacement of this methodology by direct labeling with fluorescent ligands [13, 16].

The reliability of the practical use of immunocytochemistry to predict hormone responsiveness of each individual tumour and thereby to guide management of patients has not been determined. In fact, while the predictive power of biochemical assays has been widely validated, this has not yet occurred with immunocytochemical assays.

Finally, specific receptor antibodies are now being obtained [6, 27]. Preliminary immunocytochemical studies are encouraging [26] and make them attractive probes for examining the structure and function of receptors, so that it can be envisaged that they will replace steroid antibodies in the near future.

References

1. Castaneda E, Liao S (1975) The use of anti-steroid antibodies in the characterization of steroid receptors. J Biol Chem 250: 883–888
2. Clark JH, Peck EJ (1977) Steroid hormone receptors: basic principles and measurements. In: O'Malley BW, Birnbauer L (eds) Receptors and hormone action, vol 1. Academic Press, New York, pp 383–410
3. Dubois PM, Morel G, Forest MG, Dubois MP (1978) Localization of luteinizing hormone (LH) and testosterone (T) or dihydrotestosterone (DHT) in the gonadotropic cells of the anterior pituitary by using ultracryomicrotomy and immunocytochemistry. Horm Metab Res 10: 250–252
4. Fazekas AG, MacFarlane JK (1980) Studies on cytosol and nuclear binding of estradiol in human breast cancer. J Steroid Biochem 13: 613–622

5. Fishman J, Fishman JH (1974) Competitive binding assay for estradiol receptor using immobilized antibody. J Clin Endocrinol Metab 39: 603–606

6. Greene GL, Nolan C, Engler JP, Jensen EV (1980) Monoclonal antibodies to human estrogen receptor. Proc Natl Acad Sci USA 77: 5115–5119

7. Govindan MV (1980) Immunofluorescence microscopy of the intracellular translocation of glucocorticoid receptor complexes in rat hepatoma (HTC) cells. Exp Cell Res 127: 293–297

8. Kopp F, Martin PM, Rolland PH, Bertrand MF (1979) A preliminary report on the use of immunoperoxidases to study binding of estrogens in rat uteri. J Steroid Biochem 11: 1081–1090

9. Kurzon RM, Sternberger LA (1978) Estrogen receptor immunocytochemistry. J Histochem Cytochem 26: 803–808

10. Mercer WD, Lippman ME, Wahl TM, Carlson CA, Wahl DA, Lezotte D, Teague PO (1980) The use of immunocytochemical techniques for the detection of steroid hormones in breast cancer cells. Cancer 46: 2859–2868

11. Morel G, Raynaud JP, Dubois PM (1981) Localisation ultrastructurale de l'oestradiol et du moxestrol dans les cellules gonadotropes du rat par immunocytologie après cryo-ultramicrotomie: caractérisation de la spécificité hormonale. Experientia 37: 98–100

12. Nenci I (1978) Receptor and centriole pathways of steroid action in normal and neoplastic cells. Cancer Res 38: 4204–4211

13. Nenci I (1981) Estrogen receptor cytochemistry in human breast cancer. Status and prospects. Cancer 48: 2674–2686

14. Nenci I, Beccati MD, Piffanelli A, Lanza G (1976) Detection and dynamic localization of estradiol-receptor complexes in intact target cells by immunofluorescence technique. J Steroid Biochem 7: 505–510

15. Nenci I, Beccati MD, Piffanelli A, Lanza G (1977) Dynamic immunofluorescence tracing of estradiol interactions with cytoplasmic and nuclear constituents in target cells. Res Steroids 7: 137–147

16. Nenci I, Dandliker WB, Meyers CY, Marchetti E, Marzola A, Fabris G (1980) Estrogen receptor cytochemistry by fluorescent estrogen. J Histochem Cytochem 28: 1081–1088

17. Nenci I, Fabris G, Marchetti E, Marzola A (1980) Intracellular flow of particulate steroid-receptor complexes in steroid target cells. Virchows Arch [Cell Pathol] 32: 139–145

18. Nenci I, Fabris G, Marchetti E, Marzola A (1980) Cytochemical evidence for steroid binding sites in the plasma membrane of target cells. In: Bresciani F (ed) Perspectives in steroid receptor research. Raven, New York, pp 61–72

19. Nenci I, Fabris G, Marzola A, Marchetti E (1980) Hormone receptor cytochemistry in human breast cancer. In: Iacobelli S, King RJB, Lindner HR, Lippman ME (eds) Hormones and cancer. Raven, New York, pp 227–239

20. Nenci I, Fabris G, Marzola A, Marchetti E (1980) Steroid-cell interactions revealed by immunological probes and electron microscopy. In: Genazzani E, DiCarlo F, Mainwaring WIP (eds) Pharmacological modulation of steroid action. Raven, New York, pp 99–110

21. Nenci I, Piffanelli A, Beccati MD, Lanza G (1976) In vivo and in vitro immunofluorescent approach to the physiopathology of estradiol kinetics in target cells. J Steroid Biochem 7: 883–891

22. Papamichail M, Tsokos G, Tsawdaroglou N, Sekeris CE (1980) Immunocytochemical demonstration of glucocorticoid receptors in different cell types and their translocation from the cytoplasm to the cell nucleus in the presence of dexamethasone. Exp Cell Res 125: 490–493

23. Peleg S, Deboever J, Kaye AM (1979) Replenishment and nuclear retention of oestradiol receptors in rat uteri during postnatal development. Biochim Biophys Acta 587: 67–74

24. Pertschuk LP (1976) Detection of estrogen binding in human mammary carcinoma by immunofluorescence: a new technique utilizing the binding hormone in a polymerized state. Res Commun Chem Pathol Pharmacol 14: 771–774

25. Pertschuk LP, Tobin EH, Brigati DJ (1978) Immunofluorescent detection of estrogen receptors in breast cancer. Comparison with dextran-coated charcoal and sucrose gradient assays. Cancer 41:907–911

26. Raam S, Nemeth E, O'Briain DS, Tamura H, Cohen JL (1981) Immunohistochemical localization of estrogen receptors in human breast carcinoma using anti-receptor antibodies (abstr). Proceedings of the annual meeting of AACR, Washington DC, vol 22, Washington, p 10

27. Raam S, Peters L, Rafkind I, Putnum E, Longcope C, Cohen JE (1981) Simple methods for production and characterization of rabbit antibodies to human breast tumor estrogen receptors. Mol Immunol 18:143–156

28. Sternberger LA (1979) Immunocytochemistry, 2nd edn. Wiley, New York

29. Thompson AJ, Cook MG, Gill PG (1981) Immunofluorescent detection of hormone receptors in cutaneous melanocytic tumours. Br J Cancer 43:644–653

30. Walker RA, Cove DH, Howell A (1980) Histological detection of oestrogen receptors in human breast carcinomas. Lancet 1:171–173

31. Willingham MC, Pastan I (1980) The receptosome: an intermediate organelle of receptor-mediated endocytosis in cultured fibroblasts. Cell 21:66–77

Use of Fluorescent Sex-Steroid Conjugates for the Histochemical Detection of Breast Cancer Cell Receptors: A Critique*

A. Danguy, G. Leclercq, and J. C. Heuson

Laboratoire d'Histologie, Faculté de Médicine, 2 Rue Evers, 1000 Bruxelles, Belgium

Introduction

All current techniques (autoradiography excepted) for the detection of nuclear or cytosol steroid hormone receptors require homogenization of tissue, and thereby sophisticated equipment not available at all centers. Several methods have been developed to trace estrogen (ER) and progesterone receptors (PgR) under the microscope (see [2] for review). In this regard the ligands employed so far consist of:
1. Steroid hormones linked to a carrier molecule (bovine serum albumin) which is labeled with fluorescent dyes ($\sim 2 \times 10^{-4}$ M effective bound steroids) [10, 12]
2. Fluorescein-labeled estrogen molecule, without a protein carrier ($\sim 10^{-6}$ M bound steroid) [5, 14]
Both types of ligands have been tested in our laboratory. Here we summarize our experience and present a critique of this new tool of investigation.

Materials and Methods

Fluorescent Ligands

Three steroid derivatives were used:
1. 17β-Estradiol-6-carboxymethyloxime-bovine serum albumin-fluorescein isothiocyanate (E_2-BSA-FITC). This compound was first produced by Dr. S. H. Lee. Later it was purchased from the Zeus Scientific Inc., Raritan, NJ (USA).
2. 11α-Hydroxyprogesterone hemisuccinate-bovine serum albumin-tetramethylrhodamine isothiocyanate (Pg-BSA-TMRITC) (same origin as E_2-BSA-FITC).
3. N-fluoresceyl-N'-(3-hydroxy-$\Delta^{1,3,5,10}$-estratrien-17β-yl)-thiourea (FE). This compound was synthesized by Organon (Oss, The Netherlands).

* This work was supported by the Fonds Cancérologique de la CGER (Belgium) and the FRSM (Belgium). We gratefully acknowledge the cooperation of Prof. C. Gompel (Service d'Anatomie Pathologique, Institut J. Bordet, Bruxelles, Belgium). We thank Miss P. Miroir for her excellent preparation of the manuscript

Origin of Tissues

Samples of primary carcinomas from patients aged 33−88 years were studied. They were obtained very shortly after surgical mastectomy (Dr. W. H. Mattheiem, Department of Breast and Pelvic Surgery, Inst. J. Bordet, Brussels).

Cytochemical Labeling

The details of the cytochemical technique have been described elsewhere [10−12]. Briefly, unfixed cryostat frozen sections were cut about 8−10 μm thick and mounted on microscope slides. They were rehydrated with 2% BSA in phosphate-buffered saline solution (PBS), covered with the fluorescent steroid conjugates, and incubated in a humid chamber at room temperature for 2 h. After removal of the reagents, the sections were rinsed in PBS and covered with phosphate-buffered glycerine and coverslip.

Microscopy

Improved illumination was achieved using epifluorescence with the Leitz Ploem illuminator (Ploempak 2.1.). The illumination source was a HBO 200 W high pressure mercury arc lamp used in combination with the FITC and TMRITC excitation filter modules.

Results

Ability to Bind to Cytoplasmic Estrogen Receptors and Cytochemical Labeling Potency of the Estradiol Fluorescent Conjugates

The binding ability of the estradiol fluorescent conjugates to mammary tumor ER was estimated by competitive inhibition of the binding of ^{3}H-estradiol (^{3}H-E$_2$). Tumor cytosol was incubated at room temperature (20° C) for 30 min with 5×10^{-9} M ^{3}H-E$_2$ and increasing amounts of a fluorescent conjugate. After incubation, unbound steroids were removed by a dextran-coated charcoal treatment and bound ^{3}H-E$_2$ was measured. FE produced a $\sim$ 50% inhibition of ^{3}H-E$_2$ binding at high concentration (10^{-5} M), indicating a very low binding affinity ($< 0.1\%$). E$_2$-BSA-FITC displayed only a very slight inhibition of ^{3}H-E$_2$ binding at 10^{-5} M (20%), indicating an absence of significant affinity.
Preliminary histological labeling of 16 breast cancers with FE did not display any significant fluorescence despite biochemically measurable ER. Twelve of them were labeled using the hydrophilic macromolecules (E$_2$-BSA-FITC and Pg-BSA-TMRITC).

Morphology of Mammary Tumors

Fifty-nine tumors were studied. All samples were tested with E$_2$-BSA-FITC, and many (80%) were also tested with Pg-BSA-TMRITC. In most samples epithelial cells exhibited a cytoplasmic fluorescence for both reagents. In 13 tumors, nuclear and cytoplasmic fluorescence was observed with E$_2$-BSA-FITC; in six, nuclear fluorescence only was

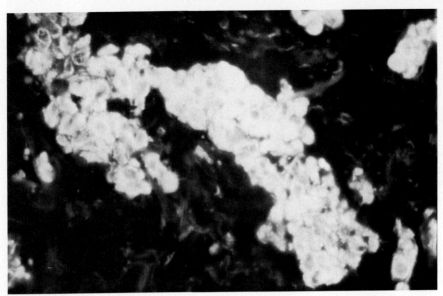

Fig. 1. Cords of duct carcinoma composed of strongly estrogen receptor-positive cells *(centre)* and estrogen receptor-negative cancer cells *(upper)* next to each other. (× 400)

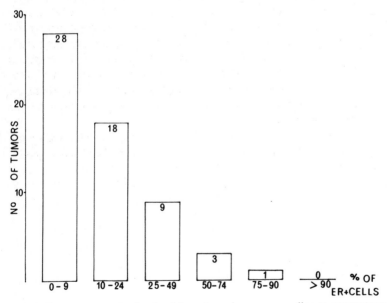

Fig. 2. Estrogen receptor levels of breast carcinomas according to percentages of ER+ cells in the cancer cell populations

observed. Remarkably, nuclear fluorescence was never found with Pg-BSA-TMRITC. Connective tissue, myoepithelial cells, and vascular smooth muscular cells were always negative. Occasionally, binding of E_2-BSA-FITC and Pg-BSA-TMRITC was observed on peripheral nerves. Furthermore, negative tumors cells often showed a membrane fluorescence as a narrow ring. This staining, probably due to retention of the steroid conjugate in these lipid-rich structures, was never considered as specific.

In all tumor samples, a considerable heterogeneity was observed in the cytoplasmic fluorescence intensity of the epithelial cells (Fig. 1). Specimens were classified according to the level of positive cells for E_2-BSA-FITC using the criteria proposed by Lee [10, 12]. Thus the most intense fluorescence in the cytoplasm of the normal ductal epithelial cells was taken as a positive arbitrary standard. Cancer cells manifesting a similar intensity of cytoplasmic fluorescence and those showing intensities of labeling above this level were defined as positive; those showing staining intensities below the normal standard were considered negative.

As shown in Fig. 2, of the 59 carcinomas none were composed of more than 90% fluorescent cells, only 7% showed more than 50% staining, and 47% were composed of less than 10% fluorescent cells. Notably, exclusion of cells exhibiting nuclear fluorescence did not modify the pattern.

Interestingly, most cells positive for E_2-BSA-FITC were also stained with Pg-BSA-TMRITC. Intensities of fluorescence were usually the same. Nevertheless, weakly estrogen-positive cells were never labeled with the progesterone reagent.

Specificity of Labeling

In several tumors addition of E_2-BSA or Pg-BSA conjugates (2×10^{-3} M bound steroids) 1 h before the addition of the fluorescent ligands produced a moderate decrease in intensity of fluorescence. In contrast, preincubation with steroids (11α-chloromethyl-estradiol, estradiol, or 11α-hydroxyprogesterone) at the maximum aquous solubilities (10^{-5} M) failed to reduce the intensity. On the other hand BSA-FITC without steroid, at the same molar concentration as the fluorescent estrogen, did not stain any cancer cells. Furthermore the fluorescent ligands failed to label nontarget tissues above the background autofluorescence (rat colon, human vermiform appendices).

Finally, breast cancer cell lines either containing (MCF-7) or lacking (EVSA-T) ER were labeled with E_2-BSA-FITC and Pg-BSA-TMRITC. Both cell lines displayed a similar intensity of fluorescence with these two reagents.

Table 1. Absence of correlation between cytochemical and biochemical ER determinations

Cytochemistry		ER determination in cytosol (fmol/mg tissue protein)
% positive cells	No. of tumors	
> 90	0	—
75−90	1	64
50−74	3	0, 36, 99
25−49	9	3×0, 29, 125, 215, 227, 351, 754
10−24	18	6×0, 19, 51, 58, 68, 96, 209, 364, 397, 406, 487, 1,160, 1,312
0− 9	28	7×0, 7, 10, 35, 51, 56, 63, 81, 121, 405, 438, 539, 579, 627, 710, 740, 825, 977, 1,011, 1,070, 1,613

Biochemical and Cytochemical Correlation

A sample of each tumor was biochemically assessed for cytoplasmic ER content [9]. Table 1 reveals a total absence of correlation between the results obtained by the cytochemical and the biochemical methods. For example, tumors cytochemically classified in the range 0–9% positive cells contained the whole range of ER concentrations. Notably, exclusion of cells exhibiting nuclear fluorescence did not modify the pattern.

Discussion

Using FE we were unable to label any tissue sections. This is not surprising if we remember that FE contains only one fluorescent dye per estradiol molecule. This labeling is certainly insufficient to visualize any estradiol binding site with the methodology here employed. Nevertheless, using another FE molecule estrogen, receptors in cryostat breast tissue sections have been reported [5, 14].

In contrast, and as reported first by Lee [10–12], the present morphological results show that E_2-BSA-FITC and Pg-BSA-TMRITC label breast cancer cells. Moreover they confirm that mammary cancers are composed of mixed fluorescent and nonfluorescent tumor cells in different proportions. Nontarget tissues failed to present any significant fluorescence with the steroid conjugates. This observation suggests some tissue specificity for the two reagents. Finally, that FITC-BSA did not stain epithelial cancer cells indicates that the steroid molecule of the reagent is required for the labeling of these cells.

These data are consistent with the view that these two ligands might detect ER and PgR in human breast cancer. However, several lines of evidence cast doubt on this interpretation. Thus preincubation with a five to tenfold excess of nonfluorescent steroids-BSA conjugates prior to the addition of fluorescent compounds did not markely suppress the staining. Furthermore, the identical pattern of staining of MCF-7 (ER+) and the EVSA-T (ER−) cell lines indicates that the reagents are inefficient in differentiating between ER+ and ER− cells in culture, although the histochemical method used was the same as described for the tissues. Finally, the total absence of correlation between the cytochemical technique and the biochemical ER evaluation strongly suggests that the binding of E_2-BSA-FITC is not attributable to the ER as defined until now.

Interestingly, a similar lack of correlation between the cytochemical and biochemical methods has also been reported by Panko et al. [15] and Berger et al. [1]. This may be explaining by our biochemical study showing a very weak binding affinity of E_2-BSA-FITC for cytoplasmic ER. Using the same biochemical technique, Humphreys et al. [7] and McCarty et al. [13] also reported a very weak binding affinity for such a compound. On the other hand, a significant affinity was reported by Rao et al. [18] using another technique (sucrose gradient centrifugation); this difference in methodology might be at the origin of this discrepancy. As far as biochemistry is concerned, several classes of estrogen binding sites have been found. ER which has a very high binding affinity for E_2 (dissociation constant of the complex, K_d is $\sim 10^{-10}$ M) has been defined as type I binder [19]. Binding sites with lower affinity (K_d $10^{-9} \sim M$) but higher capacity have been called type II [3, 4, 6, 19]. Other binding sites grouping high capacity molecules associated with the membranes, with a very great capacity ($K_d > 10^{-7}$ M), have been grouped as type III [2].

Since type I (ER) is the binder biochemically measured here, and since an absence of correlation between cytochemical and biochemical techniques is reported, we suppose that the fluorescent structures visualized by the present morphological tool could correspond to type II or III binders. Studies conducted on a variety of hormone sensitive and nonsensitive cancers may provide valuable information in this regard. The apparent specificity of the method for estrogen target tissues must also be investigated. On the other hand, in future extension of cytochemical assessment of the receptor other fluorescent ligands, such as that of Pertschuk et al. [16, 17] (E_2 linked to BSA-FITC in position 17β), could be tested. The excellent correlation between cytochemical and biochemical studies justify such a study. Another interesting cytochemical approach would be the use of specific antibodies against estrogen receptor [8].

Conclusion

With regard to clinical application of two ligands tested here, E_2-BSA-FITC and Pg-BSA-TMRITC, the following must be emphasized: Whatever sites are actually visualized they do not seem to be identical to the sex-steroid receptors as measured biochemically. It must be borne in mind that the morphological approach therefore remains purely investigational in nature and until additional information is available only biochemical assessment should be considered for the selection of the appropriate therapy.

References

1. Berger G, Frappart L, Berger N, Bremond A, Feroldi J, Rochet Y (1980) Localisation cytoplasmique des récepteurs stéroïdiens des carcinomes mammaires par histofluorescence. Arch Anat Cytol Pathol 26: 341−345
2. Chamness GL, Mercer WD, McGuire WL (1980) Are histochemical methods for estrogen receptor valid? J Histochem Cytochem 28: 792−798
3. Clark JH, Hardin JW, Upchurch S, Eriksson H (1978) Heterogeneity of estrogen binding sites in the cytosol of the rat uterus. J Biol Chem 253: 7630−7634
4. Clark JH, Markaverich B, Upchurch S, Eriksson H, Hardin JW (1979) Nuclear binding of the estrogen-receptor: heterogeneity of sites and uterotropic response. In: Leavitt WW, Clark JH (eds) Steroid hormone receptor systems. Plenum, New York, p 17
5. Dandliker WB, Brawn RJ, Hsu ML, Brawn PN, Levin J, Meyers CY, Kolb VM (1978) Investigation of hormone-receptor interactions by means of fluorescence labeling. Cancer Res 38: 4212−4224
6. Eriksson H, Upchurch S, Hardin JW, Peck EJ Jr, Clark JH (1978) Heterogeneity of estrogen receptors in the cytosol and nuclear fractions of the rat uterus. Biochem Biophys Res Commun 81: 1−7
7. Humphreys J, Westwood JH, Ormerod MG, Coombes RC, Neville AM (1980) Immunocytochemical localization of oestrogen receptors. Br J Cancer 42: 183
8. Jensen EV (1981) Hormone dependency of breast cancer. Cancer 47: 2319−2326
9. Leclercq G, Heuson JC, Schoenfeld R, Mattheiem WH, Tagnon HJ (1973) Estrogen receptors in human breast cancer. Eur J Cancer 9: 665−673
10. Lee SH (1978) Cytochemical study of estrogen receptor in human mammary cancer. Am J Clin Pathol 70: 197−203
11. Lee SH (1979) Cancer cell estrogen receptor of human mammary carcinoma. Cancer 44: 1−12
12. Lee SH (1980) Cellular estrogen and progesterone receptors in mammary carcinoma. Am J Clin Pathol 73: 323−329

13. McCarty KS Jr, Woodrad BH, Nichols DE, Wilkinson W, McCarty KS Sr (1980) Comparison of biochemical and histochemical techniques for estrogen receptor analyses in mammary carcinoma. Cancer 46: 2842–2845

14. Nenci I, Dandliker WB, Meyers CY, Marchetti E, Marzola A, Fabris G (1980) Estrogen receptor cytochemistry by fluorescent estrogen. J Histochem Cytochem 28: 1081–1088

15. Panko WR, Mattioli C, Wheeler T (1980) A histochemical assay for estrogen receptor using a 6-linked estrogen: lack of correlation with the biochemical assay. J Cell Biol 87: 166a

16. Pertschuk LP, Gaetjens E, Carter AC, Brigatti DJ, Kim DS, Fealey TE (1979) An improved histochemical method for detection of estrogen receptors in mammary cancer. Comparison with biochemical assay. Am J Clin Pathol 71: 504–508

17. Pertschuk LP, Tobin EH, Gaetjens E, Brigatti DJ, Carter AC, Kim DS, Degenshein GA, Bloom ND (1980) Histochemical assay of steroid hormone receptors. In: Bresciani F (ed) Perspectives in steroid receptor research. Raven, New York, p 299

18. Rao BR, Patrick TB, Sweet F (1980) Steroid-albumin conjugate interaction with steroid-binding proteins. Endocrinology 106: 356–362

19. Watson CS, Clark JH (1980) Heterogeneity of estrogen binding sites in mouse mammary cancer. J Recept Res 1: 91–111

Microscopic Visualization of Steroid Receptor Sites: A Mirage?

G. Daxenbichler, P. Weiss, A. Ortner, and O. Dapunt

Universitätsklinik für Frauenheilkunde, Anichstrasse 35, 6020 Innsbruck, Austria

Introduction

Histochemical assays measuring the incorporation of fluorescent or enzyme labeled steroids, steroid antibodies, or receptor antibodies have provoked enormous interest, especially among pathologists, because some authors have claimed to visualize steroid antibodies using these techniques. Histochemical methods, although not quantitative and not characterizing the binding component, would have some advantages over the radioligand assay, as they require only a minimum of tissue or dispersed cells and relatively inexpensive equipment. Furthermore, they would allow evaluation of each cell separately and could be performed by the pathologist, who has easy access to tissue and in-depth knowledge of tissue morphology and pathology.

Although the literature on histochemical receptor methods is extensive, the question still remains as to whether we are really determining receptors or hormone sensitive cells by these methods? To answer this we developed a theoretical model based on the biochemical receptor assay and determined whether the results obtained with fluorescent labeled steroids fitted this model. Basic experiments concerning the sensitivity of the method, the uptake of ^3H steroids into cells, and the validity of published methods were performed.

Summary of Published Methods and Results

Indirect Immunohistochemical Techniques

According to this method, receptors are saturated with the corresponding steroid, which is then detected by specific steroid antibodies and fluorescent or enzyme labeled anti-IgG [1–10]. Selective staining of certain cells, translocation of the stain into the nucleus, and predominant localization in the nucleolus after incubation with the steroid at elevated temperature could be observed. Nevertheless, the basic mechanism of these processes remains obscure, particularly since it was found that a steroid cannot be linked to a receptor and an antibody at the same time [11, 12]. If the steroid dissociates from the receptor prior to linkage with the antibody, as assumed by some authors, how can it then immobilize or localize the receptor? Under conditions at which no cytoplasmic receptor should be present, Chamness could still observe fluorescence in the cytoplasm [13].

Recent Results in Cancer Research. Vol. 91
© Springer-Verlag Berlin · Heidelberg 1984

Polyestradiol phosphate [14] − as a substitute for estradiol − would not be expected to work because of its extremely low affinity to the receptor and the antibody.

Direct Immunohistochemical Methods

At least three authors have claimed to localize receptors using purified or biotin labeled monoclonal antibodies against the receptor [15−17] which themselves were visualized with fluorescein or enzyme labeled anti-IgG or with fluorescein labeled avidin. Provided the sensitivity of these methods is high enough, they would represent the most elegant way of localizing receptors.

Direct Histochemical Techniques

Steroid-Albumin (BSA) Conjugates. Pertschuk [18−21], Lee [22−24], and others [10, 25−27] used methods detecting the incorporation of steroid-albumin conjugates labeled with fluorescein, rhodamine or peroxidase. The affinity of these compounds for their corresponding receptor is low, showing ∼ 0.1% relative binding affinity compared with the native steroid [27−29].

The principal steps of the method consist in preparing frozen sections and incubating them with the fluorescent reagents ($10^{-6}-10^{-5}$ M) in buffer. After extensive washing and fixation, the sections are evaluated microscopically. Occasionally fluorescence uptake can be inhibited by a 100- to 1,000-fold excess of synthetic steroids [10, 18] or unlabeled steroid albumin conjugates [22]. The correlation between the results obtained by histochemical methods and by biochemical analysis varies between weak [23, 30, 31] and excellent [27, 32, 33] when only distinguishing between positive and negative. Pertschuk [33] found response to hormonal treatment in 52% of the histochemically positive stage IV mammary carcinomas, whereas poor binding correlated with failure to respond in over 90%.

Steroid Fluorescein Conjugates. Steroids directly bound to fluorescein were applied by Dandliker and Rao [34−36], Barrows and Stroupe [37], and our group [38−40]. The relative binding affinities for their corresponding receptors are higher than for the steroid-BSA conjugates [36, 39]. Their low molecular weight allows penetration through the intact cell membrane. Correlation with biochemical methods in mammary carcinoma samples was found by Rao to be satisfactory [36]. Translocation of the compound into the nucleus at elevated temperature has been reported [36, 37].

Summary of Our Methods and Results

The fluorescent steroid derivatives of estradiol (E_2-Fl), desoxycorticosterone (DOC-Fl), dihydrotestosterone (DHT-Fl), and prednisolone (Pr-Fl) used in our laboratory are shown in Fig. 1. All the conjugates displayed relatively high affinity for their corresponding receptors, i.e. between 3% and 30% compared with that of the naturally occurring steroid. Their affinity for other receptors was negligible. Staining was performed by incubating small tissue fragments, cryostat sections, or dispersed cells with a 10^{-7} or 10^{-6} M solution of

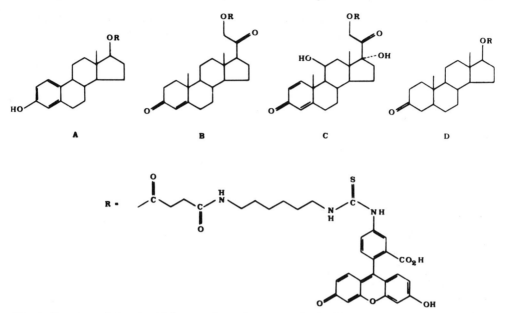

Fig. 1. Structure of the steroid fluorescein conjugates synthesized in our laboratory. *A*, E$_2$-Fl; *B*, DOC-Fl; *C*, Pr-Fl; *D*, 5αDHT-Fl

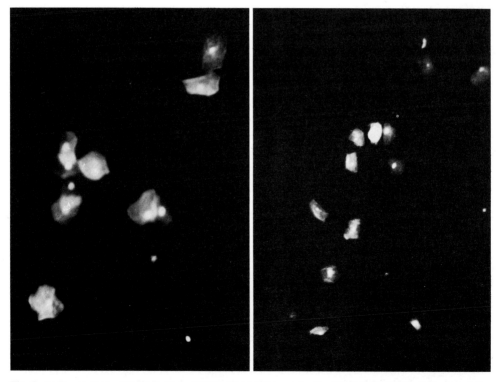

Fig. 2. Accumulation of E$_2$-Fl *(left)* and DOC-Fl *(right)* in vaginal epithelial cells of the 15th day of the menstrual cycle. Incubation was performed with 10^{-6} *M* of fluorescent conjugate for 2 h at 4° C

each fluorescent steroid. To achieve possible inhibition of fluorescence uptake, samples were preincubated with a 250-fold excess of the unlabeled natural steroid.

Cellular incorporation of E_2-Fl and DOC-Fl was observed in endometrium, myometrium, prostate, endometrial and ovarian carcinoma. Increasing the concentration of fluorescent derivatives resulted in an increased uptake. No saturation was observed. Both cytoplasm and nuclei were stained but not necessarily to the same extent [38, 40]. Quantitative evaluation of staining and of a partial inhibition of staining by the native steroid was difficult. The autofluorescence of some tissues, especially of elastic fibres and blood vessels, caused problems of interpretation. Incorporation of E_2-Fl and DOC-Fl into vaginal epithelial cells is shown in Fig. 2. In many of the cells nuclear staining was predominant and occurred at 4° C and 37° C.

Staining patterns for E_2-Fl and DOC-Fl were not always the same and varied throughout the menstrual cycle. Preincubation with a 100-fold excess of estradiol or progesterone in some cases inhibited fluorescence uptake but in other cases led to even greater staining.

Approaches to Test the Validity of the Histochemical Methods

To prove that the histochemical methods mentioned above allow the determination of receptors, the following questions have to be answered:

1. Does the receptor remain in the microscopic section during the histochemical procedure?
2. What concentration of receptor or how many receptor sites can we expect in a hormone sensitive cell?
3. Is the microscopic fluorescein detection sensitive enough to detect the expected receptor concentration?
4. To how many sites/cell does the fluorescence observed correspond?
5. Does the incorporation follow the characteristics of receptor binding?
6. Can a competitive inhibition, characteristic for receptors, be achieved?
7. What is the contribution of other binding components at the assay conditions applied?
8. Is a comparison of histochemical staining results and the biochemically obtained receptor values meaningful?

Extraction of Receptors During Incubation

When we incubated 4-μm-thick frozen sections of calf uterine tissue for 10 min in buffer at room temperature or at 4° C, conditions that are applied in histochemical methods, we found a complete loss of receptor activity in the sections but the presence of binding sites in the incubation buffer (Table 1). This was also the experience of others [30, 41].

Concentrations of Binding Sites in Cell Preparations and Compartments

For the hypothetical case presented in Table 2, the concentration of receptor sites in this extremely receptor-rich cell are presented in Table 3. If receptors are located in microscopically distinguishable nuclear compartments, theoretically one would reach local

Table 1. Extractions of receptors from 4-μm frozen sections during incubation with phosphate buffered saline (pH 7.4) for 10 min

Sample	ER (fmol/mg protein)	$K_d \times M$
Cytosol of frozen sections before incubation	246	1.4×10^{-9}
Cytosol of frozen sections after incubation at 4° C	< 5	
Cytosol of frozen sections after incuabtion at 37° C	< 5	
Incubation buffer (4° C)	174	1.6×10^{-10}
Incubation buffer (37° C)	96	2×10^{-9}

Table 2. Assumptions for the calculation of receptor concentrations

Receptor concentration in cytosol:	1 nM
Protein concentration:	2 mg/ml
Receptor concentration:	500 fmol/mg protein

10% of the cells contain receptors
Cell volume: 4,000 μm^3
Cell diameter: 20 μm
Volume of the nucleus = 1/10 of cell volume
Nuclear compartment has 1/10 of nuclear volume

Table 3. Concentration of steroid receptors for the hypothetical case described in Table 2

Tissue homogenate	$10^{-9}\ M$
Mixed cell sap	$10^{-8}\ M$
Receptor containing cell	$10^{-7}\ M$
Nuclei of receptor containing cell	$10^{-6}\ M$
Nuclear organelles	$10^{-5}\ M$

concentrations as high as $10^{-5} M$. To express the receptor concentration of this cell ($10^{-7} M$) in terms of sites/cell, one must perform the following calculation: 10^{-7} mol/l = 4×10^{-19} mol/4,000 μm^3 or per cell. Multiplying the moles/cell by Avogadro's number ($4 \times 10^{-19} \times 6 \times 10^{23}$) gives 240,000 sites/cell.

Sensitivity of the Microscopic Fluorescein Determination

A 4-μm layer of a solution of increasing concentrations of one of our mono-fluorescein-labeled steroid conjugates in buffer, wax, or gelatine was placed under the microscope. The lowest concentration visible in all three cases was ~ $10^{-6} M$ (Fig. 3). According to the calculations just mentioned, $10^{-6} M$ would correspond to 2,400,000 sites/cell if the binding sites were distributed uniformly throughout the cell. Therefore we should be unable to specifically detect cytoplasmic receptors, even if the steroid were

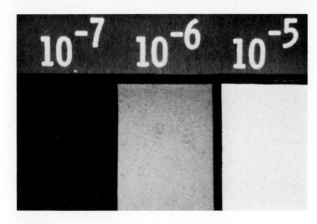

Fig. 3. Sensitivity of the microscopic visualization of fluorescein. A 4-μm layer of a solution of E_2-Fl at concentrations indicated in the figure was observed at a 160-fold magnification in a Reichert Biovar microscope

labeled with five molecules of fluorescein. If all receptors were translocated into the nucleus, minimal staining of the nucleus due to receptors would be possible. But it should be emphasized that in this model the receptor concentration is at the upper limit of reality.

Translation of Fluorescence into Sites/Cell

The "beautiful" cytoplasmic staining observed by us and by others, especially when applying the commercially available estradiol and progesterone BSA-fluorescein or rhodamine derivatives, corresponds to more than 5,000,000 binding sites/cell.

Characteristics of the Uptake of ^3H Steroids and Fluorescent Steroid Derivatives into Cells

To investigate whether the uptake of steroids into tissue sections is characteristic for steroid receptor binding, we incubated sections of calf uterine tissue either with ^{3}H-estradiol or E_2-Fl. The tritiated steroid was extracted with ether whereas the incorporation of the fluorescent conjugate was evaluated microscopically. The uptake of ^{3}H steroids at the various concentrations in the medium is presented in Fig. 4. No saturation could be observed. We are dealing with low affinity–high capacity binding not even saturable at the high concentrations normally applied in histochemical assays (10^{-6}–10^{-5} M). As already mentioned, uptake of fluorescent derivatives was also not saturable. 10^{-7} M for intact cells and 10^{-6} M for 4-μm tissue sections were the minimal concentrations necessary to observe uptake of fluorescence.

Inhibition of Incorporation

The uptake of ^{3}H-estradiol and E_2-Fl could not at all or could only partially be inhibited by a 100-fold excess of steroids. Theoretically, a concentration of $10 \times K_d$ of the ligand in the

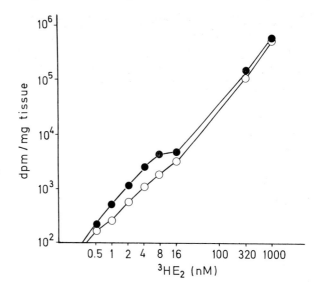

Fig. 4. Uptake of ^{3}H-estradiol into 4-μm frozen sections after incubation for 10 min at room temperature and brief washing with buffer.
●————● ^{3}H-estradiol alone;
○————○ ^{3}H-estradiol plus a 250-fold excess of estradiol

incubation medium would occupy 90% of receptor sites. Under these conditions $100 \times K_d$ of natural steroid ($10^{-7} M$) should be sufficient to inhibit 90% of binding. But with none of the methods was it possible to inhibit incorporation with $10^{-7} M$ of the native steroid. Even a 100-fold excess ($10^{-5}-10^{-4} M$) was not always sufficient, and even if it were, would not allow us to conclude that we are dealing with receptors, because binding to other entities is also compatible with an excess of unlabeled ligand.

Contribution of Low Affinity–High Capacity Binding Sites to the Incorporation of Steroids and Steroid Derivatives

Fluorescent derivatives have a lower affinity for their receptors, with relative binding affinities of 10%–0.1% compared with those of active steroids. This indicates the need for a 10- to 1,000-fold concentration of ligand compared with that of the active steroid in order to saturate most of the receptor sites. Thus concentrations up to $10^{-5} M$ are necessary. Unfortunately, therefore, we are confronted with other binding phenomena in addition to receptor binding, e.g. so-called type II binding (K_d of complex with steroids $\sim 10^{-8} M$) [42] and low affinity binding (K_d of complex with steroids $\sim 10^{-6}-10^{-5} M$). These binding entities are present in cells in a 10- to 100-fold excess compared with the receptors. One has to assume that at least the low affinity binding has a similar capacity for both naturally occurring steroids and steroid derivatives. Figure 5 illustrates the contributions of the various binding entities to the total binding of steroids and steroid derivatives at the concentration of ligand necessary to occupy 90% of receptor sites. At the appropriate concentration of derivatives with low affinity for the receptor (e.g., steroid-BSA conjugates), the contribution of receptors to the incorporation would be less than 5%. In other words, receptor and low affinity binders for these conjugates cannot be distinguished because their affinity for the fluorescent ligands are too similar.

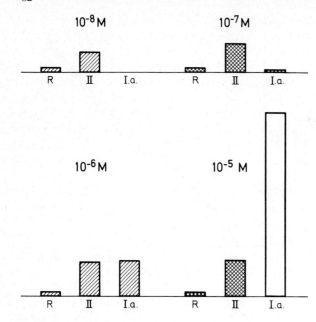

Fig. 5. Contribution of receptor (R) type II and low affinity (l.a.) binding sites to the total binding at the ligand concentrations indicated. The assumption was made that type II binding is present in a 10-fold and low affinity binding in a 100-fold excess compared with the receptor

Correlation Between Histochemically Staining Properties and Biochemically Obtained Receptor Values

These correlations are doubtful because of the arbitrary choice of "cut-off points", the distinction between positive and negative only, and the intrinsic errors in both microscopic and histochemical methods caused by the subjective evaluation of microscopic samples and by the heterogeneity of tissue respectively. A good correlation cannot alone be proof of the validity of histochemical methods.

Summary and Discussion

Although microscopic "receptor" assays are already practiced in many pathology laboratories, their validity has not yet been proven. Our results with fluorescent labeled steroids agreed with the theoretical considerations and with basic experiments of ^{3}H steroid uptake into intact cells and offered several facts countering the possibility of visualizing receptor sites.

Briefly: When manipulating frozen sections the receptor is washed out. The sensitivity of the methods was found to be too low to detect receptor. The intensity of staining observed by us and other authors is $50-100$ times more than it should be due to receptor sites. The incorporation of steroid conjugates is not saturable and cannot be inhibited with the appropriate amount of native steroid, and thus does not show the characteristics of receptor binding. At the high concentrations of ligand necessary to saturate receptor sites and to observe incorporation, low affinity binding sites, present in at least a 100-fold excess compared with receptors, are filled. Finally, "good" correlation between results obtained by histochemical and biochemical methods cannot be an argument for the validity of the histochemical assay in detecting receptors.

Although we are persuaded that the histochemical methods described up to now do not actually visualize receptors, there is some evidence that in spite of this they may be able to localize hormone-sensitive cells. Cells known to be hormone dependent, i.e., epithelial cells of endometrium, mammary gland, prostate, and vagina are preferentially stained. In the case of vaginal epithelial cells, changes in the nuclear incorporation of our fluorescent E_2 and DOC conjugates were observed during the menstrual cycle. Fluorescent steroid conjugates are reportedly incorporated more frequently into cells of mammary tumors containing receptors (reported as "good correlation" between biochemical and histochemical methods), and finally, Pertschuk et al. could find good agreement between response to hormonal therapy and the uptake of steroid BSA-fluorescein conjugates in mammary cancer.

At present, however, we do not know which binding entity could possibly lead to this labeling. Is it a specific low affinity−high capacity binding, e.g., an enzyme or type II receptor, or is it a nonspecific binding, e.g., a preferential adsorption due to specific physical properties of the intracellular compartments of cells assumed to be hormone sensitive. Our results in vaginal epithelial cells support the former assumption as the staining properties are different with E_2-Fl compared with DOC-Fl at the period of ovulation.

On the other hand, the commercially available estradiol- and progesterone-BSA conjugates are generally both incorporated into the same cells and to the same extent in mammary cancer tissues, which disagrees with the biochemical receptor determination and supports the hypothesis of a nonspecific binding.

In conclusion, we want to answer the question posed by the title of this article affirmatively. The question about the histochemical detection of hormone-sensitive cells cannot, in our opinion, be answered at this time. Therefore these methods are not a valid alternative to the traditional biochemical receptor assays, especially when clinical decisions are based on them, e.g., the selection of therapy in mammary cancer. We consequently believe that the advertisement and commercial sale of kits containing steroid fluorescein derivatives for use in histochemical receptor assays is at present both presumptuous and premature.

References

1. Nenci I, Beccati MD, Piffanelli A, Lanza G (1976) Detection and dynamic localisation of estradiol receptor complexes in intact target cells by immunofluorescence technique. J Steroid Biochem 7: 505
2. Nenci I, Piffanelli A, Beccati MD, Lanza G (1976) In vivo and in vitro immunofluorescent approach to the physiopathology of estradiol kinetics in target cells. J Steroid Biochem 7: 883
3. Nenci I (1978) Receptor and nucleolar pathways of steroid action in normal and neoplastic cells. Cancer Res 38: 4204
4. Malan IB, Janss DH (1978) Demonstration of estrogen-binding protein in human and rat mammary epithelial cultures by fluorescent antibody staining. In Vitro 14: 399
5. Mercer WD, Carlson CA, Wahl TM (1977) Identification of estrogen receptors in human breast cancer cells by immunofluorescence and immunoperoxidase techniques. Proc Soc Exp Biol Med 2: 13
6. Mercer WD, Carlson CA, Wahl TM (1978) Identification of estrogen receptors in mammary cancer cells by immunofluorescence. Am J Clin Pathol 70: 330
7. Mercer WD, Carlson CA, Wahl TM (1978) Identification of estrogen receptors in human breast cancer cells by immunological techniques. Fed Proc. 37: 1312

8. Kurzon RM, Sternberger LA (1978) Estrogen receptor immunochemistry. J Histochem Cytochem 26: 803

9. Ghosh L, Ghosh BC, Das Gupta TK (1978) Immunocytological localization of estrogen in human mammary carcinoma cells by horseradish-antihorseradish peroxidase complex. J Surg Oncol 10: 221

10. Walker RA, Cove DH, Howell A (1980) Histological detection of estrogen receptor in human breast cancer. Lancet 1: 171

11. Castaneda E, Liao S (1975) The use of anti-steroid antibodies in the characterization of steroid receptors. J Biol Chem 250: 883

12. Fishman J, Fishman JH (1974) Competitive binding assay for estradiol receptor using immobilized antibody. J Clin Endocrinol Metab 39: 603

13. Chamness GC, Mercer WD, McGuire WL (1980) Are histochemical methods for estrogen receptor valid? J Histochem Cytochem 28: 792

14. Pertschuk LP, Tobin EH, Brigati DJ, Kim DS, Bloom ND, Gaetjens E, Berman PJ, Carter AC, Degenshein GA (1978) Immunofluorescent detection of estrogen receptors in breast cancer. Comparison with dextran-coated charcoal and sucrose gradient assays. Cancer 41: 907

15. Papamichail M, Tsokos G, Tsawdaro-Glou N, Sekeris CC (1980) Immunocytochemical demonstration of glucocorticoid receptors in different cell types and their translocation from the cytoplasm to the cell nucleus in the presence of dexamethasone. Exp Cell Res 125: 490

16. Allan TC, Jensen EV (1982) Immunohistochemical analysis of MCF-7 receptor using monoclonal antibody to human estrophilin. In: Wittliff JL, Dapunt O (eds) Hormone-cell interaction in reproductive tissues. New York

17. Raam S, Tamura H, Nemeth EJ, O'Brian DS, Cohen JL (1981) Comparison of localization of estrogen receptors in human mammary carcinomas using anti-receptor antibodies and FITC-conjugated BSA-estradiol. 11th Int Congr of Clinical Chemistry, 30 Aug−5 Sept 1981, Vienna. Abstr in: Ber Oesterr Ges Klin Chem 4: 202

18. Pertschuk LP, Gaetjens E, Carter AC, Brigati DJ, Kim DS, Fealey TE (1979) An improved histochemical method for detection of estrogen receptor in mammary cancer. Am J Clin Pathol 71: 504

19. Pertschuk LP, Carvounis EE, Tobin EH, Gaetjens E (1980) Renal glomerular steroid hormone binding. Detection by fluorescent microscopy. J Steroid Biochem 13: 1115

20. Pertschuk LP, DiMaio MFAC, Gaetjens E (1980) Histochemical demonstration of steroid hormone binding sites in the lung. J Steroid Biochem 13: 1121

21. Pertschuk LP, Gaetjens E (1980) Synthesis of fluorescein labeled steroid hormone-albumin conjugates for the fluorescent histochemical detection of hormone receptors. J Steroid Biochem 13: 1001

22. Lee SH (1978) Cytochemical study of estrogen receptor in human mammary cancer. Am J Clin Pathol 70: 197

23. Lee SH (1979) Cancer cell estrogen receptor of human mammary carcinoma. Cancer 44: 1

24. Lee SH (1980) Cellular estrogen and progesterone receptors in mammary carcinoma. Am J Clin Pathol 73: 323

25. Brigati DJ, Bloom ND, Tobin EH, Kim DS, Gaetgens E, Degenshein EA, Pertschuk LP (1978) Morphologic methods of steroid hormone receptor analysis in human breast cancer. A review. Breast 5: 27−33

26. Gaetjens E, Pertschuk LP (1980) Synthesis of fluorescein labelled steroid hormone-albumin conjugates for the fluorescent histochemical detection of hormone receptors. J Steroid Biochem 13: 1001

27. Böhm M, Binder B, Kolb R, Jakesz R, Rainer G (1982) Comparison of the staining properties of several estrogen conjugates with respect to receptors specificity: Measurement of their competition against ^{3}H-E$_2$ using dextran-coated charcoal adsorbtion. In: Wittliff JL, Dapunt O (eds) Hormone-cell interactions in reproductive tissues. Masson, New York

28. Poortman J (1981) 2nd Innsbruck winter conference, Innsbruck Igls, 29−31 Jan

29. Rao BR, Patrick TB, Sweet F (1980) Steroid-albumin conjugate interaction with steroid-binding proteins. Endocrinology 106: 356

30. Hawkins RA, Penney GC (1981) Histochemical detection of estrogen receptors: the Edinburgh experience. 11th int congr of clinical chemistry, 30 Aug–5 Sept 1981, Vienna. Abstr. in: Ber Oesterr Ges Klin Chem 4:203

31. Remmele W, Heicke B, Heine M, Frank K, Keogh HJ, Schmitt A (1982) Bestimmung der Steroid-Rezeptoren im Tumorgewebe von Mammakarzinomen – Methodik und Empfehlung für die Praxis. Dtsch Ärztebl 4:25

32. Walker R (1981) The use of peroxidase-labelled hormones in the study of steroid binding in breast carcinomas. 11th Int congr of clinical chemistry, 30 Aug–5 Sept 1981, Vienna. Abstr. in: Ber Oesterr Ges Klin Chem 4:203

33. Pertschuk LP (1981) Immunohistochemical detection of estrogen receptors with monoclonal antibodies. Steroid binding by histochemistry: Biochemical and clinical correlation in breast and prostate cancer. 11th Int congr of clinical chemistry, 30 Aug–5 Sept 1981, Vienna. Abstr. in: Ber Oesterr Ges Klin Chem 4:202

34. Dandliker WB, Hicks AN, Levson SA (1977) A fluorescein-labeled derivative of estradiol with binding affinity toward cellular receptors. Biochem Biophys Res Commun 74:538

35. Dandliker WB, Brawn RJ, Hsu ML, Brawn PN, Levin J, Meyers CY, Kolb M (1978) Investigation of hormone-receptor interactions by means of fluorescence labeling. Cancer Res 38:4212

36. Rao BR, Fry CG, Dandliker WB (1978) Fluorescent probe for rapid detection of steroid receptors. J Steroid Biochem 9:837

37. Barrows GH, Stroupe, S, Riehm JD (1980) Nuclear uptake of a 17β-estradiol-fluorescein derivative as a marker of estrogen dependence. Am J Clin Pathol 73:330

38. Daxenbichler G (1981) Histochemischer Nachweis hormonsensitiver Zellen. In: Jonat W, Maass H (eds) Steroidhormonrezeptoren im Carcinomgewebe. Emke, Stuttgart

39. Daxenbichler G, Grill HJ, Domanig R, Moser E, Dapunt O (1980) Receptor binding of fluorescein labeled steroids. J Steroid Biochem 13:489

40. Daxenbichler G, Weiß P, Grill HJ, Dapunt O (1982) Histochemical detection of steroid receptors: an evaluation. In: Wittliff JL, Dapunt O (eds) Hormone-cell interactions in reproductive tissues. Masson, New York

41. Chamness GC, McGuire WL (1981) Histochemistry of steroid receptors from a biochemical viewpoint. 11th Int congr of clinical chemistry 30 Aug–5 Sept 1981, Vienna. Abstr. in: Ber Oesterr Ges Klin Chem 4:203

42. Clark JH, Hardin J-W, Upchurch S, Eriksson H (1978) Heterogeneity of estrogen binding sites in the cytosol of the rat uterus. J Biol Chem 253:7630

Part I: A Critical Summary

R. J. B. King

Hormone Biochemistry Department, Imperial Cancer Research Fund,
P. O. Box 123, Lincoln's Inn Fields, London WC2A 3PX, United Kingdom

Introduction

Two questions must be asked of the methodologies described in the preceding chapters of this section, namely, what is the assay measuring and what is its clinical significance? My overview will discuss the chapters in the context of those questions. As the articles fall into the category of cytochemical or biochemical analysis, my comments will be likewise divided.

Biochemical Methods

The biochemical papers in this section deal with three important aspects, namely, improving the prognostic value of receptor measurements by the inclusion of additional assays, receptor assay in small samples and methods of calculating results.

What Are the Assays Measuring?

There is now an enormous literature attesting to the fact that the various methods are indeed measuring the relevant receptor although debate continues as to the accuracy of the methods. Thus Leclercq points out that the use of oestradiol as a ligand may result in over-estimation at low receptor values and that moxoestrol might be better ligand. Braunsberg's chapter makes the strong point that methodological discussion must encompass calculation methods. This is clearly not a trivial matter when identical raw data can be transformed into very disparate final values depending on the mathematical method employed.

The isoelectric focussing method described by Wrange is more time consuming than the standard dextran/charcoal routine but is finding increasing use where small amounts of tissue are available. Its use in this area is discussed by Silfverswärd. Isoelectric focussing gives comparable results to those obtained with other methods with the possible exception of progesterone receptor, where there is disagreement as to whether dextran charcoal results correlate with the $8\,S$ [9] or $8 + 4\,S$ [1, 7] molecular forms. Wrange's evidence suggests that the focussing method correlates with the $8\,S$ receptor. On the other hand, because of the trypsin treatment prior to focussing, the RE assay measures both 8- and 4-S forms of that receptor.

Recent Results in Cancer Research. Vol. 91
© Springer-Verlag Berlin · Heidelberg 1984

The article by Cowan on nuclear oestradiol receptor attempts to define those tumours with cytosol receptor but with a defective nuclear transfer machinery. The as yet unresolved question here is whether it is really nuclear receptor that is being assayed. The question must be asked because of the ability to label at 4° C and the answer must await further data on whether or not nuclei contain unoccupied receptors as opposed to contamination of nuclei with extranuclear components [5, 6].

Clinical Relevance

The importance of tumour sampling at the time of surgery has not received the attention it deserves and I strongly endorse the view expressed in Nicolo's chapter as to the central role of the pathologist at this stage of processing. I am less enthusiastic about his suggestion of putting the tumours into ice rather than solid carbon dioxide or liquid nitrogen and, for the reasons given below, his recommendation of cytochemical staining.

One of the major limitations of dextran/charcoal assays is that they cannot be performed on needle biopsies because of the small amounts of tissue so obtained. The use of isoelectric focussing in this context as described by Wrange and by Silfverswärd therefore represents a significant methodological advance. As both Silfverswärd and Magdelènat in his treatise on drill biopsy material emphasise, good histological assessment of these small samples is vital to the correct interpretation of such assays.

The theory behind the use of nuclear oestradiol receptor assays is confirmed by the clinical data on their prognostic value for both disease-free interval and response to endocrine therapy (see article by Cowan). As the clinical reason for wanting this type of assay is the same as for progesterone receptor it will be interesting to see whether the two assays complement each other or simply indicate the same thing [2].

Finally, it is clear from Braunsberg's data that if receptor values are to be incorporated into multicentre clinical trials, a common method of calculation is desirable.

Cytochemical Methods

There is general agreement that such methods are urgently required and that research in this area should be actively pursued; however, at the present time it would be prudent not to let desirability override scientific validation of the methods. My reading of the literature makes me concur with the views expressed by both Daxenbichler and Danguy in their chapters urging caution in the interpretation of cytochemical results obtained with either fluorescent steroids or fluorescent- or peroxidase-labelled derivatives thereof.

What Are the Assays Measuring?

Both Daxenbichler and Machetti place emphasis on the criteria that must be satisfied before concluding that a given method is measuring recpetor rather than some other binding protein. There is general agreement, based on a large biochemical literature, as to what those criteria are and it is therefore of interest that these two groups do not come to the same conclusions. Danguy and Daxenbichler present data indicating that the staining is not due to classical receptors whilst Marchetti suggests that it is. There is straightforward conflict of data between Marchetti and the other two authors as to whether the cytochemical binding is inhibited at meaningful concentrations of steroid, a conflict that is reflected in other publications [3]. This may partly be due to a point omitted from any of the present chapters, namely the presence of free steroid in some derivatized samples [4]. The above comments apply primarily to the fluorescence methods but caution must also be exercised when the ligand is stained by a peroxidase method [10]. Other areas of disagreement concern assay sensitivity, ability of antibodies to steroids to recognise those steroids when the latter are bound within a receptor protein and the ability of the receptor to withstand the processing necessary for the cytochemical methods. The one point of agreement is that some cell specificity of staining exists at both nuclear and extranuclear levels. My overall conclusion is that the cytochemical methods are displaying something of biological interest but that that something is unlikely to be receptor.

Clinical Relevance

All of the data relating endocrine response of human breast cancer to oestradiol and progesterone receptor levels have been obtained with biochemical assays. Therefore any new methods must be either thoroughly validated against the biochemical assay or independently tested against clinical response; neither has yet been achieved in a reproducible manner. Both Daxenbichler and Danguy present data indicating lack of correlation between cytochemical and biochemical methods whilst Marchetti quotes contrary data and further indicates a reasonable association between cytochemical results and response to endocrine treatment [8].

My conclusion is that we need to know more about the cytochemical assays and I would emphasise Daxenbichler's statement that ". . . the advertisement and commercial sale of kits containing steroid fluorescein derivatives for use in histochemical receptor assays is at present both presumptuous and premature."

References

1. Anderson KM, Bonomi P, Marogil M, Hendrickson C, Economou S (1980) Comparison of dextran-coated charcoal and sucrose density gradient analyses of estrogen and progesterone receptors in human breast cancer. Cancer Res 40: 4127−4132
2. Barnes DM, Skinner LG, Ribeiro GG (1979) Triple hormone-receptor assay: a more accurate predictive tool for the treatment of advanced breast cancer. Br J Cancer 40: 862−865
3. Cancer 46 (1980) (Supplement on steroid receptors in breast cancer)
4. Chamness GC, Mercer WD, McGuire WL (1980) Are histochemical methods for estrogen receptor valid? J Histochem Cytochem 28: 792−798
5. Edwards DP, Martin PM, Horwitz KB, Chamness GC, McGuire WL (1980) Subcellular compartmentalization of estrogen receptors in human breast cancer cells. Exp Cell Res 127: 197−213
6. Levy C, Mortel R, Eychenne B, Robel P, Baulieu E-E (1980) Unoccupied nuclear oestradiol-receptor sites in normal human endometrium. Biochem J 185: 733−738
7. Namkung PC, Petra PH (1981) Measurement of progesterone receptors in human breast tumors: comparison of various methods of analysis. J Steroid Biochem 14: 851−854
8. Pertschuk LP, Tobin EH, Tanapat P, Gaetjens E, Carter AC, Bloom ND, Macchia RJ, Eisenberg KB (1980) Histochemical analyses of steroid hormone receptors in breast and prostatic carcinoma. J Histochem Cytochem 28: 799−810
9. Powell B, Garole RE, Chamness C, McGuire WL (1979) Measurement of progesterone receptor in human breast cancer biopsies. Cancer Res 39: 1678−1682
10. Zehr DR, Satyaswaroop PG, Sheehan DM (1981) Nonspecific staining in the immunolocalization of estrogen receptors. J Steroid Biochem 14: 613−617

Part II. Quality Control

Quality Control of Estrogen and Progesterone Receptor Analyses in Denmark

S. M. Thorpe, K. Olsen, K. O. Pedersen, H. S. Poulsen, and C. Rose*

The Fibiger Laboratory, Ndr. Frihavnsgade 70, 2100 Copenhagen, Denmark

Three Danish laboratories presently perform estrogen and progesterone receptor analyses[1]. All three laboratories utilize the dextran-coated charcoal (DCC) assay method recommended by EORTC in 1981 [2] with minor modifications. Data are analyzed by Scatchard plot analysis [3].

Efforts to standardize the ER and PgR analyses have been made within the European community through participation of one of the Danish laboratories (The Fibiger Laboratory) in the EORTC standardization group. More recently, in an effort to standardize the steroid hormone receptor analyses within Denmark, a receptor committee has been established under the auspices of the nationwide Danish Breast Cancer Cooperative Group (DBCG) [1]. The first quality control investigation that this group has conducted utilized the standard EORTC lyophilized calf uterine cytosol powders used for the 1981 EORTC quality control trial. The laboratory participating in the EORTC trial received 30 vials (9, 9, 9, and 3 vials of powders A, B, C, and D respectively), while the other two Danish laboratories received 6 vials (2 vials each of powders A, B, and C). The powders were produced so that the receptor content was in a ratio of 6 : 3 : 1 for powders A, B, and C, respectively. The contents of the vials were unknown to those participating in the investigation until all results had been reported.

The results of the first Danish quality control investigation are shown in Table 1. For purposes of comparison, the values reported for the laboratory also participating in the EORTC trial are derived from results obtained the two first consecutive times each powder A, B, and C was analyzed. Owing to dilution of two cytosols prior to analysis in laboratory III, the results are given as fmol/mg cytosol protein rather than as fmol/ml cytosol, which permits a more direct comparison of the receptor assay. Each laboratory performed the assays and computed the data in the manner that was routinely used in the given laboratory.

---

* The authors are members of the Danish Breast Cancer Cooperative Group receptor committee: S. M. Thorpe, The Fibiger Laboratory, Copenhagen; K. Olsen, Dept. of Oncology, Herlev; K. O. Pedersen, Dept. of Clinical Chemistry, Ålborg Hospital, Ålborg; H. S. Poulsen, The Institute of Cancer Research, Århus; C. Rose, The Fibiger Laboratory, Copenhagen

1 The Fibiger Laboratory, Dept. of Clinical Physiology, The Finsen Institute, Copenhagen; The Institute of Cancer Research, Århus; and the Dept. of Clinical Chemistry, Ålborg Hospital, Ålborg

Table 1. Results of the first Danish quality control investigation

	Powder	Laboratory		
		I	II	III
Estrogen receptor (fmol/mg cytosol protein, coefficient of variation)	A	432 (11%)	308 (21%)	142 (5%)
	B	194 (2%)	171 (6%)	110 (30%)
	C	68 (8%)	87 (8%)	56 (41%)
Progesterone receptor (fmol/mg cytosol protein, coefficient of variation)	A	937 (1%)	558 (17%)	612 (36%)
	B	419 (6%)	530 (7%)	270 (26%)
	C	128 (16%)	596 (80%)	83 (35%)
Protein determination[a] (mg/ml cytosol, coefficient of variation)	A	3.7 (12%)	2.7 (11%)	3.6
	B	3.8 (0%)	2.9 (3%)	3.8 (7%)
	C	3.1 (5%)	2.7 (8%)	3.3
K_d for ER ($\times 10^{-10}$ M, coefficient of variation)	A	0.6 (13%)	2.9 (20%)	0.4 (106%)
	B	1.9 (67%)	2.9 (15%)	0.6 (47%)
	C	1.6 (1%)	7.9 (24%)	4.2 (101%)
K_d for PgR ($\times 10^{-10}$ M, coefficient of variation)	A	2.2 (35%)	29 (72%)	7.4 (2%)
	B	7.2 (2%)	71 (1%)	9.3 (27%)
	C	11 (44%)	82 (66%)	10 (57%)

[a] Protein contents and coefficients of variation for laboratory III are only given for data derived from undiluted cytosol

The ratio of 6 : 3 : 1 in ER content was only apparent in laboratory I; laboratory II found a 3.5-fold difference and laboratory III a 2.5-fold difference between powders A and C. With respect to PgR analyses, both laboratories I and III found approximately a 6 : 3 : 1 ratio, while laboratory II quantitated the same number of progesterone receptors in all three powders. The coefficients of variation for the duplicate determinations are generally higher in laboratory III than in the other two laboratories.

The protein content of the vials was found to be approximately 20% lower in laboratory II than in laboratories I and III.

The K_d values for both receptors showed great intra- and interlaboratory variation.

It could be concluded from the data that further efforts to standardize both the protein determinations and the steroid hormone receptor analyses were necessary. To accomplish this end, it was agreed that as of 1 January 1982 all laboratories would use the same methods. Furthermore, vials of standard lyophilized calf uterus cytosol powder are being prepared and distributed among the laboratories. The standard cytosol is being routinely analyzed in each assay, and the results collected and reported upon bimonthly.

References

1. Andersen KW, Mouridsen HT, Castberg TH, Fischerman K, Andersen J, Hou-Jensen K, Brinker H, Johansen H, Henriksen E, Rørth, M, Rossing N (1981) Organization of the Danish adjuvant trials in breast cancer. Dan Med Bull 28: 102–106
2. EORTC Breast Cancer Cooperative Group (1980) Revision of the standards for assessment of hormone receptors in human breast cancer: report of the second EORTC workshop held on 16–17 March, 1979 in the Netherlands Cancer Institute. Eur J Cancer 16: 1513–1515
3. Scatchard G (1949) The attractions of proteins for small molecules and ions. Ann NY Acad Sci 51: 660–672

Results of External Quality Control Trials Performed by the German Cooperative Group for Receptor Assay Standardization

H. Bojar

Abteilung für Onkologische Biochemie, Institut für Physiologische Chemie II,
Medizinische Einrichtungen, Universität Düsseldorf,
Moorenstrasse 5, 4000 Düsseldorf, FRG

Within the scope of a project aimed at supporting clinical research in the field of medical oncology, the Government of the Federal Republic of Germany encouraged multidisciplinary cooperative therapeutic studies at a national level. In this context the outlines of a National Breast Cancer Study Group emerged in 1979. The plan for a national adjuvant study in breast cancer in which estrogen and progestin receptor status are to be used for selecting hormone-dependent neoplasias necessitated the formation of a committee for standardization of the assessment of hormone sensitivity. The committee was established in 1979 and consists of the following members (given in alphabetical order):

Prof. Dr. H. Bojar, Abteilung für Onkologische Biochemie, Physiologische Chemie II, Universität Düsseldorf
Priv.-Doz. Dr. Geyer, Universitätsfrauenklinik, Freiburg
Dr. H.-O. Hoppen, Max-Planck-Institut für Experimentelle Endokrinologie, Hannover
Dr. W. Jonat, Zentralkrankenhaus St.-Jürgen-Straße, Frauenklinik, Bremen
Dr. K. Klinga, Universitätsfrauenklinik, Heidelberg
Prof. Dr. Kuß, Laboratorium für Klinische Chemie, Spezialuntersuchungen, I. Frauenklinik der Universität, München
Prof. Dr. K. Pollow, Frauenklinik der Johannes-Gutenberg-Universität, Mainz
Prof. Dr. G. Trams, Universitätsfrauenklinik, Hamburg
Dr. C. de Waal, I. Universitätsfrauenklinik, München
Dr. Hannelore Würz, Universitätsfrauenklinik, Köln

The committee agreed on the necessity of determining of both the cytoplasmic estrogen and progestin receptors. The multiple point dextran-coated charcoal assay analyzed by the method of Scatchard was selected as the standard procedure, with the option of using more refined techniques when they are available. At two conferences held at the University of Düsseldorf in 1979 and 1980 the details of the experimental procedure were specified; it was decided that the methodological recommendations of the EORTC Breast Cancer Cooperative Group should be followed in order to facilitate international (European) cooperation in this field. Three members of the national committee (W. Jonat, H.-O. Hoppen, and H. Bojar) also belong to the EORTC committee for steroid receptor assay standardization.

The members of the national committee agreed on the need to establish an efficient quality control system. For this purpose the Department of Biochemical Oncology, Düsseldorf, has produced vacuum-sealed lyophilized calf uterine tissue powder. At the "Consensus

Recent Results in Cancer Research. Vol. 91
© Springer-Verlag Berlin · Heidelberg 1984

Meeting on Steroid Receptors in Breast Cancer" (Bethesda, Maryland, USA) in 1979 our laboratory presented data on the thermostability of estrogen, progestin, androgen and glucocorticoid receptors in the freeze-dried material. As has been published in detail elsewhere [1], we were able to demonstrate, for example, that storage even at the high temperature of +80° C for 16 h resulted in a loss of only 36% in the estrogen binding capacity and less than 30% for the other binding proteins. Storage of the lyophilized powder at +20° C for several months did not reduce the binding activity. We concluded from our data that the freeze-dried uterine powders can be useful quality control specimens for receptor assays.

After having developed the quality control resource we started our external quality control trials in 1979. The Department of Biochemical Oncology has served as producer and distributor of the control samples and has also evaluated the binding data. In order to avoid abuse of the results and to encourage less experienced laboratories to participate in these experiments it was decided that the reported binding data would be compiled without entering the name of the institution. As can be seen in Table 1, three quality control trials have been performed in Germany. Participation in these trials was not restricted to the charter members of the group. For each of the annual trials a separate batch (K-EP-001−K-EP-003) of quality control specimens was prepared. All participants received samples of the same batch. The binding capacities as estimated at the Department of Biochemical Oncology, Düsseldorf, are shown at the top of Table 1. The participating laboratories are coded A-M. Each horizontal line represents the binding data reported by an individual laboratory in the annual trials. Unless otherwise indicated, multiple point dextran-coated charcoal assay was used. Ten laboratories participated in the trial of 1979. The mean of the binding capacities assessed by our laboratory (Düsseldorf) while using the material in daily internal quality control for 23 working days was calculated and found to be 155 fmol/mg cytosol protein for the estrogen receptor and 2491 fmol/mg for the progestin receptor. Under these conditions the variation coefficients were determined to be less than 8%. Variation coefficients calculated for quality control samples (exclusively for those analyzed in our laboratory) of both subsequent trials (1980 and 1981) were found to be within the same limit. In the trial of 1979 nine out of ten laboratories reported the presence of estrogen receptors in the samples. One laboratory failed to demonstrate specific estrogen binding. The statistical data were as follows (negative results included): mean ($\bar{X}$) of the binding capacities (fmol/mg cytosol protein) and variation coefficient (V; %): $\bar{X} =$ 104.9, V = 56 [binding data evaluated by recommended standard procedure (STP) only]; $\bar{X} =$ 105.4, V = 49 [binding determined by standard plus optional procedures (STP + OP)].

In the same trial eight of the ten laboratories succeeded in demonstrating specific progestin binding, while two failed. *Statistical analysis:* $\bar{X} = 662$, V = 126 (STP); $\bar{X} = 774$, V = 122 (STP + OP). In the 1979 trial estrogen receptor determination was found to be significantly more reliable than progestin receptor analysis.

The quality control experiment performed in 1980 resulted in an improvement of the reliability of progestin receptor determination. Only one laboratory reported false-negative results concerning the estrogen receptor. Analyses of progestin binding did not produce false-negative data. *Statistical analysis:* (a) estrogen receptor: $\bar{X} = 95.5$, V = 75 (STP); $\bar{X} = 106.9$, V = 63 (STP + OP); (b) progestin receptor: $\bar{X} = 960.4$, V = 65 (STP); $\bar{X} = 800.7$, V = 76 (STP + OP).

In the trial of 1981 all of the 13 participants agreed on an estrogen receptor-positive status. One laboratory failed to detect specific progestin binding components in the quality control sample. *Statistical analysis:* estrogen receptor: $\bar{X} = 310.6$, V = 81.1 (STP); $\bar{X} = 295.5$,

Table 1. Results of external quality control trials performed by the German Cooperative Group for Receptor Assay Standardization

Receptor laboratory	1979 (K-EP-0001) Binding capacity (fmol/mg cytosol protein)		1980 (K-EP-0002) Binding capacity (fmol/mg cytosol protein)		1981 (K-EP-0003) Binding capacity (fmol/mg cytosol protein)	
	Estrogen receptor	Progestin receptor	Estrogen receptor	Progestin receptor	Estrogen receptor	Progestin receptor
Düsseldorf	155	2,491	125	1,337	243	703
A	170	240	122	2,100	504	880
B	117/107[a]	1,800/2,830[a]	150/147[a]	850/580[a]	205[a]	573[a]
C	160	Negativ	75	523	115	625
D	98[a]	523[a]	Negativ[a]	346[a]		
	106[b]	685[b]	Negativ[b]	453[a]	265	1,070
	104	645	Negativ	383		
E	Negativ	Negativ	240	1,400	960	Negativ
F	101[a]	38[a]	168/139[a]	184/195[a]	314/169[a]	93/24[a]
	106[b]	43[b]	224/185[b]	295/286[b]	252/142[c]	115/28[c]
			133/89[c]	160/207[c]		
G	46.7	463	35.9	804	325	626
H	91	331	81.7	912	128	771
I	113	470	142	–	413	766
			27	224		
K	Not participated		Not participated		96	589
L	Not participated		Not participated		116	500
M	Not participated		Not participated		252	674

The quality control experiments were performed using lyophilized calf uterine tissue powders sealed in a vacuum [1]. Specific steroid binding was estimated by multiple point dextran-coated charcoal assay (analyzed by the method of Scatchard) alone or in addition to:
[a] Agar gel electrophoresis
[b] A single concentration of radiolabeled ligand
[c] Sucrose gradient centrifugation
Two laboratories (B and F) have not as yet used the standardized assay procedure

$V = 78.8$ (STP + OP); progestin receptor: $\bar{X} = 654.9$, $V = 40.7$ (STP); $\bar{X} = 603$, $V = 48.6$ (STP + OP).
The results of the annual quality control trials may be summarized as follows:
1. When starting the experiments in 1979 a fairly good agreement in the reported estrogen binding capacities was observed. No further improvement of the estrogen receptor assay could be demonstrated.
2. In contrast, a significant improvement in the quality of the progestin receptor assay could be seen.
3. Using a threshold value of $10-20$ fmol/mg cytosol protein for the definition of receptor-positive breast cancer specimen, 94% of estrogen receptor assays and 91% of progestin receptor assays would be in agreement as far as clinical consequences are concerned.

Despite points 2 and 3, the data also show that more work has to be done to improve the quality of receptor assays. The fourth German quality control trial is now in progress; in this trial various batches of lyophilized calf uterus cytosols which differ in receptor content have been used.

Lyophilized cytosols have the advantage over freeze-dried powders that the total protein content in samples of the same batch is not expected to differ significantly. Therefore the binding data of cytosolic quality control samples can be reliably expressed on a volumetric basis and in relation to protein content, thus allowing separate quality control of receptor assay and protein determination.

Reference

1. Bojar H, Staib W, Beck K, Pilaski J (1980) Investigation of the thermostability of steroid hormone receptors in lyophilized calf uterine tissue powders. Cancer 46: 2770–2774

British Interlaboratory Quality Assessment of Steroid Receptor Assays*

S. Cowan and R. E. Leake

Department of Biochemistry, University of Glasgow, Glasgow G12 8QQ, United Kingdom

Introduction

Interlaboratory quality assessment of steroid receptor assays began in 1977 with a small study initiated through the Christie Hospital, Manchester (Dr. D. Barnes). This study was extended to include nine laboratories in 1979, since when each laboratory has participated regularly (see Part VII). With centres in Birmingham (Dr. A. Hughes), Cardiff (Drs. R. Nicholson and D. Wilson), Edinburgh (Dr. A. Hawkins), Glasgow (Dr. R. Leake), London (Drs. H. Braunsberg, R. King and A. Wilson) and Manchester (Drs. D. Barnes and A. Howell), the country is reasonably well covered, although additional groups continue to show an interest in the study. We are also fortunate to have an additional control through the participation of the Nijmegen group.

The initial objectives of the study included identification of major sources of variation in quantitative estimates of receptor content, both in methodology and in subsequent handling of the data. It was also of interest to see whether samples purporting to contain a low concentration of receptor were actually uniformly reported as receptor positive or negative.

Materials and Methods

All samples were lyophilised material. The source of material in each case is shown in Table 1. Samples were aliquoted into 5-ml vials, lyophilised and then capped.

Oestrogen and progesterone receptor content of the lyophilised material remained unaltered, within experimental error, throughout the period of the study (Fig. 1).

Vials were distributed to the participating laboratories by ordinary post; so far, only one has been lost and none damaged. Each vial was accompanied with a questionnaire designed to establish storage time, precise reconstitution conditions and all relevant details of the assays for both progesterone and oestrogen receptor. The completed questionnaires containing the calculated receptor concentration data were returned, whenever possible with the original Scatchard plots, to the co-ordinating centre.

* The British Quality Assessment study is entirely dependent on the goodwill and efforts of each participating laboratory. In addition to the people named in the Introduction, we are very grateful to Elizabeth Lloyd, Graham Groom and, particularly, Ton Koenders for advice and suggestions

Table 1. Source of lyophilised assay material

Sample no.	Tissue
1	Calf uterus
2	DMBA-induced rat mammary tumour
3	Benign human breast tumour
4	Human myometrium
5	Human myometrium

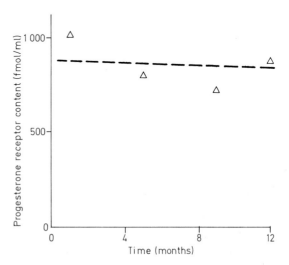

Fig. 1. Storage stability of progesterone receptor in lyophilised material. Equal volumes of solution were aliquoted into vials, lyophilised and then assayed for progesterone receptor content after the storage time indicated. Oestrogen receptor was found to be at least as stable over the same time period

Results

Oestrogen and progesterone receptor content of the various samples, as determined by each laboratory, is summarised in Table 2. Results are given in fmol/mg protein. For this reason the protein content of each sample is also shown.

On first inspection the results in Table 2 suggest that very serious differences in both quantitative and qualitative assessment of samples can occur. On closer inspection of the data it is apparent that multiple assays of the same sample within a single laboratory always gave very similar results. However, the final concentration of receptor reported could vary considerably between laboratories. For example, sample 1 was assayed on three separate occasions and one group reported 122, 127 and 131 fmol/mg protein for oestrogen receptor, whereas another reported 66, 65, and 70 fmol/mg protein. Since the data in Table 2 show such a large variation in the reported protein content of each sample, they were re-expressed as fmol/ml. The same results were then 476, 483 and 643 fmol/ml and 389, 374 and 376 fmol/ml. Thus the difference in reported receptor concentration can be explained in part, but not entirely, on the basis of differences in measured protein content.

Small differences between laboratories occurred in the assay procedures and the methods of calculation (Tables 3, 4). It was a qualitative impression that different final concentrations for charcoal led to different results, although this was not quantified. Dextran coating of the charcoal improved removal of free and loosely bound steroid from solution. It also decreased the possibility that, after centrifugation, charcoal particles could

Table 2. Mean concentration of oestrogen and progesterone receptors determined in lyophilised material

Sample	Oestrogen receptors: fmol/mg protein			Progesterone receptors: fmol/mg protein			Protein: mg protein/ml		
	Range (n)	Mean ± SD	C of V (%)	Range (n)	Mean ± SD	C of V (%)	Range (n)	Mean ± SD	C of V (%)
1	48–408 (15)	131 ± 93	71	0–228 (13)	95 ± 75	79	1.76– 5.9 (15)	4.75 ± 1.24	26
2	0– 77 (25)	25 ± 21	84	0–161 (22)	(17 ± 40)	235	3.2 –12.12 (24)	7.73 ± 2.35	30
3	0– 36 (16)	(4 ± 9)	225	0– 19 (15)	(4 ± 7)	175	0.9 – 8.0 (16)	4.33 ± 1.58	36
4	0– 67 (26)	28 ± 18	64	0–239 (23)	87 ± 75	86	2.15– 7.9 (25)	5.00 ± 1.45	29
5	0– 44 (26)	18 ± 12	67	0–220 (24)	60 ± 47	78	2.5 – 8.92 (26)	5.32 ± 1.88	35

n, number of assays; SD, standard deviation; C of V, coefficient of variation

Table 3. Assay conditions used by the participating laboratories

Labo-ratory	Cytosol (μl)	Incubation vol/final vol (μl)	Final concen-tration DCC[a]	Time (min)	Protein assay Method	Standard
1	150	200/1,100	0.05 0.08	15	Lowry	BSA
2	50	60	0.16	10	Lowry	BSA
3	200	250 E_2 260 prog.	0.14 0.13	10 5	Lowry	BSA
4	100 E_2 200 prog.	1,200 1,300	0.04 0.04	15	Bradford	BSA
5	100	200	0.25	15	Lowry	BSA
6	100	200	3.57	10 E_2 20 prog.	Lowry	BSA
7	200	400	0.25	30	Lowry	BSA
8	(Steroid ppt with polyethylene glycol)				Lowry	BPA
9	100	200	0.25	30	Lowry	BSA

[a] DCC, dextran-coated charcoal. Figure given is the final concentration of charcoal expressed as %

Table 4. Interlaboratory methods for determining specific binding and analysing data

Labo-ratory	Oestrogen receptor Calculation	Competitor	Progesterone receptor	^{3}[H] ligand	Competitor
1	Sc. Pl.	D.E.S.	Sc. Pl.	Prog.	Prog. + cort.
2	Sc. Pl.	D.E.S.	Sc. Pl.	R-5020	R-5020
3	S.D. 5 nM	D.E.S.	S.D. 10 nM	Prog.	Nor + cort.
4	Sc. Pl.	E_2	Sc. Pl.	Org 2058	Org 2058
5	Sc. Pl.	D.E.S.	Sc. Pl.	Prog.	Nor
6	Sc. Pl.	D.E.S.	Sc. Pl.	R-5020	R-5020
7	S.D. 1.8 nM	E_2	S.D. 7.6 nM	R-5,020	R.5,020
8	Sc. Pl.	H.D.	Sc. Pl.	Prog.	H.D. + cort.
9	Sc. Pl.	D.E.S.			

Sc. Pl., Scatchard plot; *S.D.,* single dose assay; *Nor,* norethisterone; *H.D.,* heat denaturation; *cort.,* cortisol
All laboratories used ^{3}H-oestradiol-17β for oestrogen receptor assay. R-5020 and Org 2058 are synthetic progestins. The radiochemical ligands were obtained from NEN and The Radiochemical Centre, respectively

be picked up in the aliquot removed for counting. A charcoal : dextran ratio of 100 : 1 seemed to give consistent results.

In view of the variation in protein content results, we subsequently attempted to establish a uniform assay using the Bradford procedure [1]. Unfortunately, the results of a single round of assays (Table 5) confirm our earlier conclusion that adopting a uniform protein

Table 5. Oestrogen and progesterone receptor content of common samples assayed using the Bradford protein method

Sample no.	Receptor protein content (fmol/mg)			
	Oestrogen receptor		Progesterone receptor	
	Range (n)	Mean ± SD	Range (n)	Mean ± SD
1	13–145 (9)	89 ± 33	12–271 (8)	114 ± 86
3	0– 13.4 (9)	2.8 ± 4.5	0– 28 (8)	5 ± 10
4	13– 43 (9)	26 ± 10	17–179 (8)	106 ± 58
5	10– 48 (9)	24 ± 12	20–149 (8)	103 ± 52

assay does not rule out interlaboratory variation. This continued discrepancy may be explained in part by the differences in methods of analysis of raw data. Laboratories carrying out single dose assays produce more variable data than those generating a Scatchard plot of specifically bound material. However, there is no significant difference between the mean values obtained by the two methods for those samples which have been measured at least four times each.

Discussion

The objective of any quality assessment study is to identify any sources of weakness or variability in an assay. However, the biological integrity of the answer must be maintained. We do not wish to obtain a uniform but incorrect answer!

In the case of this particular study, each laboratory analysed common lyophilised samples using the routine assay already existing in that laboratory. The biggest single variant was protein content (Table 2), although most groups used the same Lowry method. Even when all laboratories used the same protein assay method (Bradford), a standard source of dye and an agreed standard, protein receptor concentration for common samples was still very variable although qualitative agreement on receptor-positive and receptor-negative tissue was very good (Table 5).

To determine the importance of the different calculation methods (and computer programs) in generating the variation in reported results, a common set of raw data is now being analysed by each laboratory. We are also collecting the raw data on a common sample from each laboratory with a view to putting it through a common computer program. Since individual laboratories already generate very similar answers for a single lyophilised sample when the sample is assayed at different times over a period of months, it is reasonable to expect that the incorporation of a common protein assay and common results analysis will lead to good general agreement. Nevertheless, to get reproducible data on receptor content of tumour tissue one has to establish a common procedure for handling tissue and, most importantly, a uniform approach to tissue homogenisation.

Even if the outcome of quality control is that interlaboratory results become truly comparable, there is still the major problem of intratumoral variation in receptor content [2–5]. However, there are good prospects that in the near future assays in different participating laboratories will be strictly comparable and a receptor-positive tumour will be reported as such by all laboratories. Uniform cut-off points of receptor concentration, above which response to therapy can be expected, should soon be established.

References

1. Bradford MM (1976) A rapid and sensitive method for the quantitation of microgram quantities of protein utilizing the principle of protein-dye binding. Anal Biochem 72:248−254
2. Hawkins RA, Roberts MM, Forest APM (1980) Oestrogen receptors and breast cancer: current status. Br J Surg 67:153−169
3. Leake RE, Laing L, Smith DC (1979) A role for nuclear oestrogen receptors in prediction of therapy regime for breast cancer patients. In: King RJB (ed) Steroid receptor assays in human breast tumours: methodological and clinical aspects. Alpha Omega, Cardiff, pp 73−85
4. Silverswärd C, Skoog L, Humla S, Gustafsson SA, Nordenskjold B (1980) Intratumoral variation of cytoplasmic and nuclear oestrogen receptor concentrations in human mammary carcinoma. Eur J Cancer 16:59−65
5. Tilley WD, Keightley DD, Cant LM (1978) Inter-site variation of oestrogen receptors in human breast cancer. Br J Cancer 38:544−546

Quality Control Program for Estradiol Receptor Determination: The Italian Experience

A. Piffanelli, S. Fumero, and D. Pelizzola

Istituto di Radiologia dell'Università, Corso Giovecca 203, Ferrara, 44100 Italy

Introduction

The main objective of the Italian interlaboratory quality control program was to evaluate the methods applied by the numerous laboratories that determine estradiol receptor in tumors, in order to achieve both standardized methods and consequently more reliable and comparable data.

The quality control program consisted in assays of lyophilized animal uterus cytosol. Estradiol receptor in these preparations proved stable in time [4, 6].

The use of lyophilized supernatant permits identification of variations due to the final steps of the ER determination method. Future phases of the Italian quality control program will deal with the homogenization and centrifugation steps.

Since no reference samples of known content are available, we prepared a series of lyophilized cytosols at scalar receptor concentrations in order to cull as much information as possible about the intra- and interlaboratory variability. Part of these results have recently been published [4].

Preparation of the Lyophilized Calf Uterus Cytosols

The uterus of one young calf was homogenized with phosphate buffer pH 7.4 5 mM, containing 0.15 g/l of dithioerythrol, with an Ultraturrax for 30 s at 4° C. The homogenate was centrifuged at 28,000 g for 1 h at 0°−4° C. The calf uterus supernatant was diluted 1 : 2 (preparation no. 4) with a pool of female human serum diluted 30-fold with physiologic solution. The calf uterus supernatant was further diluted 1 : 2, 1 : 4, and 1 : 8 with the same diluted serum. This diluted serum was also used as negative cytosol (preparation no. 8). One milliliter of each preparation was placed in a lyophilizing vial and lyophilized overnight (Edwards Modulyo Freeze Dryer). The vials were vacuum sealed. The lyophilized samples, stored at 4° C, were dispatched by normal mail to the collaborating laboratories. Each dispatch was accompanied by a form giving indications of how to dissolve the lyophilized powder, and requesting that the laboratory specify the features of the method it used.

Methods

Each laboratory dissolved the lyophilized substance with 5 ml of the recommended eluent (phosphate buffer) and determined the estradiol receptor by the dextran-coated charcoal method (DCC) [1−3]. The essential features of the methods followed by the participating laboratories are reported in Table 1.

Generally, the receptor concentration was evaluated by Scatchard analysis without correction.

Since preparations nos. 5, 6, and 7 were obtained by scalar dilutions of preparation no. 4, it was possible to make a variance analysis of each laboratory's linear regression and of the mean values of all laboratories.

Results and Discussion

Table 2 gives the results that the participating laboratories reported after determining estradiol receptor concentration, expressed as fmol/ml and as fmol/mg of protein, and after determining protein level in each of the lyophilized preparations. In the same table are reported the mean values, the standard deviations and the variation coefficients of these results.

One laboratory (F) reported that its determinations on samples nos. 6 and 7 were lost. Only one laboratory (D) considered the result obtained on preparation no. 7 (the one with the lowest receptor content) as borderline.

The variation coefficient of the results of estradiol receptor, expressed as fmol/ml, ranges from 25% to 46%, while the same expressed as fmol/mg protein, ranges from 36% to 43%. The highest variation coefficient proved to be for the sample with the lowest receptor content.

Data expression as fmol/ml markedly lowers the variability of the results, because a factor that increases variability is constituted by protein determination, the variation coefficient of which ranges from 35% to 42%.

Considerable variability is also evident in the K_d values given in Table 3.

Statistical analysis of the receptor content in these preparations of the scalar concentration permits identification of intramurally variable parameters, identification of the systematic factors among the participating laboratories, and, finally, a better estimation of receptor content obtainable by similar methods in different laboratories.

The regression coefficient for each laboratory ranges from 0.9850 to 0.9994.

The regression of mean values of estradiol receptor expressed as fmol/ml is in excellent agreement with the theoretical scalar dilutions, with a highly significant coefficient (0.9993).

A first (qualitative) goal of any quality control program concerns the response that the assay can provide on a sample by classifying it as positive or negative for the presence of the receptor, and the Italian program amply achieved this goal. The positive/negative distinction is, for the present, still the cardinal factor for selecting the therapy appropriate to each case. Every laboratory, in fact, defined all samples containing receptor as positive, and all laboratories classified the only negative sample as such.

A second qualitative objective concerning the concentration response obtainable from the assay was met with variability. When the concentration was expressed in fmol/ml, the variability was still acceptable, except for sample 7, which had the lowest concentration.

Table 1. Features of methodologies used by laboratories participating in the Italian quality control program (1980)

Labo-ratory	Date of determina-tion	Protein assay method	Protein standard	Range of ^{3}H-E$_2$ concentration	Specific activity of ^{3}H-E$_2$ (Ci/mmol)	DES concen-tration (nM)	Dextran percentage in final incubation	Charcoal percentage in final incubation	DCC contact time (min)	Incubation time/temperature
A	9. 7. 80	Lowry	BSA	1.8 Sc 4.62 S	115	360	0.14	0.0014	10	18 h, −4° C
B	17. 2. 81	Bio-Rad	5% HSA− 3% IgG	0.15−2.3	100	230	0.31	0.031	10	18 h, −4° C
C	31. 7. 80	Bio-Rad	BSA	0.13−4.17	110	834	0.28	0.028	10	16 h, −4° C
D	29. 8. 80	Bio-Rad	KABI	0.13−4.17	101	834	0.31	0.031	15	16 h, −4° C
E	17. 7. 80	Bio-Rad	BSA	n.r.−4.17	108	4,170	0.28	0.028	30	16 h, −4° C
F	14. 7. 80	Bio-Rad	BSA	n.r.−3.33	101	666	0.25	0.025	10	16 h, −4° C
G	15. 7. 80	Lowry	HSA	0.06−0.4	91	40	0.25	0.025	30	2 h, +15° C
H	9. 9. 80	Bio-Rad	BSA	0.09−5.0	85	2,500	0.25	0.025	15	18 h, −4° C
I	29. 9. 80	Lowry	BSA	0.62−20	91	2,000	0.5	0.05	10	18 h, −4° C
L	9. 80	Lowry	BSA	0.065−4.16	91	830	0.31	0.031	10	18 h, −4° C
M	19. 5. 81	Bio-Rad	BSA	0.06−4.17	112	800	0.62	0.031	15	18 h, −4° C

n. r., not reported

Table 2. Estradiol receptor concentration expressed as fmol/ml and as fmol/mg protein in the five lyophilized calf uterus cytosols used in the Italian quality control program (1980)

Laboratory	Prep. no. 4 (100%)			Prep. no. 5 (50%)			Prep. no. 6 (25%)			Prep. no. 7 (12.5%)			Prep. no. 8		
	a	b	c	a	b	c	a	b	c	a	b	c	a	b	c
A	355	135	2.5	168	55	2.9	72	23	3.1	44	14	3.1	0	0	3.0
B	200	200	1.0	90	72	1.2	43	31	1.4	26	18	1.4	0	0	1.5
C	326	233	1.4	130	86	1.5	46	31	1.5	25	16	1.5	0	0	1.6
D	225	225	1.0	129	129	1.0	63	58	1.1	32	27	1.2	0	0	1.4
E	361	425	0.8	145	145	1.0	63	53	1.2	31	25	1.2	0	0	1.2
F	201	102	1.9	90	41	2.2	Lost			Lost			0	0	1.0
G	361	230	1.5	132	66	2.0	44	28	1.5	24	14	1.7	0	0	2.0
H	380	344	0.9	180	133	1.2	86	63	1.3	47	28	1.6	0	0	1.9
I	184	205	0.9	70	70	1.0	43	39	1.1	17	17	1.0	0	0	0.5
L	300	250	1.2	137	106	1.3	83	69	1.2	22	11	2.1	0	0	n.m.
M	272	323	0.8	150	113	1.3	64	43	2.4	29	15	1.9	0	0	n.m.
Mean	287	242	1.26	129	92.3	1.50	60.7	43.8	1.58	26.8	16.0	1.67	0	0	1.56
SD	74.5	92.3	0.53	33.7	34.7	0.60	16.3	16.0	0.65	12.5	6.9	0.60	–	–	0.70
VC	25.9	38.1	42.0	26.1	37.5	40.0	26.8	36.5	41.1	46.6	43.6	35.9	–	–	44.8

a, fmol/ml; b, fmol/mg protein; c, protein mg/ml; n.m., not measurable

Table 3. Dissociation constant values ($K_d \cdot 10^{-10}$ M) obtained for estradiol receptor in the five lyophilized calf uterus cytosols used in the Italian quality control program (1980)

Laboratory	Prep. no. 4	Prep. no. 5	Prep. no. 6	Prep. no. 7	Prep. no. 8
A	0.19	0.56	1.63	2.04	–
B	1.23	1.63	2.84	2.66	–
C	0.39	1.30	2.41	1.31	–
D	0.17	1.40	1.60	n.d.	–
E	1.08	1.09	1.70	5.16	–
F	1.60	1.60	Lost	Lost	–
G	2.80	2.90	2.50	4.40	–
H	1.00	3.00	2.90	2.20	–
I	13.00	4.38	3.70	5.80	–
L	1.72	1.57	1.50	2.15	–
M	1.13	2.70	2.70	2.00	–
Mean	2.21	2.01	2.35	3.08	–
SD	3.66	1.10	0.73	1.61	–

But variability rose markedly when the concentration was expressed as fmol/mg protein, this being directly dependent on the high variability in the protein determination.

While other European quality control programs [5] have reported similar variability levels, it is a matter of concern that the protein assay represents one of the major sources of variability in receptor determination. The distribution of K_d values was also rather wide. As the receptor concentration decreases, the K_d tends to increase. A further investigation ought to ascertain whether this trend is due to the lyophilized preparations themselves or to some other factor yet to be identified.

An overview of Italian program as it has been implemented up to now indicated that there is good intramural reproducibility, as the single correlation coefficients demonstrate: from analysis of these regressions, the systematic intramural variables can be identified.

Very probably, quality control conducted on lyophilized tissue including the homogenization and centrifugation phases, which in the initial Italian experience were not required, would produce increased variability in terms of concentration found. So, before this second phase of the Italian program is undertaken, further efforts are necessary to pinpoint the variability parameters and to standardize methods that can guarantee greater uniformity of responses. Only then can the numerous variables in the homogenization and centrifugation phases be appropriately dealt with.

References

1. EORTC Breast Cancer Cooperative Group (1973) Standards for the assessment of estrogen receptors in human breast cancer, 1st workshop. Eur J Cancer 9: 379–381
2. EORTC Breast Cancer Cooperative Group (1980) Standards for the assessment of estrogen receptors in human breast cancer, 2nd workshop, Amsterdam, 1979. Eur J Cancer 16: 1513–1515
3. Koenders A, Thorpe, SM on behalf of EORTC Receptor Group (1983) Standardization of steroid receptor assay in human breast cancer. I. Reproducibility of Estradiol and Progesterone receptor assays. Eur J Cancer Clin Oncol 19: 1221–1229

4. Fumero S, Berruto GP, Mondino A, Pelizzola D, Grilli S, Buttazzi C, Di Fronzo G, Bertuzzi A, Bozzetti C, Mori P, Concolino G, Marocchi A, Robustelli della Cuna G, Zibera C, Cerrutti G, Ros A, Piffanelli A (1981) Results of the Italian interlaboratory quality control program for estradiol receptor assay. Tumori 67: 301–306
5. King RJB, Bames DN, Hawkins RA, Leake RE, Maynard PV, Roberts MM (1978) Measurements of estradiol receptors by five institutions on common tissue samples. Br J Cancer 38: 428–430
6. Koenders AJ, Geurts-Maespots J, Kho KH, Benraad ThJ (1978) Estradiol and progesterone receptor activities in stored lyophilized target tissue. J Steroid Biochem 9: 947–950

Participating Laboratories

Istituto di Radiologia, Università di Ferrara (Pelizzola D., Piffanelli A., Giovanni G.)
Istituto Ricerche Biomediche 'Antoine Marxer' RBM, Ivrea (Fumero S., De Bortoli M.)
Istituto Cancerologia Università di Bologna (Grilli S., Buttazzi C.)
Istituto Nazionale Tumori di Milano (Di Fronzo G., Ronchi E., Capelletti V.)
Servizio Oncologia Ospedali Riuniti di Parma (Bozzetti C., Cocconi G.)
Clinica Medica Generale V, Università di Roma (Concolino G., Marocchi A.)
Divisione Oncologia Fond. Clinica Lavoro, Università di Pavia (Robustelli della Cuna G., Zibera C.)
Clinica Ostetrica Università di Padova, Sede di Verona (Costanzo C., Ros A.)
Istituto Patologia Generale, Facolytà Medica I, Università Napoli (Sica V., Puca G.)
Istituto per lo Studio e la Cura dei Tumori, Genova (Nicolò G., Esposito M.)
Istituto Farmacologia, Università Palermo (D'Alessandro N., Sanguedolce R.)

Quality Control of Steroid Receptor Assays in the Netherlands

A. Koenders and T. J. Benraad

Department of Experimental and Chemical Endocrinology, Medical Faculty, University of Nijmegen, 6500 HB Nijmegen, The Netherlands

Introduction

In 1977 a quality control program for steroid receptors, performed in breast cancer tissues, was initiated in The Netherlands. Presently 18 laboratories are participating in this program. During the first three trials lyophilized tissue powders were used as reference samples, because this type of preparation showed no loss of receptor binding when stored for at least 3 months at 4° C and for several weeks at room temperature [1]. Recently, the usefulness of lyophilized samples for daily control of steroid receptor assays within laboratories and for comparison and standardization of measurements between laboratories has been reviewed [6]. In the first trials of this quality control program large variations in receptor values between laboratories were observed, although the participants agreed on the classification of the reference samples as estradiol receptor (ER) positive [5]. The tissue powders used in those trials contained intermediate or high receptor values. These variations in reported results were ascribed to the variety of methodological techniques employed by the participants, including the use of several different protein assays [5]. These methodological factors caused laboratories to score rather consistently high or low on the various reference samples. In assessing these results, it was noted that variation in protein values could be minimized if all laboratories used the same type of protein assay in addition to the same protein standard. Therefore all participants agreed to measure the protein content of the cytosol by the method of Bradford [2], using Kabi human albumin as a protein standard. In addition it was decided to analyze lyophilized reference cytosols in the forthcoming trials in order to eliminate interlaboratory differences in the preparation of the cytosol and to permit easier delineation and standardization of the most important steps involved in the receptor binding assay itself. These include incubation conditions, determination of the nonspecific binding, separation conditions of bound and free steroid, and calculation of receptor binding parameters. The stability of steroid receptors in lyophilized uterine and breast tumor cytosols under various storage conditions has recently been evaluated [6].

Preparation of Lyophilized Reference Cytosols

Tissue specimens frozen in liquid nitrogen were pulverized in the frozen state to a fine homogeneous powder by means of a Thermovac tissue pulverizer and a Microdismem-

---

* The authors are indebted to Gail Janes for carefully correcting this manuscript

brator. The tissue powder was stirred with buffer (0.02 M Na_2HPO_4/NaH_2PO_4, 1.5 mM EDTA, 3.0 mM NaN_3, pH 7.4) and centrifuged at 50,000 g for 0.5 h at 2° C. The tissue weight : buffer volume ratios for calf uterine tissue (reference sample A), DMBA-induced rat mammary tumors (reference sample B), and benign human breast tumor tissue (reference sample C) were 1 : 8, 1 : 4, and 1 : 6, respectively. It may be noted that tumor tissues had been stored at −70° C for more than 3 years before the specimens were lyophilized. During this period the DMBA tumors had lost all their original progesterone receptor (PgR) activity. The obtained cytosols were filtered and 3.5-ml aliquots were measured into glass vials immersed in liquid nitrogen and then lyophilized for 48 h. Following this, the vials were stoppered under vacuum while still inside the lyophilization chamber, and stored at 4° C until shipment.

Instructions to Participants

The three reference samples were dispatched to the participating institutions by mail without any precautions regarding temperature control. It had been demonstrated previously that receptor binding sites do not decline during storage for 2 weeks at room temperature [6]. After arrival the vials were stored at 4° C. The participants received the following instructions:
1. Tap vials so that lyophilized cytosol is on the bottom of the vial and remove caps very carefully to release vacuum
2. Place the opened vials on ice and introduce into each vial exactly 3.5 ml of ice cold (0°−4° C) distilled water
3. Carefully swirl the vials and then place them back on ice for 10 min to allow the lyophilized material to go into solution
4. Immediately thereafter, i.e., without centrifugation, analyze the obtained cytosols for steroid receptor binding activity
5. Express the results as fmol/ml cytosol and classify the sample as receptor positive or negative

In addition the participants were requested to fill in a questionnaire concerning the exact methodology of their respective receptor assays and to report all raw data.

Results

All receptor assays were performed within 4 weeks of mailing to the participants. The stability of the reference cytosols was investigated by storing the vials first at room temperature for 3 days (to simulate the mailing period) and then in the refrigerator at 4° C. Figure 1 shows only the receptor-positive results. No loss of receptor activity was observed during a period of 5 weeks. Please note that in this figure and in the following tables the results are expressed as fmol/ml cytosol to avoid variations in protein values. The average receptor and protein values obtained over the 35-day period are summarized in Table 1.

The actual ER values and the receptor-negative and borderline classifications reported by the 15 participating laboratories are collected in Table 2. A large range of values was reported, although all participants agreed on the receptor status of sample A. The interlaboratory coefficient of variation (CV) was 35% (274 ± 95 fmol/ml cytosol, mean ± SD of 15 assays). Of 15 laboratories, 4 (27%) reported control cytosol B as ER

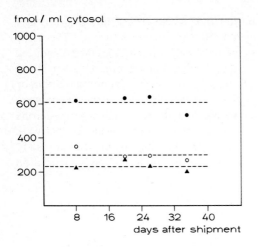

Fig. 1. Stability of steroid receptor binding in lyophilized reference cytosols stored at 4° C. Calf uterus cytosol: ER (○) and PgR (●). DMBA-induced rat mammary tumor cytosol: ER (▲)

Table 1. Characteristics of lyophilized reference cytosols

	Cytosol A		Cytosol B		Cytosol C
Estradiol receptor binding					
fmol/ml cytosol	300	± 34[a]	236	± 33	Negativ
fmol/mg protein	181	± 14	39	± 9	
Progesterone receptor binding					
fmol/ml cytosol	608	± 49	Negativ		Negativ
fmol/mg protein	368	± 30			
Cytosolic protein[b]					
mg/ml cytosol	1.66 ± 0.16		6.1 ± 0.52		3.51 ± 0.08

Reference cytosol A = lyophilized calf uterus cytosol
Reference cytosol B = lyophilized DMBA-induced rat mammary tumor cytosol
Reference cytosol C = lyophilized benign human breast tumor cytosol
[a] Mean ± standard deviation of four determinations performed over a period of 35 days
[b] The protein content of the cytosol was determined by the method of Bradford using Kabi human albumin as a reference protein

negative, while the remaining laboratories reported values between 35 and 295 fmol/ml cytosol or between 6 and 41 fmol/mg protein. As observed before [5], laboratories relatively consistently reported high or low values on the various reference samples ($r_{Spearman} = 0.66$; $P < 0.05$, $n = 11$; negative assays omitted). The majority of ER assays performed on reference sample C were classified as negative or borderline. Nevertheless, 4 out of 15 laboratories (27%) reported this benign human breast tumor cytosol as receptor positive (10–21 fmol/mg protein). Two (labs A and C) disagreed with the majority of the participants on the receptor status of both cytosol B and C. Moreover these two laboratories both reported very low ER values on control cytosol A.

The progesterone receptor results are presented in Table 3. For each reference cytosol the majority of nine participants agreed on the receptor positivity or negativity of the sample. The overall agreement on receptor status was 88% if receptor-borderline classifications

Table 2. Estradiol receptor values of lyophilized reference cytosols obtained by 15 laboratories participating in The Netherlands quality control program

Laboratory	Cytosol A	Cytosol B	Cytosol C
A	70[a]	Negativ	65
B	140	135	Negativ/positiv
C	150	Negativ	80
D	210	35	Negativ/positiv
E	255	285	Negativ
F	265	160	Negativ
G	270	160	Negativ
H	300	240	Negativ
I	340	Negativ	Negativ
J	340	235	30
K	350	200	60
L	365	265	Negativ
M	370	Negativ	Negativ
N	380	295	Negativ
Reference laboratory	300 ± 34[b]	236 ± 33	Negativ

[a] All values are expressed as fmol/ml cytosol
[b] Mean ± standard deviation of four determinations performed over a period of 35 days

Table 3. Progesterone receptor values of lyophilized reference cytosols obtained by nine laboratories participating in The Netherlands quality control program

Laboratory	Cytosol A	Cytosol B	Cytosol C
F	130[a]	500	Negativ
N	405	320	Negativ
E	575	Negativ	Negativ
H	635	Negativ	Negativ
L	745	Negativ	Negativ
K	800	Negativ	90
I	925	Negativ	Negativ/positiv
J	960	Negativ/positiv	Negativ
Reference laboratory	608 ± 49[b]	Negativ	Negativ

[a] All values are expressed as fmol/ml cytosol
[b] Mean ± standard deviation of four determinations performed over a period of 35 days

were omitted. The PgR values obtained on sample A ranged between 130 and 960 fmol/ml cytosol. With the exception of the lowest value, the results agreed reasonably well; $n = 8$, 708 ± 185 with a CV of 26% (omitting lab F). Two receptor assays performed on cytosol B were reported as receptor positive (labs F and N). One of these laboratories (lab N) used a single concentration of R-5020. Several other laboratories employing multiple concentrations of this ^{3}H ligand demonstrated that this compound was not bound with high affinity and therefore this sample was classified as receptor negative. This example confirms the fact discussed by Clark and Peck [3], that one-point assays can lead to erroneous results. Interestingly, the other of the two labs (lab F), using the tritiated Organon compound 2058,

Table 4. Summary of protein results obtained by the method of Bradford using Kabi human albumin as the standard

	Cytosol A	Cytosol B	Cytosol C
Range[a]	1.1−2.75	3.9−12.0	2.8−6.0
Mean	1.75	6.85	3.75
SD	0.45	2.03	0.77
CV	26%	30%	20%

[a] Expressed as mg protein/ml cytosol

reported a PgR value of 500 fmol/cytosol or 40 fmol/mg protein. However, one additional participant (lab J) reported this sample as borderline, also using Organon 2058. All laboratories except one scored control cytosol C as negative or borderline. Laboratory K measured a value of 90 fmol/ml cytosol (30 fmol/mg protein) with a K_d value of 3.1×10^{-9} M. For comparison, the K_d values obtained on the calf uterus cytosol ranged between 1.2 and 4.0×10^{-9} M.

In this trial all participating laboratories measured the protein content of the cytosols by the Bradford procedure, employing the same protein standard (Kabi human serum albumin). In our laboratory the protein values observed with this method are about 70% of the values obtained using the Lowry procedure with BSA. Two- to threefold differences in protein values were observed between laboratories (Table 4). The various laboratories consistently measured low, intermediate, or high values in relation to the other participants; e.g., the highest protein values observed on the three reference samples were reported by the same laboratory.

During this trial all participants employed a dextran-coated charcoal separation of bound and free steroid. Some further details of the various ER assays are listed in Table 5; additional features of the various receptor assays are described in the literature [5]. From this particular trial emerged the following methodological factors which may contribute to the interlaboratory variations in receptor results:

1. *The ratio of cytosol volume to the total volume during the charcoal treatment.* Three participants (labs A−C) used cytosol volumes of 50 µl per incubation tube, whereas the total volume (including the volume of the charcoal suspension) varied between 600 and 1,050 µl, resulting in ratios ranging from 0.083 to 0.048. All other groups utilized ratios of 0.2 or higher. From Table 2 it can be seen that laboratories A−C reported the lowest receptor values on sample A and that two of these laboratories disagreed on the receptor status of samples B and C.

2. *The type of competitive inhibitor used for the determination of nonspecific binding.* Comparison of Tables 5 and 2 reveals that laboratories using nafoxidine generally reported lower values than those using diethylstilbestrol or estradiol; e.g., the mean ± SD of these two groups calculated for sample A was 218 ± 96 ($n = 6$) and 312 ± 76 ($n = 9$), respectively.

3. *The concentration and volume of the dextran-coated charcoal suspension.* Laboratories utilizing a 0.5% charcoal : 0.05% dextran suspension and volumes of 300 µl or more obtained lower values than laboratories adding 150 µl or less of a 0.25% charcoal : 0.025% dextran suspension; e.g., sample A 184 ± 78 ($n = 6$) and 331 ± 30 ($n = 5$), respectively.

Table 5. Description of estradiol receptor methods employed by participating laboratories

Laboratory	Determination of nonspecific binding	DCC 0.5%[a]	0.25%[b]	Calculation of results Single dose	Scatchard
A	Nafoxidine	300 µl		4.95 nM[d]	
B	DES	300 µl		5.9 nM	
C	Nafoxidine	500 µl		3.2 nM	
D	Nafoxidine	500 µl		2.0 nM	
E	DES	120 µl			0.3– 7.0 nM
F	Nafoxidine	500 µl		2.0 nM	
G	Nafoxidine	500 µl		2.0 nM	
H	E_2		100 µl		1.0– 8.0 nM
I	Nafoxidine	200 µl			0.4– 1.6 nM
J	E_2		100 µl		0.5–16.0 nM
K	DES		100 µl		1.0– 8.0 nM
L	DES		150 µl		0.5–18.0 nM
M	E_2		500 µl[c]		0.3– 8.9 nM
N	DES	90 µl		7.0 nM	
Reference laboratory	DES		100 µl		1.0– 8.0 nM

[a] 0.5% charcoal/0.05% dextran
[b] 0.25% charcoal/0.025% dextran
[c] 0.25% charcoal/0.05% dextran
[d] Concentration(s) of ^{3}H-estradiol employed

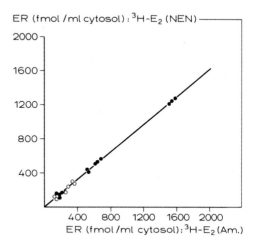

Fig. 2. Comparison of estradiol receptor binding sites determined with ^{3}H-estradiol obtained from Amersham (*Am*) or New England Nuclear (*NEN*) in lyophilized reference samples (●) and human breast tumor specimens stored in liquid nitrogen (○). ^{3}H-estradiol (Amersham): specific activity 106 Ci/mmol; ^{3}H-estradiol (*NEN*): specific activity 111 Ci/mmol

4. *The calculation of binding sites from one (single-point assay) or multiple concentrations (Scatchard analysis) of ^{3}H-estradiol.* The group of participants performing single-point assays reported lower ER values than those laboratories calculating the number of receptor binding sites according to the method of Scatchard; e.g., sample A 212 ± 104 ($n = 7$) and 328 ± 39 ($n = 8$), respectively. Three participants (labs D, F, and G) incubated the cytosol with multiple concentrations of ^{3}H-estradiol, but nevertheless

calculated the concentration of receptor binding sites at one fixed concentration of radioactive ligand. From their raw data it could be estimated that the number of binding sites calculated by Scatchard analysis was 10%−15% higher than the values calculated at one fixed concentration of ^{3}H-estradiol.

5. *The type of ^{3}H-estradiol used.* In a recent study in our laboratory ER binding was measured simultaneously with ^{3}H-estradiol supplied both by Amersham and by New England Nuclear. The number of receptor binding sites obtained with both batches of ^{3}H-estradiol correlated very well ($r = 0.99$, Fig. 2). However, the receptor values observed with the NEN tracer were consistently 20% lower than the values found with the Amersham tracer. K_d values and nonspecific binding were similar for both tracers. The observed differences may occur because of small errors in the values of the specific activities given by the suppliers and/or impurities (labeled or unlabeled) of the tracers.

6. *The type of protein assay, if results are expressed as fmol/mg protein.*

Discussion

The existence of large interlaboratory variations in estradiol receptor assays is now well acknowledged [8]. In the trial described here, CVs of 34% and 37% were obtained for the lyophilized reference cytosols prepared form calf uterus and rat mammary tumors, respectively. The use of lyophilized control cytosol allowed the expression of the results as fmol/ml cytosol, thereby eliminating variations in protein results. This resulted in lower CVs than had previously been reported for lyophilized reference tissues [5]. It may be noted that most participants obtained values that agreed reasonably well, whereas a few laboratories reported values consistently lower than the mean. As an example, if the two lowest ER and PgR values reported on the various reference samples are omitted, the CVs decrease to 20%−23%. There were several possible methodological sources for the observed variations, which may be related to the various dextran-coated charcoal techniques employed by the participants. Generally more than one unfavorable methodological factor was applied simultaneously by the various investigators (Table 5). Therefore the influence of separate factors could not be established. In future trials evaluation of these methodological differences and standardization are imperative in order to establish optimum assay conditions. For the forthcoming trials consensus was achieved about determination of the nonspecific binding with diethylstilbestrol. This compound was given preference over nafoxidine as a competitive inhibitor because of its much higher affinity for the estradiol receptor. In many receptor assays the use of nafoxidine resulted in overestimation of the nonspecific binding, leading to curved Scatchard plots, whereas a normal linear plot was obtained with diethylstilbestrol. Moreover Fig. 2 demonstrates that the batch of ^{3}H-estradiol may be a source of variability in estradiol receptor assays. Therefore it was decided to perform a trial in which differences in reagents will be eliminated as completely as possible. To achieve this, all groups will be supplied with the same batch of tracer, will use the same charcoal and dextran, and will determine the nonspecific binding in the presence of $10^{-6} M$ diethylstilbestrol. Furthermore, identical reagents for the protein assay will be employed and the accuracy of the counting efficiency used for the receptor calculations will be checked.

In this and previous trials it appeared that participants agreed on the ER positivity of lyophilized reference samples with high receptor values [5]. Reference samples with low receptor values are, however, frequently misclassified as ER negative. In this study four out of 15 groups (27%) misclassified reference cytosol B as ER negative. Raam et al. [7] reported for the Eastern Cooperative Oncology Group (ECOG) that 29% of the assays of a low content tissue powder were reported as ER negative when 3 fmol/mg protein was accepted as the cut-off value for positivity or 42% when 10 fmol/mg protein was accepted as a positive value. King [4] also concluded that disagreement in receptor status was predominantly confined to samples with low ER content. Comparison of the raw data in our study revealed that at least some of the disagreements in receptor status were due to different cut-off values being applied by those laboratories that performed a single-point assay, and to varying interpretations of the obtained Scatchard plots. For example, one laboratory performing a single point assay reported a receptor value of 120 fmol/ml cytosol or 14 fmol/mg protein obtained on sample B as receptor negative on the basis of a receptor positivity cut-off value of 27 fmol/mg protein. On the other hand, another laboratory reported a value of 35 fmol/ml cytosol or 6 fmol/mg protein as receptor positive. This laboratory calculates the receptor content at one fixed concentration of the ^{3}H-estradiol and, in addition, constructs a Scatchard plot as an additional criterium to classify tumor samples as receptor positive or negative. The influence of the interpretation of Scatchard plots is illustrated by the next example. A Scatchard plot indicating a receptor value of 315 fmol/ml cytosol or 49 fmol/mg protein with a K_d value of 1.8×10^{-9} M (sample B; six concentrations of ^{3}H-estradiol; $r = 0.73$) was regarded as receptor negative, whereas a Scatchard plot showing a value of 60 fmol/ml cytosol or 21 fmol/mg protein with a K_d value of 2.6×10^{-9} M (sample C; six concentrations; $r = -0.52$) was reported as ER positive. Uniformity in the analysis and interpretation of raw data is therefore highly desirable in order to avoid unnecessary disagreements on receptor status.

In the ECOG trial, Raam et al. [7] concluded that determination of the cytosol protein content by a single control laboratory fails to reduce the interlaboratory variation in receptor values. In that study the ratio of protein values obtained by each participant to that measured by the reference laboratory varied from 0.79 to 1.35. Previously, we reported that protein values can differ as much as sixfold from one laboratory to another [5]. Standardization of the protein assay and the protein standard reduced the variation between the laboratories. Nevertheless the range of values observed (a two- to threefold difference between the highest and lowest value) was still unacceptably wide. Future trials will evaluate the question of whether additional standardization will further reduce the variation in protein values.

References

1. Benraad T, Koenders A (1980) Estradiol receptor activity in lyophilized calf uterus and human breast tumor tissue. Cancer 46: 2762–2764
2. Bradford MM (1976) A rapid and sensitive method for the quantitation of microgram quantities of protein utilizing the principle of protein dye-binding. Anal Biochem 72: 248–254
3. Clark JH, Peck EJ (1977) Steroid hormone receptors: basic principles and measurement. In: O'Malley BW (ed) Receptors and hormone action. Academic, London, pp 383–410
4. King RJB (1980) Quality control of estradiol receptor analysis: The United Kingdom experience. Cancer 12: 2822–2824
5. Koenders A, Geurts-Moespot J, Hendriks T, Benraad T (1981) The Netherlands inter-laboratory quality control program of steroid receptor assays in breast cancer. In: Sarfaty GA, Nash AR, Keightley DD (eds) Estrogen receptor assays in breast cancer. Laboratory discrepancies and quality assurance. Masson 69–82

6. Koenders A, Benraad T (1981) Preparation of lyophilized reference samples for quality control of steroid receptor measurements. Ligand Rev 3 (4): 32–39
7. Raam S, Gelman R, Cohen JL (1981) Estrogen receptor assay: Interlaboratory and intralaboratory variations in the measurement of receptors using dextran-coated charcoal technique: A study sponsored by ECOG. Eur J Cancer 17: 643–649
8. Sarfaty GA, Nash AR, Keightley DD (eds) (1981) Estrogen receptor assays in breast cancer. Laboratory discrepancies and quality assurance. Masson, New York

Participating Institutions

Hospital "de Lichtenberg", Amersfoort
Antoni van Leeuwenhoek Hospital, Amsterdam
Foundation Medical Laboratories, Breda
Foundation of Cooperative Hospitals Delft (SSDZ), Delft
Catharina Hospital, Eindhoven
Hospital "de Stadsmaten" and "Ziekenzorg", Enschede
Academic Hospital, Groningen
"De Wever" Hospital, Heerlen
Laboratory of Public Health, Leeuwarden
Department of Pathological Chemistry, Academic Hospital, Leiden
Department of Experimental and Chemical Endocrinology, St. Radboud Hospital Nijmegen
Scientific Development Group, Organon International B.V., Oss
Department of Biochemistry II, Erasmus University, Rotterdam, Rotterdam
Rotterdam Radio-Therapeutic Institute, Dr. Daniel den Hoed Clinic, Rotterdam
Institute of Oncology, Dr. Bernard Verbeeten, Tilburg
Department of Endocrinology, Academic Hospital, Utrecht
Laboratory for Nuclear Medicine, "Voorburg", Vught
Sophia Hospital, Zwolle

Quality Control of Clinical Steroid Receptor Assays in Sweden

J. F. Sällström and K. Björkqvist

Department of Pathology, University of Uppsala, Sjukhusvägen 10, 751 85 Uppsala, Sweden

Introduction

In Sweden two to three thousand estrogen (ER) and progesterone receptor (PgR) determinations on primary and metastatic breast cancer are performed every year. At present there are six laboratories in regional or university hospitals receiving samples for analysis, but their service does not yet cover the whole country. However, further laboratories are to start steroid receptor analysis in the near future.

Approximately twice yearly, representatives from the above-mentioned six centers and from the Radiumhospitalet in Oslo, Norway, meet in an effort to coordinate steroid receptor determinations. The meetings are organized by the "Coordinating Group for Clinical Steroid Receptor Research", which is sponsored by the Swedish Cancer Society.

Standardization

The coordinating group has issued the following recommendations: Adequate tumor samples for the biochemical analyses should be selected, preferably by a pathologist, adjacent to the samples taken for histopathology. The isoelectric focusing method described by Wrange et al. [4] is uniformly used for ER assay. Furthermore, the analogous method for PgR determination [6] is being used or is under evaluation. It has also been agreed that the receptor content of the sample should be related to the DNA content of the tumor sample as determined by Burton's method [1]. An internal standard should be included in each isoelectric focusing assay, e.g., a pool of homogenized calf uterus. Standard schemes for the mentioned methods have been distributed.

Quality Control

Twice yearly frozen quality control samples are distributed to the various laboratories. These include tissue samples for ER and PgR analyses and DNA standards. We distribute coursely ground tissue that needs homogenization in an effort to include this critical procedure in the comparison.

Results and Discussion

As is evident from Tables 1 and 2, the results show a marked variation between the laboratories. The intra-assay variation is known to be less than 10% (Wrange et al. [5] demonstrated 4.6% intra-assay variation). Repeated analyses of internal standards show that the interassay variation is in the order of 10%−30%. It is apparent that the variation between the laboratories is much higher, sometimes more than 50%, making further standardization desirable. However, this interlaboratory variation should be correlated to the more than three orders of magnitude of difference in receptor content between tumors that can be detected with the isoelectric focusing procedure. If the material is arbitrarily grouped in negative, weakly positive (< 0.1), positive (0.1−1), and strongly positive (> 1 nmol receptor/g DNA) tumors, there is a good correlation between the analyses in the different laboratories.

Table 1. ER values (nmol/g DNA) of 10 control samples analyzed by different laboratories. Both tissue samples and their corresponding cytosol preparations were distributed. *CV*, coefficient of variation

Control sample	Number of testing laboratories	Tissue sample				Corresponding cytosol			
		Lowest value	Mean value	Highest value	CV (%)	Lowest value	Mean value	Highest value	CV (%)
1	4	1.1	2.5	3.2	33	0.7	2.6	4.0	46
2	3	1.7	1.7	1.8	3	1.2	2.8	4.9	47
3	5	1.2	1.9	3.3	41	0.3	2.0	3.0	51
4	5	0.3	0.5	1.3	8	0.1	0.7	0.9	5
5	4	< 0.1	< 0.1	< 0.1		0	< 0.1	< 0.1	
6	5	0	0	0		0	< 0.1	0.1	
7	5	0	< 0.1	< 0.1		0	0	0	
8	5	0	< 0.1	< 0.1		< 0.1	< 0.1	< 0.1	
9	5	2.4	5.6	8.8	46	1.5	1.9	2.2	15
10	4	0.6	1.3	2.8	68	0.5	0.9	1.5	48

Table 2. DNA values (mg/g tissue) of eight control samples analyzed by different laboratories. *CV*, coefficient of variation

Control sample	Number of testing laboratories	Lowest value	Mean value	Highest value	CV (%)
1	4	1.3	1.9	2.6	27
2	3	0.1	0.2	0.2	44
3	4	1.4	1.9	2.5	21
4	3	0.1	0.2	0.3	50
5	3	2.4	3.0	4.0	24
6	2	0.2	0.2	0.2	1
7	3	1.8	2.1	2.6	16
8	2	0.1	0.1	0.1	11

By this kind of control we detected a systematic error in one laboratory. It was found that the reason for this was that the gel slices were allowed to stand overnight before scintillation fluid was added and the extraction of steroid from the gel was initiated. The Swedish data appear to compare favorably with the results of similar, larger quality control studies [2, 3].

At the meetings of the coordination group we also compare median values and statistical distribution of values obtained in different laboratories and during different time periods.

It is reasonable to expect that our control system and our uniform technology will yield receptor values for which the laboratory variation is much less than the threefold variation registered within a given mammary carcinoma [7].

References

1. Burton K (1956) A study of the conditions and mechanism of the diphenylamine reaction for the colorimetric estimation of deoxyribonucleic acid. Biochem J 62: 315−323
2. King RJB (1980) Quality control of estradiol receptor analysis: the United Kingdom Experience. Cancer 66: 2822−2824
3. Raam S, Gelman R, Cohen JL et al. (1981) Estrogen receptor assay: interlaboratory and intralaboratory variations in the measurement of receptors using dextran-coated charcoal technique: a study sponsored by E.C.O.G. Eur J Cancer 17: 643−649
4. Wrange Ö, Nordenskjöld B, Gustafsson J-Å (1978) Cytosol estradiol receptor in human mammary carcinoma: an assay based on isoelectric focusing in polyacrylamide gel. Anal Biochem 85: 461−475
5. Wrange Ö, Ramberg I, Gustafsson J-Å, Nordenskjöld B (1978) Estradiol receptor analysis in human breast cancer tissue by isoelectric focusing in polyacrylamide gel. LKB application note no. 313
6. Wrange Ö, Humla S, Ramberg I, Gustafsson SA, Skoog L, Nordenskjöld B, Gustafsson J-Å (1981) Progestin-receptor analysis in human breast cancer cytosol by isoelectric focusing in slabs of polyacrylamide gel. Steroid Biochem 14: 141−148
7. Silfverswärd C, Skoog L, Humla S, Gustafsson SA, Nordenskjöld B (1979) Intratumoral variation of cytoplasmic and nuclear estrogen receptor concentrations in human mammary carcinoma. Eur J Cancer 16: 59−65

Participating Laboratories

Sweden

Regionsjukhuset, Linköping (Dr. R. Boll)
Hospital of Lund, Lund (Dr. M. Färnö)
Karolinska Sjukhuset, Stockholm (Dr. S. Humla)
Hospital of Umeå, Umeå (Dr. S. Marklund)
Jubileumskliniken Sahlgrenska Sjukhuset, Göteborg (Dr. A. Nilsson)
University of Uppsala, Uppsala (Dr. J. F. Sällström)
Allmänna Sjukhuset, Malmö (Dr. J. Thorell)

Norway

Det Norske Radiumhospital Montebello, Oslo (Dr. O. Børmer)

Interlaboratory Variability in the Determination of Estrogen Receptor and Progesterone Receptor Content in Human Breast Tumors: Quality Control in Switzerland

D. T. Zava

Ludwig Institut für Krebsforschung, Inselspital, 3010 Bern, Switzerland

Introduction

Analysis of estrogen receptor (ER) and progesterone receptor (PgR) in breast tumor biopsies has become routine practice in many clinical laboratories, primarily for two reasons: first, to help the clinician select the most effective therapy for patients with breast cancer, and, second, to compare the hormone receptor status of patients' tumors with other disease-related parameters. For such retrospective comparisons within large study groups contributing data to common trials to be meaningful, it is essential that the interlaboratory differences in receptor data gathering be reduced to a minimum. Quality control studies are therefore necessary to recognize and eliminate the differences in interlaboratory methodology in order to be able to statistically compare with confidence the hormone receptor data with other disease parameters.

This report details a quality control study which was designed to help identify factors which might contribute to the interlaboratory variations in ER and PgR assay results among six Swiss laboratories (SAKK Study Group) contributing hormone receptor data to common breast cancer trials.

Materials and Methods

Preparation and Distribution of Frozen Tumor Powders

Breast tumors for this study were derived from the residual portion of frozen ($-70°$ C) biopsies which had been previously assayed for ER and PgR. Frozen tissues were pooled from three categories of ER and PgR binding profiles: those tumors containing (a) less than 10, (b) 20–50, and (c) greater than 50 fmol ER and/or PgR/mg cytosol protein; these frozen tissue samples will be referred to as samples A, B, and C. The frozen powders of each category were coded and then dispatched on solid CO_2 to each of five participating laboratories.

Processing of Powders by Participants

The participants were requested to process the tumor powders within 2 weeks of receipt as follows:

Recent Results in Cancer Research. Vol. 91

1. Store the tissue at $-70°$ C until the assay.
2. Process 1 g of each sample by the methods normally used in the laboratory concerned.
3. Return to the reference laboratory 0.5 g of the original powder (on solid CO_2) from each of the three coded samples.
4. Assay half of the cytosol prepared from the 1 g of each powder (see above) and then snap-freeze (liquid nitrogen) the remaining half and return it to the reference laboratory with the 0.5 g of residual tumor powder (see 3 above).

Specific details of the assay methods and all raw results (calculations etc.) were to be returned to the reference laboratory.

Standard ER and PgR Assay Procedures Used by the Reference Laboratory and Other Participants

One gram of frozen pulverized tissue was homogenized in 3 ml of Tris buffer (0.01 M Tris: HCl, pH 7.4 at 4° C, 0.0015 M EDTA, 10% glycerol, 0.001 M monothioglycerol). Cytosol resulting from the high-speed (100,000 g) centrifugation of crude homogenate was diluted to 10 ml with Tris buffer. The protein concentration of diluted cytosols was determined by the method of Lowry et al. [2] with BSA as a standard protein.

The concentrations of ER and PgR in the diluted cytosols were assessed from the dextran-coated charcoal (DCC)-resistant radioactivity resulting from the incubation of 100 µl cytosol (in duplicate) with 100 µl of five doses of ^{3}H-estradiol (0.4–6 nM) or ^{3}H-promegestone (1–10 nM) with and without a 100-fold excess of diethylstilbestrol (DES) or R-5020, respectively.

After incubation at 4° C for 3 h, a 500-µl suspension of DCC (2.5 mg Norit A activated charcoal, 25 mg dextran in 1 ml Tris buffer, pH 8.0, 4° C) was added to each tube. After 30 min of constant agitation, the charcoal was sedimented by centrifugation at 4° C for 5 min at 2,000 rpm. The supernatant was combined with 3 ml of Beckman Ready-Solv scintillation fluid and radioactivity was determined in a Beckman Model LS8100 liquid scintillation counter with a counting efficiency of about 38%. The ER and PgR data were analyzed by the method of Scatchard [1] to determine the dissociation constant (K_d) and concentration of ER and PgR of each tumor powder. Data were expressed as femtomoles receptor per milligram of cytosol protein.

The distinguishing features of the methods used by each of the five participants (I–V) relative to the reference laboratory are illustrated in Table 1.

Interlaboratory Variations in Data Analysis

To check for interlaboratory differences in methods of calculating the raw ER and PgR binding data, each of the participants was presented a questionnaire listing the unprocessed binding data for a five-dose Scatchard analysis. Included was other pertinent information (assay volume, volume of DCC added, volume counted, protein concentration, efficiency of scintillation counter, specific activity of radiolabeled ligands used) necessary to make the appropriate calculations. Each laboratory was requested to calculate by their routine methods the following information: (a) the concentrations of ER and PgR in fmol/mg cytosol protein and (b) the binding constant (K_d) for each sample. Any comments concerning the binding plots (Scatchard analysis) were to be recorded on the questionnaire to help clarify discrepancies in results.

Table 1. Methods used by participants

| Center | Ligands (dose)[a] | Protein assay[b] | Cyt. vol. (ml) | Protein (mg/ml)[c] | | | Inc. vol.[d] (ml) | Inc. time[e] (ER/PgR) | DCC (ml)[f] (Time ER/PgR) |
				A	B	C			
Ref. lab.	E + DES (0.2–3 nM) R 5,020 ± R 5,020 (0.4–6 nM)	Lowry	0.1	RL) 1.5 RL) 1.5	1.6 1.7	1.3 1.3	0.2	3 h	0.5 (30/30)
I	E + DES (0.13–2 nM) R 5,020 ± Pg (0.5–8 nM)	Biorad	0.1	I) 1.2 RL) 2.7	1.9 –	2.1 3.0	0.1	Overnight	0.2 (10/10)
II	E + DES (0.1–2 nM) R 5,020 ± Pg (0.5–8 nM)	Lowry	0.1	II) 2.0 RL) 3.1	2.0 2.5	2.0 2.7	0.1	4 h	0.2 (15/15)
III	E + DES (0.13–2 nM) R 5,020 ± Pg (0.5–8 nM)	Lowry	0.1	III) 2.0 RL) 1.9	2.0 1.9	2.0 2.0	0.1	4 h	0.2 (30/30)
IV	E + DES (0.05–1 nM) R 5,020 ± R 5,020 (0.6–5 nM)	Lowry	0.1	IV) 2.0 RL) 1.7	2.0 1.6	2.0 1.6	0.2	22/4 h	1 (30/30)
V	E + E (0.15–3 nM) R 5,020 ± R 5,020 (0.15–3 nM)	Turbid- imetry	0.1	V) 2.2 RL) 2.7	1.9 2.4	1.8 2.7	0.2	Overnight	0.25 (30/30)

Ref. lab., Ludwig Institute for Cancer Research, Inselspital, Bern; *I*, Dept. of Gynecology and Research, Basel; *II*, Dept. of Medicine, Zürich; *III*, Ticino Institute of Pathology, Locarno; *IV*, Dept. of Medicine, Lausanne; *V*, Center for Oncology-Hematology, Geneva

[a] Final concentration of ligand

[b] BSA was used as a standard protein in all laboratories

[c] Final diluted concentration of protein added to incubation assayed by participant and subsequently by reference laboratory (RL)

[d] Total incubation volume

[e] Incubation time at 0°–4° C

[f] Volume of DCC suspension (concentration as indicated in text) added to incubation tubes, and time of exposure

Results

Intralaboratory Variability in ER and PgR Assays

The results of Table 2 reveal that the low, medium, and high concentrations of tumor ER, but not of PgR, could be clearly distinguished whether the tissue remained in the reference laboratory (category 1), was returned to the reference laboratory by the participants in the same frozen powder originally delivered to them (category 2), or was returned to the reference laboratory in the form of cytosol prepared from the frozen powder by the participants (category 3). The results of these three categories negate any possibility that ER was destroyed in the frozen powders during transport or that differences in receptor concentration were attributable to the methods used for preparing cytosols (i.e., buffer, homogenization, centrifugation techniques, etc.). It is apparent from Table 2 that during transport the PgR content of tumors was subject to greater loss than was the ER content, especially in the form of frozen cytosols (category 3).

Interlaboratory Variability in ER and PgR Assays

Although there was little intralaboratory variation in the ER and PgR content of tumor powders measured in the reference laboratory five consecutive times over a 1-month period (category 1), the interlaboratory concordance (category 1 vs category 4) was not as uniform. Quantitatively the mean values of ER and PgR were either in close agreement with (participants III and IV) or higher than (participants I, II, and V) those reported by the reference laboratory. Although there was not a definite consensus among the

Table 2

Category	Assay laboratory	Estrogen receptor[a] sample			Progesterone receptor[a] sample		
		A	B	C	A	B	C
1	Ref. lab.[b]	6 ± 5	39 ± 12	115 ± 17	2 ± 2	94 ± 37	253 ± 62
2	Ref. lab.[b, c]	6 ± 3	36 ± 5	110 ± 32	2 ± 3	78 ± 35	205 ± 170
3	Ref. lab.[b, d]	6 ± 3	32 ± 8	105 ± 37	0	41 ± 22	92 ± 31
4	Part. I	4/2[e]	115/−	281/196	41/31	134/−	168/119
	Part. II	3/2	64/51	295/218	7/5	118/94	365/263
	Part. III	5/5	26/26	75/75	5/5	75/75	227/227
	Part. IV	5/6	25/31	105/131	0/0	76/95	109/136
	Part. V	26/21	85/67	326/218	0/0	61/48	100/67
	Mean ± SD[f]	9 ± 9/	63 ± 35/	216 ± 105/	11 ± 15	93 ± 28/	192 ± 93/
	Mean ± SD[e]	7 ± 7	44 ± 16[g]	167 ± 56	8 ± 12	78 ± 19[f]	162 ± 72

[a] fmol/mg cytosol protein
[b] Mean values ± standard deviation for five assays (category 1, Table 2)
[c] Tumor powders returned by participants and then assayed by reference laboratory
[d] Tumor cytosols returned by participants and then assayed by reference laboratory
[e] Second value indicates that receptor content is readjusted according to cytosol prepared by participant, but assayed for protein by the reference laboratory
[f] Mean values ± standard deviation for participants, excluding Ref. lab.
[g] Participant I not included in calculations for mean values

laboratories about the quantitative content of ER and PgR in the tumor powders, all groups (exceptions: participant I, PgR sample A, and participant V, ER sample A) were generally able to qualify each tumor as containing low-, medium-, or high-range ER and PgR, even though some overlap in medium- and high-range binding did exist. Most important was that no laboratories reported either false-positive ER or PgR values using the Scatchard plot and a cut-off value of 10 fmol/mg cytosol protein for definition of negative receptor status. There were no significant group differences in the binding constants (K_ds) reported, indicating that the ER and PgR binding sites were of high affinity and limited capacity.

Standardization of ER and PgR Values According to the Cytosol Protein Assayed in the Reference Laboratory

When the cytosols were prepared and analyzed for protein content in the reference laboratory, the results (Table 1) revealed an obvious discrepancy in the protein values of laboratories I, II, and V relative to the reference laboratory, thus accounting, in part, for the higher receptor values reported by these groups. The ER and PgR contents of each tumor based on the readjusted protein values are illustrated in Table 2.

Interlaboratory Variations in Methods for Processing Data

Differences in tumor ER and PgR concentrations could not be attributed to differences in the methods for processing the binding data since each of the participating institutions which calculated receptor binding sites and binding constants from unprocessed data were in close agreement (data not shown), with the exception of one sample. The discrepancies arising from this sample were due to the difficulty in evaluating the Scatchard plot. These results ruled out the possibility that the interlaboratory differences in receptor content reported by the various participants were due to the methods of data processing.

Discussion

The objectives of this study were to determine whether the Swiss laboratories which routinely assay steroid hormone receptor in breast tumor biopsies could accurately identify homogeneous frozen breast tumor samples containing low, medium, and high concentrations of ER and PgR and, if not, for what reasons.

It is clear that the differences in ER and PgR values reported by the participants in this study cannot be attributed to decay of receptor during transport, to the methods of cytosol preparation, or to differences in data processing. The results do indicate, however, that the source of error leading to the quantitative discrepancies in the ER and PgR binding sites among the participating laboratories are a consequence of differences in the methods for quantitating the cytosol protein content and in the incubation conditions employed for the assay system. When the ER and PgR binding values were readjusted relative to the protein concentration determined by the reference laboratory, the interlaboratory variation was significantly reduced but not eliminated entirely, revealing that the incubation conditions were primarily responsible for the quantitative discrepancies among the participating groups. The only apparent differences in methodology of the laboratories (I, II, and IV) that reported the higher receptor values were a longer incubation period (overnight for participants I and V, as opposed to only 3−4 h for other laboratories) and a shorter exposure time to DCC (10−15 min for participants I and II relative to 30 min for the other participants).

Other quality control studies carried out among national and international breast cancer trial groups [3−6] have revealed that interlaboratory variations in the concentrations of ER in frozen calf uterus do exist. These studies, however, failed to identify the reasons for the discrepancies in receptor binding sites. This study is in accord with other reports but in addition elucidates at least some of the reasons for the interlaboratory variabilities in the measurement of not only ER but also of PgR in *human* breast tissue.

In view of this study and the quality control reports of other cooperative groups [3−6], it is clear that the interlaboratory differences in the quantitation of steroid hormone receptors will probably persist among laboratories which participate in common trials. To expect such laboratories to reproduce ER and PgR binding data with strict conformity may be unreasonable. However, it should be possible to reduce significantly the interlaboratory variability in receptor results by standardizing the methods of protein analysis and the methods of incubation with radiolabeled ligands. This should permit groups participating in common trials to qualify tumor ER or PgR content into the categories of low, medium, or high binding.

Although the present report focused primarily on the technical problems of the assay methods which are potential causes of interlaboratory variations in the ER and PgR binding values, it should be recognized that other factors may dwarf these assay problems. For example, the steroid hormone receptors in some tumor specimens may rapidly degrade before the tumors reach the steroid hormone receptor laboratory if proper cooling procedures are not practiced. In addition, assay of a section of tumor not representative of the tumor bulk may lead to erroneous receptor results. Both factors may significantly influence the final concentration of tumor receptor reported by the hormone receptor laboratory and should be recognized as contributing factors to the variability of steroid hormone receptor content in breast tumors.

References

1. Scatchard G (1951) The attraction of proteins for small molecules and ions. Ann NY Acad Sci 51: 660−672
2. Lowry DH, Rosenbrough WJ, Farr AL, Randall PJ (1961) Protein measurement with the folin phenol reagent. J Biol Chem 193: 265−275
3. Jordan VC, Zava DT, Eppenberger U, Kiser A, Sebek S, Dowdle, E, Krozowski Z, Bennett RC, Funder J, Holdaway IM, Wittliff JL (1983) Reliability of steroid hormone receptor assays: an international study. Eur J Cancer Clin Oncol 19: 357−363
4. Raam S, Gelman R, Cohen JL, Bachrach A, Fishchinger AJ, Jacobson HI, Keshgegian AA, Konopka SJ, Wittliff JL (1981) Estrogen receptor assay: interlaboratory and intralaboratory variations in the measurement of receptors using dextran-coated charcoal technique: a study sponsored by ECOG Eur J Cancer 17: 643−649
5. King RJB (1980) Quality control of estradiol receptor analysis: the United Kingdom experience. Cancer 46: 2822−2824
6. Zava DT, Wyler-von Ballmoos A, Goldhirsch A, Roos W, Takahashi A, Eppenberger U, Arrenbrecht S, Martz G, Losa G, Gomez F, Guelpa C (1983) A quality control study to assess the interlaboratory variability of routine estrogen and progesterone receptor assays. Eur J Cancer Oncol 18: 713−721

Participating Institutions

Ludwig Institute for Cancer Research, Bern (Dr. D. T. Zava)
Department of Gynecology and Research, University Women's Clinic, Basel (Dr. U. Eppenberger)
Department of Medicine, Universitätsspital, Zürich (Dr. S. Arrenbrecht)
Ticino Institute of Pathology, Locarno (Dr. G. Losa)
Department of Medicine, C.H.U.V., Lausanne (Drs. Lemarchand-Bertrand and F. Gomez)
Center for Oncology-Hematology, Geneva (Dr. G. Rosset)

Standardization of Steroid Receptor Analysis in Breast Cancer Biopsies: EORTC Receptor Group

A. Koenders and T. J. Benraad*

Department of Experimental and Chemical Endocrinology, Medical Faculty, University of Nijmegen, 6500 HB-Nijmegen, The Netherlands

Introduction

In 1972 several members of the EORTC Breast Cancer Cooperative Group agreed on the potential value of estrogen receptor (ER) determinations in human mammary carcinoma for therapeutic guidance [3]. During that workshop standards for the assessment of these assays were proposed. The charcoal adsorption technique was recommended as a first standard procedure, and the receptor concentration was to be calculated according to Scatchard. In 1978 the EORTC Breast Cancer Cooperative Group decided that the ER content of the tumor would determine the entry of breast cancer patients into some of the future clinical trials. To achieve adequate and uniform methodology of the ER assay, a workshop was held in 1979 [4]. The purpose of this workshop was to discuss practical aspects of techniques of measuring ER and moreover to decide upon a single standardized receptor assay. Some of the most important steps agreed upon with regard to the receptor binding assay can be summarized as follows:

1. The composition of the extraction buffer (10 mM HPO$_4$/H$_2$PO$_4$, 1.5 mM EDTA, 3 mM NaN$_3$, 10 mM monothioglycerol, 10% v/v glycerol; pH 7.5).
2. High-speed centrifugation, resulting in particle-free extracts, is preferred over low-speed centrifugation.
3. The cytosol protein concentration should not be less than 1 mg/ml.
4. The minimal purity of the radioactive ligands should be 95%.
5. The recommended ligands for the ER determination are estradiol and moxestrol, while R-5020 or Org-2058 should preferentially be used for the progesterone receptor (PgR) assay.
6. The nonspecific binding is to be determined in the presence of a 100-fold excess of unlabeled diethylstilbestrol for the ER assay and R-5020 or Org-2058 for the PgR assay.
7. The charcoal adsorption technique combined with Scatchard analysis was to be retained as the standard procedure.
8. The receptor concentration is expressed as fmol/mg protein. Protein is measured according to Bradford [2], using Kabi human albumin as a protein standard. The Coomassie-blue reagent is obtained from Bio-Rad.

---

* The authors thank Gail Janes for reviewing the manuscript

Finally, the participants agreed on the establishment of a quality control system. Because of their thermostability, lyophilized samples were to be used as reference preparations. The present report summarizes the results of the first three quality control trials organized in 1979 and 1980.

Analysis of Lyophilized Reference Preparations

Trial 1. Lyophilized calf uterine tissue powder was used in the first round (Table 1). In order to evaluate the homogeneity of the tissue powder, each laboratory received seven identical vials. Almost all participants analysed these seven vials in one assay, making calculation of the intra-assay variation possible. It was recommended that they add 1.2 ml buffer per 10 mg of lyophilized tissue powder. Tissue powder and buffer were mixed by repeated (10 times) aspiration and discharge through a pasteur pipette, followed by centrifugation. The results were expressed as fmol/mg protein.

Trial 2. Lyophilized tissue powders were prepared from calf and bovine uterine tissue as described previously [1, 5]. From each reference preparation the participating laboratories obtained two identical vials. In this trial 10 mg tissue powder was added to 1.0 ml buffer and the powder was again drawn back and forth into a pasteur pipette to allow thorough mixing. Again the results were standardized against the protein content of the cytosol.

Trial 3. To avoid both interlaboratory differences in the preparation of cytosols from tissue powders and also variations in protein results, lyophilized cytosols were prepared (Table 1). The lyophilized cytosols contained very different receptor levels (negative, low, medium, and high) and each participant performed a single determination on each sample. The laboratories received the following instructions for the preparation of cytosols: remove caps very carefully to release vacuum. Place the opened vials on ice and introduce into each vial exactly 5.0 ml of ice cold $(0°-4° C)$ water containing 10% (v/v) glycerol. The contents of the vials will dissolve completely when left on ice for $10-15$ min with regular swirling. Analyze the reconstituted cytosols without delay and without centrifugation. Report your results as fmol/ml cytosol.

Table 1. Lyophilized reference preparations analyzed in 1979 and 1980

Sample no.	Type of tissue	Identical vials analyzed	Trial no.
1	Lyophilized calf uterine tissue	7	1: May 1979
2	Lyophilized calf uterine tissue	2	2: Jan 1980
3	Lyophilized bovine uterine tissue	2	2: Jan 1980
4	Lyophilized pig uterine cytosol	1	3: July 1980
5	Lyophilized benign human breast tumor cytosol	1	3: July 1980
6	Lyophilized calf uterine cytosol	1	3: July 1980
7	Lyophilized bovine uterine cytosol diluted with receptor-negative human breast tumor cytosol	1	3: July 1980

Results, Conclusions, and Comments

The lyophilized reference samples were mailed to the participating laboratories without any precautions regarding temperature control. On arrival, the vials were stored at $0°-4°$ C until assay. As a control for shipping conditions several vials were placed at ambient temperature for at least 3 days and subsequently stored in the refrigerator ($0°-4°$ C). At various time intervals during the analysis period employed by the participating laboratories, these vials were assayed to check the stability of the receptor binding sites. The results of a typical experiment (trial 2; reference preparations 2 and 3) are collected in Fig. 1. ER and PgR levels appeared to be stable during the entire investigation period of 35 days. In addition these reference preparations were kept at room temperature for a period of 2 weeks. During this time five sequential assays were performed (days 2, 5, 8, 11, and 14). The values observed at this temperature were similar to the values observed at $4°$ C: i.e., sample 2: ER 442 ± 10 and PgR 632 ± 36; sample 3: ER 62 ± 4 and PgR 295 ± 8 fmol/mg protein.

The ER, PgR, and protein results of the seven different lyophilized reference preparations analyzed are summarized in Tables 2-4. With regard to the results of these first three trials the following comments can be made: Agreement between laboratories was excellent on the receptor status of lyophilized reference samples having high receptor values. Only 1 of 87 receptor assays performed on samples with a mean value above 50 fmol/mg protein was reported as receptor negative (one negative PgR result on sample 7). The number of false-negative or false-positive assessments of receptor status on samples with low values or on receptor-negative samples was also small. That is, 3 of 22 ER assays (14%) performed on samples 4 (43 ± 20 fmol/mg protein) and 7 (41 ± 18 fmol/mg protein) were reported as receptor negative, while one laboratory classified sample 5 as receptor positive.

For all reference samples, large interlaboratory variations in ER as well as PgR values were noted. These observed differences in receptor results may be related to the following sources of variability:

1. *Heterogeneity of the tissue powders employed in trials 1 and 2.* This possible source of variability was studied in trial 1 by analysing seven identical vials in one assay. The intra-assay coefficients of variation of the ER assay, which ranged between 2.5% and 10.5%, indicated that the various vials contained identical lyophilized tissue powders.

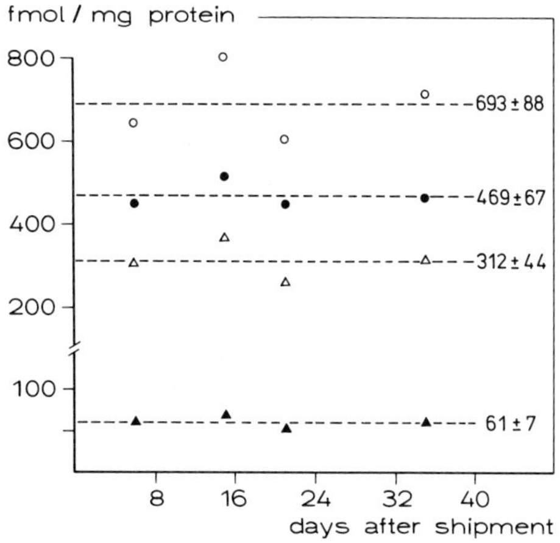

Fig. 1. Stability of steroid receptor activity on lyophilized calf uterine tissue (ER ●; PgR ○) and lyophilized bovine uterine tissue (ER ▲; PgR △) analyzed during trial 2. After shipment, samples were placed at room temperature for 3 days and subsequently stored at $4°$ C

Table 2. Summary of ER results

	Sample no.						
	1[a]	2[a]	3[a]	4[b]	5[b]	6[b]	7[b]
Participants	10	8	8	11	11	11	11
Range	114−537[c]	88−525	12−90	Negativ−226	Negativ−39	272−1,891	Negativ−104
Mean	364	379	51	131 (10)[d]	39 (1)[d]	1,289	80 (9)[d]
SD	155	171	23	49	−	489	21
CV[e]	43%	45%	45%	38%	−	38%	26%

[a] Expressed as fmol/mg protein
[b] Expressed as fmol/ml cytosol
[c] One laboratory omitted
[d] Number of positive results i.e., negative classifications omitted
[e] Interlaboratory coefficient of variation

Table 3. Summary of PgR results

	Sample no.						
	1[a]	2[a]	3[a]	4[b]	5[b]	6[b]	7[b]
Participants	6	7	7	10	10	10	10
Range	183−1,210	123−730	49−376	68−882	Negativ−51	545−4,007	Negativ−385
Mean	642	451	224	474	51 (1)[c]	2,335	167 (9)[c]
SD	288	220	120	297	−	1,224	122
CV	45%	49%	53%	63%	−	52%	73%

[a] Expressed as fmol/mg protein
[b] Expressed as fmol/ml cytosol
[c] Number of positive results i.e., negative classifications omitted

Table 4. Summary of protein results[a]

	Sample no.						
	1	2	3	4	5	6	7
Participants	7[b]	7[b]	7[b]	11	11	11	
Range	1.7−3.6[c]	1.1−6.4	1.2−5.3	2.3−4.0	2.4−5.2	2.3−4.15	1.6−3.8
Mean	2.22	2.89	2.56	3.20	3.16	3.14	2.14
SD	0.29	1.55	1.33	0.48	0.79	0.61	0.66
CV	13%	54%	52%	15%	25%	19%	31%

[a] All results are expressed as mg protein/ml cytosol
[b] Protein values were included only if the recommended ratio of tissue weight: buffer volume was used
[c] One laboratory which reported protein values between 11.1 and 18.7 mg cytosol was omitted

2. *Differences in receptor extraction during the preparation of the cytosol.* Wagner and Jungblut [7] have studied the influence of the homogenization procedure and the presence of dithiothreitol in the extraction buffer and concluded that standardization of the receptor extraction is at least as important as standardization of the receptor assay itself. However, these two factors probably do not play an important role in this study because the composition of the extraction buffer used by the participants in trials 1 and 2 was identical, whereas in trial 3 the lyophilized reference cytosols were reconstituted with distilled water containing 10% glycerol. Rather, the fact that not all participants employed the recommended procedure for the preparation of the tissue homogenate (trials 1 and 2) and furthermore applied various centrifugation speeds and times may have contributed to the variations in receptor results, expressed on a protein basis.

3. *Methodological factors related to the dextran-coated charcoal techniques used by the participating groups.* By means of a questionnaire, detailed information as to the exact methodologies of the various participants was obtained. Differences were noted in (a) the ratio of cytosol to the incubation volume and/or the total volume during charcoal treatment; (b) determination of the nonspecific binding; (c) the type of radioactive ligand used, e.g., ^{3}H-R-5020, ^{3}H-Org-2058, or ^{3}H-progesterone; (d) the composition and volume of the dextran-coated charcoal suspension added; (e) the contact time with the charcoal suspension (10−90 min); and (f) the calculation of receptor-binding sites from a single-point assay or by means of Scatchard analysis.

In a similar quality control program organized in The Netherlands by our department, several unfavorable methodological factors, which may be partly responsible for low receptor results, were recognized (see chapter entitled "Quality Control of Steroid Receptor Assay in The Netherlands"). These methodological factors may cause laboratories to report receptor values consistently higher or lower than the mean value calculated from the results of all participants. As an example, the receptor values of the control samples 2 and 3, which were assayed in one run, are compared in Fig. 2. It should be noted that the rank order of the receptor values of the various laboratories

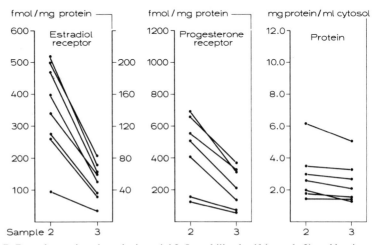

Fig. 2. Variation in ER, PgR, and protein values during trial 2. Lyophilized calf (sample 2) and bovine uterine tissue samples (samples 3) were analyzed in one assay. Drawn lines join values obtained by the various laboratories on samples 2 and 3

was similar for both samples 2 and 3. Although the receptor results were sometimes obscured by variations in protein values (trials 1 and 2), the same trend was noted when receptor results obtained by the various laboratories in all three trials were compared. Therefore the calculation of an adjustment factor for each laboratory, as suggested by Raam et al. [6], certainly will reduce the variations in assay results. According to this procedure, an arbitrary value of 100% was assigned to the individual ER values obtained for sample 2 by the participating laboratories. Adjusted to this percentage, the receptor values of sample 3 ranged between 12.9% and 17.7% of the values reported for sample 2, while the coefficient of variation decreased from 45% (Table 2) to 14%.

4. *Variations in protein results, if receptor levels are divided by mg protein.* The protein results summarized in Table 4 show that for the various control samples, the protein values differed 1.6- (sample 4) to 5.8-fold (sample 2) from one laboratory to another. Even with the elimination of differences in cytosol preparation, a wide range of protein results was registered in trial 3 (samples 4−7). Attention is drawn to the fact that during these trials a minority of laboratories used the recommended Bradford procedure and the Bio-Rad protein standard, which may have contributed to the observed variation. Figure 2 illustrates the tendency of the various groups to measure consistently high or low protein concentrations, in comparison with the other participating institutions. However, the scatter of receptor values between laboratories was only slightly smaller if receptor levels were expressed as fmol/ml cytosol instead of fmol/mg protein, indicating that the observed variations in receptor levels, expressed per mg protein, are only partly due to the variations in protein results. Nevertheless, standardization of the protein determination is imperative for quality control of steroid receptor assays, since the ability of individual laboratories to accurately measure receptor levels in reference tissue preparations (expressed as fmol/mg protein) may be obscured by the estimated cytosolic protein concentration. It is apparent that participants may report receptor levels which are in agreement or disagreement with those of other laboratories because of a too high or too low protein value.

Agreements for the 1981 Trial

Lyophilized Uterine Cytosols. Each participant was to receive 30 vials. These vials were to be assayed on 10 consecutive working days. On each working day three vials would be analyzed.

Radioactive Ligands. ^{3}H-estradiol and ^{3}H-Org-2058 were to be used as labeled ligands. Every participant was to employ the same batch of radioactive steroid, supplied by the Max-Planck-Institut für Experimentelle Endokrinologie (Prof. Dr. P. W. Jungblut). The commercially available ^{3}H-estradiol (twin-labeled) was to be purified by the Max-Planck-Institut.

Determination of the Nonspecific Binding. 10^{-6} M diethylstilbestrol and 10^{-6} M Org-2058, added before the labeled steroids, were to be used as competitive inhibitors.

Scatchard Analysis. The following concentrations of radioactive ligands were to be employed: $1 \times$, $1.5 \times$, $2 \times$, $4 \times$, $6 \times$, and 8×10^{-9} M. Incubation was to be overnight.

Charcoal Adsorption of Free Steroid. The composition of the charcoal suspension was to be 0.25% charcoal (Norit A) and 0.025% dextran T70 prepared in the phosphate extraction buffer. Norit A had to be sieved through 25 μm nylon netting. The charcoal exposure time would be 10 min.

Protein Assay. The protein concentration was to be determined by the Bradford technique (Coomassie Brilliant Blue) using the Kabi protein standard. Both reagents were to be supplied by the Max-Planck-Institut.

References

1. Benraad T, Koenders A (1980) Estradiol receptor activity in lyophilized calf uterus and human breast tumor tissue. Cancer 46: 2762–2764
2. Bradford MM (1976) A rapid and sensitive method for the quantitation of microgram quantities of protein utilizing the principle of protein dye-binding. Anal Biochem 72: 248–254
3. EORTC Breast Cancer Cooperative Group (1973) Standards for the assessment of estrogen receptors in human breast cancer. Eur J Cancer 9: 379–381
4. EORTC Breast Cancer Cooperative Group (1980) Revision of the standards for the assessment of hormone receptors in human breast cancer. 2nd EORTC workshop, 16–17 March, 1979. Eur J Cancer 16: 1513–1515
5. Koenders AJ, Geurts-Moespot J, Kho KH, Benraad TJ (1978) Estradiol and progesterone receptor activities in stored lyophilised target tissue. J Steroid Biochem 9: 947–950
6. Raam S, Gelman R, Cohen JL (1981) Estrogen receptor assay: Interlaboratory and intralaboratory variations in the measurement of receptor using dextran-coated charcoal technique: a study sponsored by ECOG. Eur J Cancer 17: 643–649
7. Wagner RK, Jungblut PW (1980) Quality control in steroid hormone receptor analyses. Cancer 46: 2950–2952

Participating Institutions

Antoni van Leeuwenhoek Hospital, Amsterdam, The Netherlands (Dr. J. P. Persijn)
Frauenklinik der Freien Hansestadt Bremen, Bremen, FRG (Dr. W. Jonat)
Institut Jules Bordet, Brussels, Belgium (Dr. G. Leclercq)
Fibiger Laboratory, Copenhagen, Denmark (Cand. Scient. S. Thorpe/Dr. C. Rose)
Ist. Radiologia, University of Ferrara, Ferrara, Italy (Dr. D. Pelizzola/Prof. A. Piffanelli)
Max-Planck-Institut für Experimentelle Endokrinologie, Hannover, FRG (Dr. H. Hoppen/Prof. P. Jungblut)
Ist. di Ricerche Biomediche "Antoine Marxer", Ivrea, Italy (Dr. S. Fumero)
Imperial Cancer Research Fund, London, England (Dr. R. King)
Dept. of Experimental and Chemical Endocrinology, University of Nijmegen, Nijmegen, The Netherlands (Dr. A. Koenders/Prof. T. J. Benraad)
Centro Medico Oncologico, Ospedali Riuniti Di Parma, Parma, Italy (Dr. C. Bozetti/Dr. P. Mori)
Rotterdamsch Radio-Therapeutisch Institut, Rotterdam, The Netherlands (Dr. F. Teulings)

Part II: A Critical Summary

G. Leclercq

Institut Jules Bordet, Centre des Tumeurs de l'Université Libre de Bruxelles,
Service de Médicine, Clinique et Laboratoire de Cancérologie Mammaire,
Rue Héger-Bordet 1, 1000 Bruxelles, Belgium

In the past, estrogen (ER) and progesterone (PgR) receptors were mainly assayed for local clinical purposes, i.e., choice of the most suitable palliative treatment. As the need developed to introduce receptor evaluation into national or international study groups investigating new therapeutic approaches, so quality control programs were designed to test the feasibility of conducting receptor assays in the various institutions participating in cooperative studies. Pilot programs were developed both in the United States (NSABP, SECSG, and ECOG) and in Europe. In all trials, specific recommendations were given to participating laboratories for using one particular experimental procedure.

Both in the United States and in Europe, all trials demonstrated the feasibility of quality control programs based on the measurement of ER and PgR contents of frozen tissue powders and lyophilized tissues or cytosols. These materials could be dispatched by mail to the various laboratories without major loss of receptor binding capacity.

The papers of this section reveal that almost all European laboratories selected the dextran-coated charcoal (DCC) methodology for the receptor assays. Moreover, a large majority of the laboratories opted for a multipoint analysis (Scatchard plot analysis) rather than for a single dose assay. Only the Swedish laboratories used the isoelectric focusing method.

It is quite difficult to compare the results of these various papers in view of several differences in the experimental conditions and analyses of the data. Moreover, some trials refer only to ER assays while others refer to both ER and PgR assays. However, some major points emerge from the trials. They can be summarized as follows.

1. In general, there is a good agreement with regard to the presence of absence of the receptors in the samples, i.e., the number of false-positive or false-negative samples is low.

2. There are large interlaboratory variations with regard to the quantitative assessment of the receptors. This variability results from the receptor assays themselves as well as from the protein measurements. However, in most trials the rank order or the receptor values is the same among the various laboratories, so that a quite good correlation is obtained when the samples are arbitrarily grouped into main categories of "low", "medium", and "high" binding activities. This is, of course, of major clinical importance.

3. The interlaboratory variability has various causes (see papers by A. Koenders and T. Benraad). The use by all participants of a common methodology should improve the consistency. Unfortunately, complete agreement on uniform methodology appears utopian.

It is clear that further efforts must be made to standardize the receptor assays. The use by all participants of radioligands of the same origin as well as of the same protein reactant and standard seems a minimum recommendation. Similarly, the use of the same calculation method for analyzing the binding data should be strongly advised. In addition, regular intralaboratory quality controls should be developed in all centers. Lyophilized material is now produced by the EORTC for such controls (new samples are prepared three times a year). This service is open to all laboratories[1].

Finally, additional controls should be carried out in main centers receiving tissue samples from satellite hospitals. Regular comparative analyses of the receptor data should be performed (centers vs. satellites) to identify possible loss of binding activity during the transport of the samples from the satellite hospitals to the laboratory. These controls are necessary in view of the major importance of processing and delivery of the tumor tissues in the assessment of the receptor contents.

---

1 For further information about this service, see Eur J Cancer Clin Oncol 18: 608 (1982) or write to Dr. A. Koenders or Prof. T. Benraad, Department of Experimental and Clinical Endocrinology, Geert Grooteplein Zuid 8, 6525 GA Nijmegen, The Netherlands

Part III. Biology of the Primary Tumor

Estrogen Receptors and Distribution of Prognostic Factors in Primary Breast Cancer*

G. Andry, W. Mattheiem, S. Suciu, R. J. Sylvester, D. Pratola, A. Verhest, G. Leclercq, and J. C. Heuson**

Service de Chirurgie, Clinique de Chirurgie Mammaire et Pelvienne, Institut Jules Bordet, Rue Héger-Bordet 1, 1000 Bruxelles, Belgium

Introduction

The interest of estrogen receptor assays has been pointed out by numerous authors [1], especially with reference to the determination of potential responders to endocrine therapy among generalized breast cancer patients. The relationship between the estrogen receptor level in breast primaries and other prognostic factors remains a matter of controversy and is the subject of the following article, which is based on a series of 490 previously unreported cases.

Materials and Methods

The distribution of estrogen receptor concentration and other potential prognostic factors was studied in 490 patients who underwent radical mastectomy according to the technique described by Madden in 1965 [2]. All patients were admitted to the Institut Jules Bordet between 1 May 1969 and 31 December 1977 for primary treatment of newly diagnosed nonmetastatic breast cancer. Among the 490 patients studied, there were five males. The estrogen receptor concentration in the cytoplasm of neoplastic cells was determined in 341 patients by the technique defined by Leclercq in 1973 [3] and expressed as femtomoles (10^{-15} mol) per milligram of tissue protein.

Correlation of Receptor Concentration with Other Prognostic Factors

The distribution of estrogen receptor concentration at the time of primary treatment is shown in Table 1. Twenty-eight percent of the patients had a concentration of 10 fmol or less and were thus considered receptor negative, while 38% had a concentration of more than 100 fmol.

* This work was supported by a grant (5R10-CA11488-11) from the National Cancer Institute, Department of Health, Education, and Welfare
** This research was conducted with the collaboration of N. Legros, Sercive de Médecine, Clinique et Laboratoire de Cancérologie mammaire, Inst. J. Bordet, Brussels and M. T'Hooft, Infirmière Graduée A1, Ecole d'Infirmière, Université Libre de Bruxelles, Brussels

Table 1. Distribution of estrogen receptor concentration (fmol/mg tissue protein)

	ER negative	ER positive		Total
	0−10	11−100	102−2,000	
Number of patients	94 (28%)	116 (34%)	131 (38%)	341

Table 2. Distribution of estrogen receptor concentration by G grade

Grading	Receptor concentration			Total
	0−10	11−100	101−2,000	
G1	8 (11%)	28 (39%)	35 (49%)	71 (28%)
G2	22 (24%)	33 (35%)	38 (41%)	93 (37%)
G3	39 (43%)	23 (26%)	28 (31%)	90 (35%)
Total	69 (27%)	84 (33%)	101 (40%)	254

Kendall's Tau B $= -0.21$, $P < 0.0001$

Correlation with Histological Grade

The histological grading of the primary tumor was reviewed in 324 patients by a team of two pathologists who were unaware of the tumor's receptor contents. The histological classification employed was based on the system defined by Bloom [4] and Scarff [5]. Two hundred and fifty-four infiltrating ductal carcinomas could be classified as G1, G2, or G3 according to a decreasing degree of tumor differentiation. Table 2 presents the distribution of the G grade according to the estrogen receptor concentration and shows that 73% of the tumors were receptor positive. The correlation between grading and receptor concentration is statistically significant ($P < 0.0001$, Kendall's Tau B) [6] and indicates that as the degree of differentiation of the tumor increases, the receptor concentration also increases.

Among the 70 noninfiltrating ductal carcinomas, 73% were also estrogen receptor positive, but 91% of the 22 lobular tumors and 93% of the 14 cribriform tumors were found to be receptor positive.

Correlation with T Category and Nodal Status

As indicated in Tables 3 and 4 respectively, there is no significant correlation of the estrogen receptor concentration with either the size [7] of the primary tumor ($P = 0.14$) or the number of invaded lymph nodes ($P = 0.42$) at the time of initial treatment.

Correlation with Menopausal Status and Age

Table 5 presents the distribution of the estrogen receptor concentration by the menopausal status, excluding the five male patients and 17 patients who underwent a total hysterectomy

Table 3. Distribution of estrogen receptor concentration by T category

Size	Receptor concentration			Total	
	0–10	11–100	101–2,000		
T1	7 (19%)	15 (40.5%)	15 (40.5%)	37	(11%)
T2	50 (26%)	70 (36%)	75 (38%)	195	(59%)
T3	28 (35%)	23 (28%)	30 (37%)	81	(24%)
T4	6 (32%)	5 (26%)	8 (42%)	19	(6%)
Total	91 (27%)	113 (34%)	128 (39%)	332	

Kendall's Tau C $= -0.49$, $P < 0.14$

Table 4. Distribution of estrogen receptor concentration by number of invaded lymph nodes

No. of invaded nodes	Receptor concentration			Total	
	0–10	11–100	101–2,000		
0–3	58 (25%)	87 (38%)	85 (37%)	230	(67%)
4	36 (32%)	29 (26%)	46 (41%)	111	(33%)
Total	94 (28%)	116 (34%)	131 (38%)	341	

Kendall's Tau C $= -0.01$, $P < 0.42$

Table 5. Distribution of estrogen receptor concentration by menopausal status

Menopausal status	Receptor concentration			Total	
	0–10	11–100	101–2,000		
Pre- or peri menopausal	38 (34%)	54 (49%)	19 (17%)	111	(35%)
Post menopausal	51 (25%)	55 (26%)	102 (49%)	208	(65%)
Total	89 (28%)	109 (34%)	121 (38%)	319	

Kendall's Tau C $= 0.26$, $P < 0.0001$

prior to the diagnosis of their malignancy. Postmenopausal patients have a significantly higher level of receptor concentration than pre- or perimenopausal patients ($P < 0.0001$). Coinciding with these results, it was also found that patients over 55 years of age had a higher level of receptors than younger patients.

Summary

These results indicate that there is a significant correlation between the estrogen receptor concentration and the patient's G grade, menopausal status, and age, while no significant correlation of the receptor concentration with either the T category or the number of invaded lymph nodes was found.

Discussion

The percentage of estrogen receptor positive tumors in our patient population (72%) (defined on the basis of a concentration of more than 10 fmol/mg of cytosolic protein content) falls within the range of percentages commonly reported [1] and confirms our previous data [8]. Our data also substantiate previous reports concerning the proportion of infiltrating ductal carcinomas [9, 10] and the distribution of estrogen receptor concentration by menopausal status and age [1, 10] in such patients. The lack of correlation between the estrogen receptor concentration and both the size of the primary and the number of invaded lymph nodes has been previously observed [11, 12] and emphasizes the independence of the former relative to these other two prognostic factors.

The finding of a significant correlation between receptor concentration and grading seems to confirm the hypothesis of an increasing level of estrogen receptor among the more differentiated infiltrating carcinomas [12, 13]. Although not observed by others [14], this finding may be of value in the selection of potential responders to chemotherapeutic agents [15] in addition to the recognized importance of the estrogen receptor assay for selection of hormonal treatment.

References

1. Hawkins RA, Roberts MM, Forrest APM (1980) Estrogen receptors and breast cancer: current status. Br J Surg 67: 153–169
2. Madden JL (1965) Modified radical mastectomy. Surg Gynecol Obstet 140: 1221–1230
3. Leclercq G, Heuson JC, Schoenfeld R, Mattheiem WH, Tagnon HJ (1973) Estrogen receptors in human breast cancer. Eur J Cancer 9: 665–673
4. Bloom HJG, Richardson WW (1957) Histological grading and prognosis in breast cancer. Study of 1,409 cases of which 359 have been followed for 15 years. Br J Cancer 11: 359–377
5. Scarff RW, Torloni H (1968) Types histologiques des tumeurs du sein. Classification histologique internationale des tumeurs 2, O.M.S., Geneve
6. Afifi AA, Azen SP (1979) Statistical analysis. A computer orientated approach, 2nd edn Academic Press, New York
7. TNM Classification of Malignant Tumors, UICC 3, Geneva (1978)
8. Leclercq G, Heuson JC, Deboel MC, Mattheiem WH (1975) Estrogen receptors in breast cancer: a changing concept. Br Med J 1: 185–189
9. Silfverswärd C, Gustafsson JA, Gustafsson SA, Humla S, Nordenskjöld B, Wallgren A, Wrange O (1980) Estrogen receptor concentration in 269 cases of histologically classified human breast cancer. Cancer 45: 2001–2005
10. Kinne DW, Ashikari R, Butler A, Menendez-Botet C, Rosen PP, Schwartz MK (1981) Estrogen receptor protein in breast cancer as a predictor of recurrence. Cancer 47: 2364–2367
11. Rosen PP, Menendez-Botet CJ, Nisselbaum JS, Urban JA, Mike V, Fracchia A, Schwartz MK (1975) Pathological review of breast lesions analyzed for estrogen receptor protein. Cancer Res 35: 3187–3194
12. Maynard PV, Davies CJ, Blamey RW, Elston CW, Johnson J, Griffiths K (1978) Relationship between estrogen receptor content and histological grade in human primary breast tumors. Br J Cancer 38: 745–748
13. Meyer JS, Ramanath B, Stevens SC, White WL (1977) Low incidence of estrogen receptor in breast carcinomas with rapid rates of cellular replication. Cancer 40: 2290–2298
14. Roberts AN, Hähnel R (1981) Estrogen receptor assay and morphology of breast cancer. Pathology 13: 317–325
15. Fisher ER, Redmond CK, Liu H, Rockette H, Fisher B, Collaborating NSABP investigators (1980) Correlation of estrogen receptor and pathologic characteristics of invasive breast cancer. Cancer 45: 349–353

Influence of Intratumoral Estradiol Biosynthesis on Estrogen Receptors

K. Carlström

Department of Obstetrics and Gynecology, Huddinge University Hospital, 141 86 Huddinge, Sweden

Introduction

According to the common theory on steroid receptor mechanism, the amount of cytosol estrogen receptor, as well as the intranuclear estradiol-receptor complex, is influenced by intracellular estradiol levels [6]. Intracellular estradiol arises from two sources: from peripheral estradiol by transport into the tumor cell and by intratumoral biosynthesis from other steroids. It is well known that cytosol receptor values are invariably low in tumors from women with high (premenopausal) serum estrogens, probably owing to blockade of the receptor by endogenous estradiol. In such cases intratumoral estradiol formation will probably be less important. On the other hand, receptor-rich as well as receptor-poor tumors are found in women with low (postmenopausal) peripheral estrogens, and in such cases intratumoral estradiol biosynthesis may be of clinical importance. The following discussion will be restricted to the situation present in the postmenopausal woman and will cover three pathways of intratumoral estradiol formation: (a) reduction of estrone; (b) ring A aromatization of androgens; and (c) hydrolysis of estrogen conjugates.

Reduction of Estrone

This reaction, which also usually constitutes the final step in pathways 2 and 3, is catalyzed by the 17β-hydroxysteroid dehydrogenase (17β-OHSD) activity. This activity also catalyzes the reverse reaction, i.e., the oxidation of estradiol. Abul-Hajj et al. [2] reported higher 17β-OHSD activity in receptor-poor tumors than in receptor-rich ones, while Lübbert and Pollow [10] found no correlations in this respect. In both studies, 17β-OHSD activity was measured by oxidation of estradiol to estrone in the presence of exogenous NAD^+, which, however, reflects the enzyme activity in the same manner as does measurement of the reduction of estrone in the presence of exogenous NADH/NADPH [17]. Studies performed with intact breast cancer cells and without the addition of exogenous pyridine nucleotides have revealed similar rates of transformation for the reduction of estrone as for the oxidation of estradiol [9, 23]. Furthermore, it should be kept in mind that most neoplastic tissues have a restricted oxygen supply in which reductive conditions prevail [19]. The results of Abul-Hajj et al. may therefore reflect a blockade of the estradiol binding sites by estradiol formed from estrone by intratumoral reduction in vivo. One explanation for the diverging results obtained by Lübbert and Pollow may be their use of the microsome fraction only for the assay of 17β-OHSD activity while Abul-Hajj et al. used 1,000 g supernatants.

Ring A Aromatization of Androgens

Considerable attention has been paid to the ring A aromatization of androgens by breast tumor preparations (for references see [4, 6, and 14]). Ring A aromatization has been demonstrated in slices, homogenates, and intact cultured cells from human breast cancer tumors; however, aromatase activity does not seem to be a common property of breast neoplasms [14]. Contradictory results in this respect have even been obtained on the same line of cells. Thus MacIndoe [11] reported formation of estradiol from testosterone by cultured MCF$_7$ breast cancer cells while D'Agata et al. [3] and Rademaker et al. [18] failed to demonstrate any estrogen synthesis by this cell preparation. Contradictory results also arise when aromatase activity of the tumor is compared with the cytosol estrogen receptor content. Abul-Hajj et al. [1] reported a significant negative correlation between the rate of conversion of an androgen (dehydroepiandrosterone) into estrogens and the cytosol receptor content, while other workers failed to demonstrate such a correlation [8, 13, 20]. In the reviewer's opinion, it is doubtful whether intratumoral aromatase activity has any greater significance in vivo. Several of the in vitro studies on breast tumor aromatase have been performed under nonphysiological conditions favoring the formation of oxidative artifacts, one of which may be estrogens. Despite this, the reported rates of estrogen formation are extremely low (see below).

Hydrolysis of Estrogen Conjugates

Intratumoral estradiol formation from estrogen conjugates seems to have been studied only with respect to estrone sulfate. Estrone sulfate is the most abundant estrogen in the postmenopausal woman and its peripheral serum levels exceed other biologically active estrogens by a factor of 10. The peripheral serum levels of estrone sulfate and other estradiol precursors in postmenopausal women are given in Table 1.

Hitherto conversion of estrone sulfate into estradiol by breast tumor preparations in vitro has been demonstrated by Rochefort's group using MCF$_7$ breast tumor cells [21] and by our group using total homogenates of breast tumors [22]. In our investigation tumors from patients with low peripheral estrogen levels were studied. [^{3}H]Estrone sulfate was

Table 1. Peripheral serum levels of estradiol precursors in postmenopausal women aged 55−65 years (reference values from the reviewers laboratory). Levels of estradiol sulfate are not available for postmenopausal women but must be considered as very low (15)

Steroid	Range (nmol/l)
Estrone (unconjugated)	0.1−0.25
Estrone (total, 85%−90% estrone sulfate)	0.5−3.0
Testosterone	0.5−2.0
4-Androstene-3,17-dione	2.0−5.0
Dehydroepiandrosterone	5.0−20
Dehydroepiandrosterone sulfate	500 −5,000

converted into [³H]estrone and [³H]estradiol by homogenates of all tumors in the presence of NADH and NADPH. In a recent investigation (Wilking et al., to be published) we have also demonstrated the formation of [³H]estradiol sulfate. Thus the intratumoral formation of estradiol from estrone sulfate proceeds via two intermediates, i.e., estrone and estradiol sulfate.

The material was divided into receptor-poor ($n = 7$) and receptor-rich ($n = 16$) tumors by using the limit of 0.3 fmol [³H]estradiol bound per microgram of DNA (H. Westerberg, personal communication). The formation of estradiol from estrone sulfate was significantly higher in the receptor-poor tumors than in the receptor-rich ones: 35.95 ± 11.60 vs 5.33 ± 1.37 fmol per minute and per milligram of protein respectively, $P < 0.001$. No difference was found in the total hydrolysis of estrone sulfate, indicating that reduction of estrone or estrone sulfate may be the rate-limiting step. There was no difference in peripheral estrogen levels, while the patients with high converting, receptor-poor tumors were significantly younger than the patients with low converting, receptor-rich tumors: 58.0 ± 5.5 vs 73.1 ± 2.1 years, $P < 0.01$. This indicates an age dependency of the intratumoral 17β-OHSD activity in women with low peripheral estrogen levels, as was suggested earlier by Varela and Dao [20]. This may explain the age dependency of cytosol estrogen receptor values present even within postmenopausal women [22].

We interpret our findings as showing that a high capacity of the tumor to form estradiol from estrone sulfate will lead to high intracellular estradiol levels, extensive blockade of the hormone binding sites, and an increased intranuclear receptor level [5]. This will in turn result in low cytosol receptor values, even in patients with low peripheral estrogen levels. On the other hand, the combination of low intratumoral estradiol formation and low peripheral estrogens seems to result in high cytosol receptor values.

Our findings indicate that estrone sulfate possesses potential biological activity when tumor growth is concerned. Similar conclusions have been drawn independently by Rochefort's group in their elegant study on intact cultured MCF₇ cells [21]. They demonstrated that estrone sulfate easily entered the cell, in which a major fraction was converted into unconjugated estrone and estradiol. The proportion of unconjugated estrogens was more important in the nuclear extract and pellet than in the cytosol. Furthermore, isotopic dilution with unlabeled estrone during the incubation with [³H]estrone sulfate resulted in a strong decrease in the unconjugated [³H]estrogens recovered from the nuclear extract and pellet, while the amounts and proportions of [³H]estrogens in the cytosol were unchanged. This strongly indicates that the estrogens present in the nuclei are bound to a saturable receptor. Finally, the estrogenic activity of estrone sulfate in this system was clearly shown by the induction of well-characterized, specific estrogen-sensitive proteins. Taken together, the results obtained in different systems by Rochefort's group and our group strongly indicate that the intratumoral formation of estradiol from estrone sulfate influences the estrogen receptor values and that the main peripheral estrogen, estrone sulfate, may be important for the growth of the tumor.

Biological Significance of Intratumoral Estradiol Biosynthesis

Variations in experimental conditions preclude an exact comparison of the quantitative importance of the three different pathways for intratumoral estradiol biosynthesis studied in vitro. Most studies in this field also lack data on linearity of the assay with respect to time and to amounts of enzyme source. However, the following approximate rates of estradiol formation (femtomoles per minute and per milligram of protein) can be calculated from studies using crude preparations (slices, minces, total homogenates, or 1,000−2,000 g supernatants), exogenous cofactors, and substrate concentrations ranging from 10^{-8} to 10^{-7} M: from *4-androstene-3,17-dione,* 0−0.02 [16, 20]; from *testosterone,* 0−0.015 [8, 12]; from *dehydroepiandrosterone,* 0−0.1 [1] or no aromatization at all [7]; from *estrone,* 5−150 (Wilking et al., to be published), and from *estrone sulfate,* 0.5−100 [22]. Experiments using intact cells without exogenous cofactors have yielded similar results, with extensive transformation of estrone into estradiol [9, 23] and of estrone sulfate into estrone and estradiol [21], while aromatization of androgens has been reported in only one of three studies, and then at a very low rate [3, 11, 18].

It is likely that the superiority of estrone and its sulfate as substrates for intratumoral estradiol formation shown in vitro will be even more manifest in vivo, since the restricted oxygen supply present in neoplastic tissues [19] may favor 17β-reduction rather than ring A aromatization. The peripheral serum levels of estrone and its sulfate in the postmenopausal woman are of the same order as for the proximate aromatization precursors 4-andros-tene-3,17-dione and testosterone (Table 1). Intratumoral formation of estradiol from estrone and its sulfate may influence the estrogen receptor values in vivo in individuals with low peripheral estrogen levels, while the significance of ring A aromatization seems rather uncertain in this respect.

References

1. Abul-Hajj YJ, Iverson R, Kiang DT (1979) Aromatization of androgens by human breast cancer. Steroids 33: 205−222
2. Abul-Hajj YJ, Iverson R, Klang DT (1979) Estradiol-17β-dehydrogenase and estradiol binding in human mammary tumors. Steroids 33: 477−484
3. D'Agata R, Monaco ME, Loriaux DL (1978) Failure of breast cancer cells in long term culture to aromatize androstenedione. Steroids 31: 463−470
4. Dao TL (1979) Metabolism of estrogens in breast cancer. Biochim Biophys Acta 560: 397−426
5. Garola RE, McGuire WL (1977) An improved assay for nuclear estrogen receptor in experimental and human breast cancer. Cancer Res 37: 3333−3337
6. Hawkins RA, Roberts MM, Forrest APM (1980) Oestrogen receptors and breast cancer, current status. Br J Surg 67: 153−169
7. Li K, Foo T, Adams JB (1978) Products of dehydroepiandrosterone metabolism by human mammary tumors and their influence on estradiol receptors. Steroids 31: 113−127
8. Li K, Adams JB (1981) Aromatization of testosterone and oestrogen receptor levels in human breast cancer. J Steroid Biochem 14: 269−272
9. Lippman M, Monaco ME, Bolan G (1977) Effects of estrone, estradiol and estriol on hormone-responsive human breast cancer in long-term tissue culture. Cancer Res 37: 1901−1907
10. Lübbert H, Pollow K (1978) Correlation between the 17β-hydroxysteroid dehydrogenase activity and the estradiol and progesterone receptor concentrations of normal and neoplastic mammary tissue. J Mol Med 3: 175−183
11. MacIndoe JH (1979) Estradiol formation from testosterone by continuously cultured human breast cancer cells. J Clin Endocrinol Metab 49: 272−277
12. Miller WR, Forrest APM (1974) Oestradiol synthesis by a human breast carcinoma. Lancet 2: 866−868
13. Miller WR, Hawkins PA, Forrest APM (1979) Oestrogen biosynthesis and oestrogen receptors in human breast cancer. Cancer Treat Rep 63: 1153
14. Nisker JA, Siiteri PK (1981) Estrogens and breast cancer. Clin Obstet Gynecol 24: 301−322

15. Nunez M, Aedo A-R, Landgren B-M, Cekan SC, Diczfalusy E (1977) Studies on the pattern of circulating steroids in the normal human menstrual cycle. 6. The levels of oestrone sulphate and oestradiol sulphate. Acta Endocrinol (Kbh) 86: 621−629
16. Perel E, Wilkins D, Killinger DW (1980) The conversion of androstenedione to estrone, estradiol and testosterone in breast tissue. J Steroid Biochem 13: 89−94
17. Pollow K, Boqui E, Baumann J, Schmidt-Gollwitzer M, Pollow B (1977) Comparison of in vitro conversion of estradiol-17β to estrone of normal and neoplastic human breast tissue. Mol Cell Endocrinol 6: 333−348
18. Rademaker B, Vossenberg JBJ, Poortman J, Thijssen JHH (1980) Metabolism of estradiol-17β, 5-androstene-3β-17β-diol and testosterone in human breast cancer cells in long term culture. J Steroid Biochem 13: 787−791
19. Shapot VS (1972) Some biochemical aspects of the relationship between the tumor and the host. Adv Cancer Res 15: 253−286
20. Varela RM, Dao TL (1978) Estrogen synthesis and estradiol binding by human mammary tumors. Cancer Res 38: 2429−2433
21. Vignon F, Terqui M, Westley B, Derocq D, Rochefort H (1980) Effects of plasma estrogen sulfates in mammary cancer cells. Endocrinology 106: 1079−1086
22. Wilking N, Carlström K, Gustafsson SA, Sköldefors H, Tollbom Ö (1980) Oestrogen receptors and metabolism of oestrone sulphate in human mammary carcinoma. Eur J Cancer 16: 1339−1344
23. Willcox PA, Thomas GH (1972) Oestrogen metabolism in cultured human breast tumours. Br J Cancer 26: 453−460

Influence of Endogenous Hormone Levels on Tumor Estradiol and Progesterone Receptors*

S. Saez and C. Chouvet

Centre Leon Berard, 28 Rue Laënnec, 69373 Lyon, Cedex 8, France

Introduction

In the story of human breast cancer, two major findings markedly modified the clinical approach to treatment. Both belong to endocrinology. The first brought to light the hormone dependency of certain tumors and paved the way for ablative endocrine surgery [1]. This, however, did not help in the selection of patients before the initiation of treatment. The second was the discovery of the estrogen receptor (ER) machinery in normal target cells and the same mechanism of hormone action in tumor target tissue [5, 6]. This opened up a new area in the knowledge of breast cancer. Further investigations demonstrated that breast tumors contain receptors for other steroids, some of whose functions have still not been elucidated. Progesterone receptors (PgR) have a unique place alongside ER since their synthesis has been demonstrated to be both estrogen and estrogen receptor dependent in several target tissues, such as endometrium, and in the mammary tumor epithelial cell line [2, 3]. In view of this, it was suggested that the existence and the quantity of ER and PgR might be regulated, even in tumor tissue. To test this hypothesis we analyzed tumor receptor contents in relation to endocrine parameters, menopausal status, and plasma estrogen and progesterone levels in 621 breast cancer patients treated in our institute.

Materials and Methods

Nonradioactive ligands, diethylstilbestrol (DES), cortisol, progesterone, estrone, estradiol, and R-5020 were gifts from J. P. Raynaud or were purchased from Roussel (Romainville). Of the labeled steroids, [6,7(n)-^{3}H]estradiol (specific activity 45 Ci/mmol) was purchased from CEA (France) and ^{3}H-R-5020 and [1,2,6,7-^{3}H]progesterone (specific activity 103 Ci/mmol) from New England Nuclear GmbH (Dreieich, Germany). Labeled compounds were purified by paper chromatography every 3 weeks.

Specific antibodies against estrone and estradiol were provided by Roussel-Uclaf and antibodies against progesterone were purchased from the Pasteur Institute (Paris).

* This work was supported in part by the Institut National de la Santé et de la Recherche Médicale (ATP 24-75-47 and CRAT 76-4-490) and the Federation Française des Centres de Lutte contre le Cancer

Peripheral blood was drawn on the day of the biopsy at 8 a.m. Plasma estrogen levels were determined by a modification of the technique of Abraham, using a celite column chromatographic separation method for estrogens [11]. Plasma progesterone extraction was performed with petroleum ether. Final measurements of estrogen and progesterone were made by radioimmunoassay. All tumor samples were frozen in liquid nitrogen immediately after excision and stored until receptor determinations were performed. Cytosol ER and PgR determinations were carried out as previously described [11], using the dextran-coated charcoal competitive protein binding assay.

The assay was performed at 4° C and measured nonoccupied estradiol receptors and total cytosol progesterone receptors. The number of sites and the dissociation constant of the binding were calculated by the Scatchard method. Results were expressed as femtomoles of bound labeled ligand per milligram of cytosol protein. Protein content was measured by the method of Lowry. A positive receptor content was taken to be equal to or greater than 3 fmol and 10 fmol ligand bound per milligram cytosol protein for estradiol and progesterone respectively.

Results

Distribution of Patients

Patients included in this series were 25–93 years old, the 50- to 70-year-old patient population being the largest one. There were 185 premenopausal and 436 postmenopausal patients (Table 1), but in patients between 30 and 60 years old there was an overlap of these two cohorts owing to early castrations and late menopause. As shown in Table 2, ER+ tumors and PgR+ tumors were more frequent after the menopause, but the differences were not significant. Distribution into more precise categories of receptor content is illustrated in Table 3. The ER+ PgR+ group was similar before and after the menopause, while ER+ PgR-tumors represented only 22% of tumors in premenopausal patients but 35% in postmenopausal patients.

Table 1. Distribution of pre- and postmenopausal patients in the different age groups

	25−29	30−39	40−49	50−59	60−69	70−79	80−89	90	Total
Premenopause	4	46	91						185
Postmenopause		4	24	135	157	92	19	5	436

Table 2. Frequency of ER-positive and PgR-positive tumors in relation to menopausal status

	n	% Positive	
		ER	PgR
Premenopause	185	58	25
Postmenopause	436	66	32
		NS	NS

NS, not significant

Table 3. Distribution of tumors in the different categories of receptor content in relation to menopausal status

	Total (n)	ER + PgR+	ER + PgR−	ER + PgR−	ER + PgR−
		% of cases in each category			
Premenopause	185	36	22	3	39
Postmenopause	436	31	35	2	32

Table 4. Mean content of ER and PgR in tumors in relation to menopausal status[a]

	n	ER	PgR
		Content in fmol/mg cytosol protein	
Premenopause	185	40 ± 10 (108)	342 ± 86 (46)
Postmenopause	436	148 ± 22 (289)	336 ± 70 (139)

[a] The number of positive cases in each category is indicated in parentheses

The mean quantity of receptors measured in tumors is shown in Table 4. The mean ER content in premenopausal patients (40 ± 10 fmol/mg protein) was significantly lower than the value observed after the menopause (148 ± 22 fmol/mg protein). The mean PgR values for pre- and postmenopausal patients were 342 ± 86 and 336 ± 70 fmol/mg protein respectively.

ER and PgR in Premenopausal Patients

We evaluated the presence of receptors in relation to the day of the menstrual cycle (Fig. 1). ER positivity did not vary significantly, being 60%, 51%, and 62% at the three successive 10-day periods, whereas PgR positivity fell from 54% to 30%.
Since changes in steroid production characterize the successive phases of the menstrual cycle, we investigated receptor positivity in relation to the plasma levels of estrogens and progesterone. Figure 2 represents the distribution of tumors in relation to estrogen levels measured on the same day as the biopsy was obtained. The percentage of tumors containing ER did not vary significantly according to the increase in plasma estrogens. By contrast, PgR positivity was as low as 21% when plasma estrogen levels were below 5 ng/100 ml, while it was more than twice as high with plasma estrogen levels of 10−15 ng/100 ml.
Figure 3 represents the distribution of ER and PgR positivity in relation to plasma progesterone level. The cut-off value of 150 ng/100 ml was chosen as the maximum found during the follicular phase and in postmenopausal patients. PgR positivity was 42% when plasma progesterone was low and decreased to 24% for higher levels. This variation shows the same type of distribution as had been observed during the luteal phase of the cycle (Fig. 1). The incidence of ER did not change in relation to plasma progesterone.
Thus ER positivity is not very sensitive to the hormonal variations of the menstrual cycle. PgR positivity, on the other hand, decreases to a very low percentage when circulating estrogens are not sufficient or the plasma progesterone level is above 150 ng/100 ml.

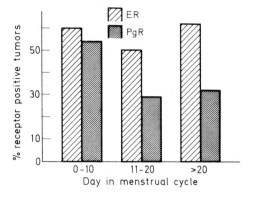

Fig. 1. Percentage of tumors containing ER and PgR at different periods in the menstrual cycle

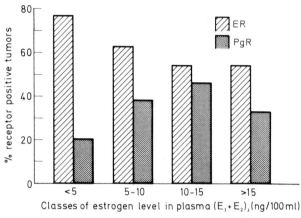

Fig. 2. Percentage of tumors from premenopausal patients containing ER and PgR in relation to the level of estrogens (estrone + estradiol, ng/100 ml) in plasma on the day of the biopsy

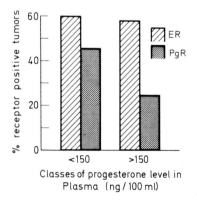

Fig. 3. Percentage of tumors from premenopausal patients containing ER and PgR in relation to the level of progesterone in plasma (below or above 150 ng/100 ml) on the day of the biopsy

ER and PgR in Postmenopausal Patients

In patients operated on during the postmenopausal period, the mean incidence of ER+ and PgR+ tumors was 66% and 32% respectively, as shown in Table 2.

The exact distribution of positivity of both receptors and the tumor receptor content were investigated in relation to age and plasma circulating steroids.

The highest incidence of both ER and PgR was observed in the 60−69 age group (Fig. 4).

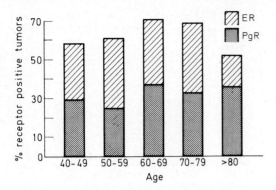

Fig. 4. Percentage of tumors containing ER and PgR in menopausal patients in relation to age

Table 5. ER content (mean ± SD) in tumors from postmenopausal patients in relation to the absence or presence of PgR and to age

Age (years)	n	Tumor ER content (pmol/mg protein) Categories of receptor content[a]	
		ER + PgR+	ER + PgR−
50−59	84	148 ± 64	116 ± 41
60−69	113	179 ± 48	122 ± 45
70−79	62	230 ± 100	117 ± 35
80	14	196	144

[a] SD was not calculated in the older class owing to the small number of cases

Table 6. Plasma estrone + estradiol (mean ± SD) in relation to the absence or presence of PgR in tumors in different age groups[a]

Age (years)	n	Plasma estrone + estradiol (ng/100 ml) Categories of receptor content		
		ER + PgR+	ER + PgR−	
50−59	74	8.35 ± 3.03	8.74 ± 1.52	NS
60−69	99	8.80 ± 3.09	7.94 ± 1.6	NS
70−79	57	10.8 ± 2.85	7.10 ± 1.74	0.05
80	11	7.6	5.4	

[a] SD was not calculated in the older class owing to the small number of patients
NS, not significant

In all age groups of postmenopausal patients the tumor ER content was higher than in the premenopausal group (Table 5). It increased in relation to age, from 50 to 79 years, but only in the ER+ PgR+ subclass. Since the synthesis of progesterone receptors in target cells is partially dependent on estrogen stimulation, circulating estrogens were measured in these patients (Table 6). The sum of plasma estrone and estradiol was taken into account since estrone, which is of adrenal origin, is the major estrogen to be produced after the menopause in breast cancer patients [12]. The level of plasma estrone + estradiol was higher than expected in all categories of postmenopausal patients, but increased with age only in the subset having PgR+ tumors.

These data confirm that the presence of PgR in tumors is related to the ER content [7] and suggest that circulating estrogen may be necessary for ER stimulation and PgR synthesis.

Discussion

Estradiol receptor is more frequently present in measurable amounts than PgR, as has been reported previously [7, 10, 11]. The quantity of receptors which is measured in tissue samples from tumors such as adenocarcinoma depends on several parameters. The pathological type of the tumor and its cellularity are responsible for parallel variations in both ER and PgR: (a) the epithelial cellularity of the tumor determines the number of sites which can be measured, and (b) if the tumor cell population is heterogeneous, the receptor content will also depend on the proportion of epithelial clones which contain receptors.

In addition, it is likely that endocrine factors regulate the precise content of receptors which can be measured in each tissue sample, provided that the cell machinery is intact. Like other workers [10, 13], we found that hormonally induced variations could be different for PgR and ER.

The presence of PgR and the quantity of ER seem to be linked to the same parameters. Our results support the hypothesis that PgR is synthesized under estrogen stimulation in human breast tumors. Thus in postmenopausal patients, the presence of PgR is related to plasma estrogens. In premenopausal patients, the highest PgR positivity is found during the first few days of the menstrual cycle, when estrogen production increases, in the absence of progesterone. Furthermore, the finding of a very small ER+ PgR-group suggests a very high degree of potential hormone dependency for tumors from premenopausal patients with ER+ tumors.

A very low rate of PgR positivity was observed in the presence of high progesterone levels during the luteal phase. We have previously shown similar results in a smaller series of patients [11]. These new data confirm the phenomenon of PgR down-regulation. But it is likely that the threshold of progesterone level at which PgR becomes unmeasurable varies with individual cases. In addition, progesterone was measured in plasma drawn on the same day that the biopsy was performed for receptor determination. It is not known if this is the most appropriate timing for recording the modifications induced by a recent hormonal event. Nevertheless, the variations of PgR positivity in relation to the cycle and to plasma progesterone remain significant. They are in agreement with the down-regulation of PgR that has been described in normal target tissue [4, 9].

Hence the absence of PgR in some tumors could be due either to inadequate estrogen stimulation or to a defect of the cells themselves. In the former case such tumors should have a good prognosis and should respond to hormone therapy in the same way as ER+ PgR+ tumors [5].

In conclusion, human breast tumor tissue which contains ER and PgR seems to mimic the function of any target tissue in which the regulation of receptors is an aspect of hormone dependency. Some correlations were found between the endocrine characteristics of patients and the receptor content of tumors. These correlations are significant when groups of patients are compared, but it is not possible to define individual values as low, normal, or high without taking into account all parameters, both pathological and endocrine.

References

1. Huggins CB, Dao TL (1953) Adrenalectomy and oophorectomy in treatment of advanced carcinoma of the breast. JAMA 151:1388–1394
2. Horwitz K, McGuire WL (1975) Predicting response to endocrine therapy in human breast cancer: a hypothesis. Science 189:726–727
3. Horwitz K, McGuire WL (1978) Estrogen control of progesterone receptors in human breast cancer. J Biol Chem 253:2273–2278
4. Janne O, Isoma V, Isotalo H, Kokko E, Vierikko P (1978) Uterine estrogen and progestin receptors and their regulation. Ups J Med Sci Suppl 22:62–70
5. Jensen E, Block GF, Smith S, Kyser K, DeSombre ER (1971) Estrogen receptors and breast cancer response to adrenalectomy. Natl Cancer Inst Monogr 34:55–70
6. Jensen EV, DeSombre ER, Jungblut P (1967) Estrogen receptors in hormone responsive tissue and tumors. In: Wissler RW, Dao TL, Wood S (eds) Endrogenous factors influencing breast tumor balance. University of Chicago Press, Chicago, pp 15–68
7. McGuire WL (ed) (1978) Hormones, réceptors, and breast cancer. Raven, New York
8. McGuire WL (1980) Steroid hormone receptors in breast cancer treatment strategy. Recent Prog Horm Res 36:135–156
9. Milgrom E, Luu Thi M, Atger M, Baulieu EE (1974) Mechanism regulating the concentration and the conformation of progesterone receptor(s) in the uterus. J Biol Chem 248:6366–6374
10. Nagai R, Kataoka M, Kobayash S, Ishihara K, Tobioka N, Nakashima K, Naruse M, Saito K, Sakuma S (1979) Estrogen and progesterone receptors in human breast cancer with concomitant assay of plasma 17β estradiol, progesterone and prolactin levels. Cancer Res 39:1835–1840
11. Saez S, Martin PM, Chouvet CD (1978) Estradiol and progesterone receptor levels in human breast adenocarcinoma in relation to plasma estrogen and progesterone levels. Cancer Res 38:3468–3473
12. Saez S (1974) Corticotrophin secretion in relation to breast cancer. In: Stoll E (ed) Mammary cancer and neuroendocrine therapy. Butterworth, London, pp 101–122
13. Vihko R, Janne O, Kontula K, Syrjala P (1980) Female sex steroid receptor status in primary and metastatic breast carcinoma and its relationship to serum and peptide hormone levels. Int J Cancer 26:13–21

Inflammatory Tumors of the Human Breast: Determination of Estrogen and Progesterone Receptors

G. Contesso, F. May-Levin, J. C. Delarue, H. Mouriesse, H. Sancho-Garnier, and M. Lemaout

Institut Gustave-Roussy, 39 Rue Camille Desmoulins, 94805 Villejuif Cedex, France

Introduction

The clinically inflammatory tumors are considered to be very severe carcinomas characterized by a particularly low rate of survival at 5 years [6, 14]. In the present study, we have simultaneously determined estrogen receptors (ER) and progesterone receptors (PgR) in these tumors and compared the results with those obtained in primary operable carcinomas. The prognostic value of ER has also been studied.

Materials and Methods

Patients

The series comprises 59 women with inflammatory tumors of the breast. Diagnosis and treatment were performed at the Institut Gustave-Roussy between March 1975 and December 1977.
Metastatic work-up included chest X-rays, mammograms, X-rays of the pelvis, and bone or liver scans. Inflammatory tumors are defined as tumors associated with inflammatory symptoms localized either in a part of or in the whole breast. The rapidly growing tumors (information obtained by careful anamnesis) were not included in the study.
Receptor measurements in these 59 cases were compared with those in 496 operable cases (T_1, T_2, or T_3 < 7 cm; N_0 or N_1; M_0 according to the TNM classification).

Receptor Assay

After biopsy under local anesthesia, tumor specimens (100−200 mg) were transported to the laboratory on ice within a few minutes. Malignancy was verified by histological examination. The samples were crushed at $0°$ C in three volumes of buffer (0.01 M Tris-HCl, 0.012 M dithiotreitol, 10% glycerol, pH 7.4) with an Ultraturrax (three 5-s bursts at 15-s cooling intervals) and homogenized in a Teflon-glass homogenizer. The homogenate was centrifuged for 1 h at 105,000 g in the 50 Ti rotor of a Beckman L_2 centrifuge. The supernatant (= cytosol) was used to determine ER and PgR by the single dose assay previously described [16]. Tumors with specific binding sites greater than 100

Recent Results in Cancer Research. Vol. 91
© Springer-Verlag Berlin · Heidelberg 1984

fmol/g tissue were considered to be ER+ PgR+. This arbitrary cut-off point corresponds to the limit of sensitivity of our technique [24]; it is comparable to those chosen by other authors [10, 27]. For positive results near the cut-off point (three results between 100 and 200 fmol/g tissue), the tumoral cell densitiy as determined by the pathologist was also taken into account: where cell density was high, results were considered negative; where it was low, results were considered positive.

Labeled steroids (estradiol for ER, R-5020 for PgR) were purchased from New England Nuclear.

Miscellaneous

We also determined:
1. Histological types, dividing tumors into three classes [4, 26]:
   a) Well-differentiated (either tubular or papillary);
   b) Pleomorphic (infiltrating ductal carcinoma with two components mixed: tubular and trabecular);
   c) Atypical (infiltrating ductal carcinoma without tubular or papillary components).
2. Histological grading according to WHO and Scarff and Bloom [1, 2].
3. Tumoral cell density (see above).

Statistical significance between groups was analyzed by the χ^2 test and the adjustment test of Boyd and Doll [3]. Disease-free survival rates were calculated by the Kaplan-Meier method [11] and curves compared by the log-rank test [23].

Results

Histological Characteristics and Hormonal Receptors

Pre- and postmenopausal women had the same distribution of histological characteristics, allowing us to combine the two populations to study the hormonal receptors.

Table 1. Relationship between histological type and ER in operable and inflammatory tumors[a]

		Histological type		
		Well-differentiated	Pleomorphic	Atypical
Operable tumors	ER⁻	8 (35%)	129 (43%)	57 (54%) } NS
	ER⁺	15 (65%)	168 (57%)	49 (46%)
Inflammatory tumors	ER⁻	1 (25%)	9 (53%)	18 (53%) } NS
	ER⁺	3 (75%)	8 (47%)	16 (47%)

[a] Sixty cases of operable tumors were not included in this classification and were classified as "other forms". In ten operable tumors and four inflammatory tumors histological type was not available

NS, not significant

A significant difference in terms of histological type ($P < 0.001$) was found between operable and inflammatory tumors – operable tumors were more often pleomorphic, inflammatory tumors more often atypical. By contrast, no significant correlation was observed in the distribution of ER among the three histological types (Table 1).

There was a significance difference ($P < 0.001$) between the two categories of tumors in terms of histological grading. However, a significant correlation ($P < 0.02$) between histological grading and ER was observed only for inflammatory tumors (Table 2): grade III inflammatory tumors were more frequently ER– and grade II more frequently ER+; no inflammatory tumor was classified as grade I.

Type of Tumor and Hormonal Receptors

Table 3 shows that the number of (ER– PgR–) cases was significantly ($P < 0.02$) higher in the inflammatory (48%) than in the operable group (28%).

Prognostic Value of Hormonal Receptors

Figure 1 shows with reference to inflammatory tumors that the number of patients presenting with metastases at the time of diagnosis was the same for ER+ tumors (11 of 28 patients) and for ER– tumors (10 of 30 patients). The disease-free curves show a more

Table 2. Relationship between histological grading and ER in operable and inflammatory tumors[a]

		Histological grading			
		I	II	III	
Operable tumors	ER–	35 (41%)	107 (47%)	87 (50%)	NS
	ER+	50 (59%)	122 (53%)	88 (50%)	
Inflammatory tumors	ER–	0	5 (29%)	25 (62%)	$P < 0.02$
	ER+	0	12 (71%)	15 (38%)	

[a] In seven operable tumors and two inflammatory tumors histological grading was not available
NS, not significant

Table 3. ER and PgR in human mammary carcinomas

Receptor status	Tumors		
	Operable	Inflammatory	
ER–, PgR–	140 (28%)	28 (48%)	
ER–, PgR+	76 (15%)	3 (5%)	$P < 0.02$
ER+, PgR–	91 (18%)	11 (19%)	
ER+, PgR+	189 (38%)	17 (28%)	

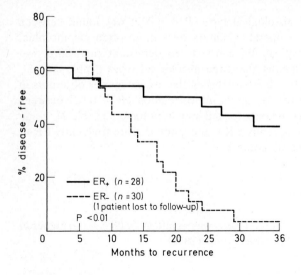

Fig. 1. ER and recurrence in all patients with inflammatory tumors

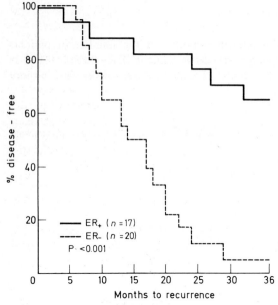

Fig. 2. ER and recurrence in patients free of metastases at the time of diagnosis of inflammatory tumor

favorable evolution for patients with ER+ tumors than for patients with ER− tumors ($P <$ 0.01). If we exlude patients with metastases at the time of diagnosis, we find a more significant difference (log-rank, $P < 0.001$) (Fig. 2).

The prognostic value of ER with regard to operable tumors is under study: we consider that a follow-up of only 36 months is not sufficient for a population with a good prognosis (80% at 5 years).

Discussion

This study confirms the high frequency of distal metastases at the time of diagnosis (21/59 or 36%) and the gravity of the inflammatory tumors.

Histological results indicate that inflammatory breast tumors constitute a separate disease entity, a large majority (62%) of atypical tumors being found. This is in agreement with the finding of Haagensen [9] that the atypical type accounted for 80% of the total population (59 cases). As opposed to our results, Martin et al. [15] found a relationship between histological type and ER distribution, provided that a two-category classification was carried out: on the one hand well-differentiated and pleomorphic tumors with more than 50% differentiation and on the other atypical and pleomorphic tumors with less than 50% differentiation.

As has already been observed [25], when grading inflammatory tumors histologically we found them to be highly malignant (70% classified as grade III, the most unfavorable group). While a significant relationship between histological grading and ER distribution could be shown only for the inflammatory tumors, such a relationship, although not statistically significant, was also seen for the operable tumors. Our results are identical to those reported by other groups [8, 12, 17, 21]. Taken together, these results confirm that ER and PgR represent an aspect of tumoral cellular differentiation.

The fact that inflammatory tumors show a higher proportion of (ER− PgR−) cases than do the operable tumors is a further argument in favor of distinguishing between these two tumor types [16, 19, 20]. These results thus seem to indicate that among this population of patients with inflammatory tumors, which overall have a very unfavorable evolution, there is a histobiological subgroup with a still worse prognosis.

The clinical progression seems to confirm these observations; indeed, the prognostic value of ER for the inflammatory tumors is in agreement with results published by other authors with respect to operable tumors [5, 7, 8, 13, 22]. Nevertheless, we must point out that patients in our study were all subjected to the same systemic treatment (chemotherapy and hormonal therapy, this latter being adapted to the hormonal status of the patient: castration in the premenopausal patient and tamoxifen in the postmenopausal patient). It is thus possible that the efficiency of hormonal treatment is at least partially responsible for the favorable evolution of ER+ tumors, which should be hormone sensitive.

In summary, we found that:

1. Inflammatory tumors constitute a very specific group in terms of biological behavior and prognosis.
2. Within this group, there is a highly malignant subgroup without estrogen receptors, the evolution of which is not influenced by any treatment. On the other hand, the ER+ tumors retain a degree of tissular differentiation and have a better prognosis.

References

1. Bloom HJG (1950) Prognosis in carcinoma of the breast. Br J Cancer 4: 259−288
2. Bloom HJG, Richardson WW (1957) Histological grading and prognosis in breast cancer. A study of 1,409 cases of which 359 have been followed 15 years. Br J Cancer 11: 359−377
3. Boyd JT, Doll R (1954) Gastro-intestinal cancer and the use of liquid paraffin. Br J Cancer 8: 231−237
4. Contesso G, Rouesse J, Petit JY, Mouriesse H (1977) Les facteurs anatomo-pathologiques du pronostic des cancers du sein. Bull Cancer 64: 525−536
5. Cooke J, George O, Shields R, Maynard P, Griffiths K (1979) Estrogen Receptors and prognosis in early breast cancer. Lancet 1: 995−997
6. Fletcher WS, Montague FO (1975) Radical irradiation of advanced breast cancer. Am J Roentgen Radium Ther Nucl Med 3: 573−584

7. Fletcher WS, Leung BS, Davenport CE (1978) The prognostic significance of estrogen receptors in human breast cancer. Am J Surg 135: 372–374

8. Furmanski P, Saunders DE, Brooks SC, Rich MA (1980) The prognostic value of estrogen receptor determinations in patients with primary breast cancer. Cancer 46: 2794–2796

9. Haagensen CS (1971) Inflammatory carcinoma. In: Diseases of the breast. Saunders, Philadelphia, p 580

10. Horwitz KB, McGuire WL, Pearson OH, Segaloff A (1975) Predicting response to endocrine therapy in human breast cancer: a hypothesis. Science 189: 726–727

11. Kaplan EL, Meier P (1958) Non-parametric estimation from incomplete observations. J Am Statist Ass 53: 457–481

12. King RJB (1980) Analysis of estradiol and progesterone receptors in early and advanced breast tumors. Cancer 46: 2818–2821

13. Knight WA, Livingston RB, Gregory EJ, McGuire WL (1977) Estrogen receptor as an independent prognosis factor for early recurrence in breast cancer. Cancer Res 37: 4669–4671

14. Lacour J, Hourtoule FG (1967) La place de la chirurgie dans le traitement des formes évolutives du cancer du sein. Mem Acad Chir 635–643

15. Martin PM, Jacquemier J, Rolland PH, Rolland AM, Toga M (1978) Correlations entre les recepteurs hormonaux stéroïdiens et l'anatomo-pathologie des tumeurs mammaires humaines. Bull Cancer 65: 383–388

16. May-Levin F, Guerinot F, Contesso G, Delarue JC, Bohuon C (1977) Etude des récepteurs cytosoliques estrogènes et progestogènes dans les carcinomes mammaires. Int J Cancer 19: 789–795

17. Maynard PV, Davies CJ, Blamey RW, Elston CW, Johnson J, Griffiths K (1978) Relationship between oestrogen-receptor content and histological grade in human primary breast tumour. Br J Cancer 38: 745–748

18. McCarty KS Jr, Barton TK, Fetter BF, Woodard BH, Mossler JA, Reeves W, Daly J, Wilkinson WE, McCarty K (1980) Correlation of estrogen and progesterone receptors with histological differentiation in mammary carcinoma. Cancer 46: 2851–2858

19. McGuire WL, Vollmer EP, Carbone PP (eds) (1975) Estrogen receptors in human breast cancer. Raven, New York

20. McGuire WL, Raynaud JP, Baulieu EE (eds) (1977) Progesterone receptors in normal and neoplastic tissues. Raven, New York

21. Millis RR (1980) Correlation of hormone receptors with pathological features in human breast cancer. Cancer 46: 2869–2871

22. Osborne CK, Yochmowitz MG, Knight WA, McGuire WL (1980) The value of estrogen and progesterone receptors in the treatment of breast cancer. Cancer 46: 2884–2888

23. Peto R, McPike, Armitage P, Breslow N, Cox DR, Howard SV, Mantel N, McPherson K, Peto J, Smith PG (1976) Design and analysis of randomized clinical trials requiring prolonged observation of each patient. Br J Cancer 34: 585–612

24. Raynaud JP, Bouton MM, Philibert D, Delarue JC, Guerinot F, Bohuon C (1977) Progesterone and estradiol binding sites in human breast carcinoma. In: Vermeulen A (ed) Research in steroids, vol 7. Elsevier, Amsterdam, pp 281–290

25. Sarrazin D, Rouesse J, Arriagada R, May-Levin F, Petit JY, Contesso G (1978) Les cancers du sein en "poussée évolutive". Rev Prat 28: 999–1009

26. Scarff RW, Torloni H (1968) Coll international histological classification of tumors no 2. WHO, Geneva, pp 204–408

27. Wittliff JL, Beatty BW, Savlov ED, Patterson WB, Cooper RA (1976) Estrogen receptors and hormone dependency in human breast cancer. In: St Arneault G, Baud P, Israel L (eds) Breast cancer: a multidisciplinary approach. Springer, Berlin Heidelberg New York, pp 59–77 (Recent results in cancer research, vol 57)

Relationship Between Estrogen Receptors and Cellular Proliferation

R. Silvestrini, M. G. Daidone, A. Bertuzzi, and G. Di Fronzo

Istituto Nazionale per lo Studio e la Cura dei Tumori, Divisione di Oncologia Sperimentale C, Via Venezian 1, 20133 Milan, Italy

Introduction

In the past few years the biology of breast cancer has been the object of intensive studies. Kinetic and hormonal characteristics have been thoroughly investigated, and their clinical relevance as prognostic factors or predictors of response to therapy has also been analyzed. The studies focused on the hormonal features of breast cancer have identified estrogen receptor (ER) status as a promising marker for predicting hormone dependence. However, whereas different studies [12, 13] have consistently shown that ER is a good discriminant in rejecting endocrinotherapy for ER-negative (ER−) tumors, other end points of hormonal action have to be identified to define the actual hormonodependence of ER-positive (ER+) tumors. The reliability of ER status in predicting clinical response to cytotoxic therapy is still controversial [3, 4, 10, 11] and remains an open problem, whereas in the past few years the prognostic relevance of ER status on the clinical course of the disease in patients submitted to surgery alone has become more evident [1, 5, 8, 9, 18]. Recent studies on cell kinetics have evidenced the prognostic significance of cell proliferative rate of the primary tumor for recurrence in patients with negative lymph node (N−) cancers submitted to surgery alone [7, 14] and radiotherapy [17]. The influence of cell kinetics on response to chemotherapy is now being studied.

On the basis of these findings it is reasonable to suppose that hormonal and kinetic features are both important for the provision of a more complete biologic characterization and for defining the biologic aggressiveness of breast cancer. A combined study of both these features and analysis of the presence and the levels of ER in relation to proliferative activity can also aid in defining homogeneous biologic subgroups of clinical relevance for adequate planning of therapy.

Materials and Methods

The study of the kinetic and hormonal characteristics of breast cancer was carried out on 357 women who underwent radical mastectomy at the Istituto Nazionale Tumori of Milan

* The authors thank Ms. L. Ventura and Mr. R. Procopio for technical assistance, and Ms. B. Johnston for editing and preparing the manuscript. This study was supported by contract no. 79.00676.96 from the Consiglio Nazionale delle Ricerche, Target Project "Control of Tumor Growth", Rome

between November 1974 and October 1979. Patients ranged in age from 25 to 78 years, with a median age of 50 years. For all the analyses patients were considered in premenopause when actively menstruating at the time of diagnosis or when less than 1 year had elapsed since the last menstrual period. Patients were considered in paramenopause if 1−5 years had elapsed since the beginning of spontaneous menopause or 0−5 years had passed since oophorectomy. Patients were considered in postmenopause if more than 5 years had elapsed since the beginning of spontaneous menopause or since oophorectomy.

The determination of the primary tumor cell proliferative rate (^{3}H-thymidine labeling index, LI) was carried out immediately after surgery, according to a previously described standardized technique [16]. The LI ranged from 0.01% to 40.7% with a median value of 2.7%. The determination of ER was performed according to the EORTC method (6), using the dextran-coated charcoal technique. Evaluation of the apparent affinity constant (K_a) and the free receptor concentration (X_0) was carried out according to Scatchard [15].

Results

The analysis of ER status and proliferative activity, carried out on 357 cases to assess the relationship between the two biologic features, showed an inverse proportionality in 230 (64%) of the cases (Table 1). More precisely, ER+ and ER− status respectively correlated with low and high proliferative rate in about 60% and 70% of the cases. It should be emphasized that a large majority of slowly proliferating tumors (147 of 179, 82%) were ER+, whereas highly proliferating tumors were equally distributed, i.e., 53% ER+ and 47% ER−.

Taking into account the influence of cell hormonal features on proliferative activity, which can be summarized by a significantly higher proliferative rate in ER− than in ER+ tumors (median LI value 5.6% vs 2% in this series, $P < 0.0001$), the influence of patients' hormonal characteristics on cell proliferation of the primary cancer was also investigated. The proliferative activity showed broad variability for tumors from all the three menopausal status groups (Fig. 1). However, the frequency distribution of LI was similar for tumors from premenopausal and paramenopausal patients, and these were both significantly different than that observed for tumors from postmenopausal patients. The median LI value was significantly higher in the first two subgroups (3.8% and 4.3%, respectively) than in tumors from postmenopausal patients (1.6%).

Since both cell and patient hormonal characteristics significantly affect the proliferative activity of breast cancer, the next step in our biologic characterization was to analyze the

Table 1. Predictive accuracy of ER with regard to proliferative activity

Receptor status	No. of cases (percentage) with an LI	
	≤ 2.7%[a]	> 2.7%
ER+	147 (60)	95 (40)
ER−	32 (28)	83 (72)

[a] 2.7%, median LI value
$P < 0.00001$ (χ^2 test)

relevance of menopausal status for the relationship between ER status and proliferative activity of the tumor (Table 2). ER− cancers proliferated significantly faster than ER+ cancers in premenopausal and postmenopausal groups, whereas only a trend was observed for paramenopausal patients. Moreover, within both ER+ and ER− cancer subgroups a grading of proliferative activity from high to low values was observed from premenopause to postmenopause. The proliferative activity of tumors from paramenopausal patients was very similar to that observed for those from premenopausal patients, but statistically differed from the proliferative rate of tumors from postmenopausal patients only for ER+ cancers. However, the results concerning the paramenopausal group may be affected by the relatively small number of cases in this group.

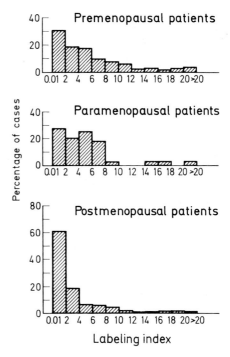

Fig. 1. Frequency distribution of labeling index in cancers from different menopausal groups: premenopausal patients (206 cases), paramenopausal patients (32 cases), postmenopausal patients (119 cases). Comparisons between frequency distribution were made by means of the χ^2 test: pre vs para, $P = 0.25$; pre vs post, $P < 0.0005$; para vs post, $P < 0.001$

Table 2. LI of primary tumors in relation to ER and menopausal status

Menopausal status	ER− tumors			ER+ tumors		
	No. of cases	LI (%)		No. of cases	LI (%)	
		Median	Range		Median	Range
Premenopause	79	6.1	0.3 −31.0	127	2.4	0.01−40.7
Paramenopause	8	6.1	0.6 −20.4	24	3.3	0.2 −30.0
Postmenopause	28	2.8	0.01−20.0	91	1.3	0.01−33.0

Comparisons between the ranked LI values were made using the Wilcoxon test
ER− vs ER+: pre ($P < 0.0001$), para ($P = 0.10$), post ($P = 0.007$)
ER−: pre vs para, $P = 0.9$; pre vs post, $P = 0.0006$; para vs post, $P = 0.17$
ER+: pre vs para, $P = 0.49$; pre vs post, $P = 0.0001$; para vs post, $P = 0.0015$

Table 3. Kinetic subgroups according to hormonal characteristics of the tumor and the patient

Group	Proliferative activity	Median LI value (%)	ER status	Menopausal status
I	High	6.1	−	Pre
		6.1	−	Para
II	Intermediate	2.4	+	Pre
		3.3	+	Para
		2.8	−	Post
III	Low	1.3	+	Post

Comparisons between the ranked LI values were made using the Wilcoxon test
High vs intermediate, $P < 0.0001$
High vs low, $P < 0.0001$
Intermediate vs low, $P < 0.0001$

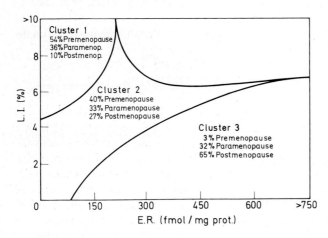

Fig. 2. Plot of cluster contours and specification of normalized cluster contents for the different menopausal groups. Normalized percentages of cluster contents were derived from the sum within the cluster of the percentages of the different menopausal groups

Taking into account these findings, three sets of tumors with statistically different median LI values were proposed (Table 3): the subgroup of tumors with a high proliferative rate included ER− tumors from premenopausal and possibly paramenopausal patients (due to the very similar median LI value); the subgroup of tumors with a low proliferative rate included ER+ tumors from postmenopausal patients; and the subgroup of tumors with an intermediate proliferative rate included all the other host and tumor hormonal situations.

A further investigation was carried out on the relationship between the degree of proliferative activity and the levels of ER in ER+ tumors. In spite of the wide ranges of ER levels observed for tumors from all the three menopausal groups, low, intermediate, and high median ER concentrations were observed in tumors from premenopausal, paramenopausal, and postmenopausal groups, respectively. A significant difference ($P = 0.0001$) was observed between median ER levels in tumors from premenopausal (31 fmol/mg protein) and postmenopausal (131 fmol/mg protein) groups as well as between median ER levels in tumors from premenopausal and paramenopausal groups (75 fmol/mg protein) ($P < 0.009$), whereas the ER levels observed in cancers from paramenopausal and postmenopausal patients were not statistically different ($P < 0.067$).

The analysis of the possible relationship between the degree of proliferative activity and ER levels in ER+ tumors showed no linear or exponential type of relation. However, the cluster analysis [2] led to the identification of three main clusters characterized by different patterns of ER and LI values, which were differently correlated with the menopausal status (Fig. 2). In spite of the presence of the three menopausal statuses in each cluster, cluster 1 showed a maximum frequency of premenopausal patients (54%) followed by para-menopausal (36%) and postmenopausal (10%) patients. An antithetical pattern was observed in cluster 3, whereas cluster 2 was equally composed of tumors from the three menopausal groups.

Conclusions

The study of the proliferative activity and the presence and levels of ER on the same tumor adds further information to the biologic knowledge of breast cancer, but at the same time clearly shows that the different biologic aspects are not simply related to each other. In fact, even if the median proliferative activity is significantly higher in ER− than in ER+ tumors, the ER status is inversely related to the rate of proliferative activity in only 64% of the cases, and the presence of such a correlation is not predictable on the basis of clinical or pathologic parameters at present available. Similarly, no relationship of a linear or exponential type was observed between ER levels and the degree of proliferative activity.

However, the combined analysis of hormonal and kinetic cell features in relation to menopausal status led to the identification of three main kinetic subgroups, which are defined by cell and patient hormonal characteristics. Moreover, an improved statistical approach led us to identify among ER+ tumors three main specific ER/LI clusters, which were significantly related to the different menopausal status. An antithetical pattern of ER and kinetic features was observed for cancers from premenopausal and postmenopausal patients, whereas tumors from paramenopausal patients presented all the possible associations of LI and ER values, with the same patterns of tumors as from premenopausal and postmenopausal patients.

Many questions still have to be answered to complete the basic knowledge of breast biology and to allow integrated use of such information for clinical purposes. For example, although we observed that ER+ tumors are not necessarily slowly proliferating, it still remains to be demonstrated whether the high proliferative activity is peculiar to the ER+ hormonodependent cell subpopulation in a condition of estrogen stimulation or to the ER− autonomous cell subpopulation. Furthermore, even if the kinetic and receptor patterns have proved to be related to biologic aggressiveness of the tumor and the latter partially indicative of hormonodependence, the improvement of the chemosensitivity tests and the identification of hormonosensitivity end points represent essential steps for rationalization of the planning of therapy.

References

1. Allegra JC, Lippman ME (1980) Estrogen receptor status and the disease-free interval in breast cancer. In: Henningsen B, Linder F, Streichele C (eds) Endocrine treatment of breast cancer. Springer, Berlin Heidelberg New York, pp 20−25 (Recent results in cancer research, vol 71)

2. Bertuzzi A, Daidone MG, Di Fronzo G, Silvestrini R (1981) Relationship among estrogen receptors, proliferative activity and menopausal status in breast cancer. Breast Cancer Res Treat 1: 253–262

3. Bonadonna G, Valagussa P, Tancini G, Di Fronzo G (1980) Estrogen-receptor status and response to chemotherapy in early and advanced breast cancer. Cancer Chemother Pharmacol 4: 37–41

4. Carter SK (1979) The dilemma of estrogen receptors and the response rate to cytotoxic chemotherapy. A problem of comparability analysis. Cancer Clin Trials 2: 49–53

5. Cooke T, George D, Shields R (1979) Oestrogen receptors and prognosis in early breast cancer. Lancet 1: 995–997

6. EORTC Breast Cancer Cooperative Group (1973) Standards for the assessment of estrogen receptors in human breast cancer. Eur J Cancer 9: 379–381

7. Gentili C, Sanfilippo O, Silvestrini R (1981) Cell proliferation in relation to clinical features and relapse in breast cancer. Cancer 48: 979

8. Hähnel R, Woodings T, Vivian AB (1979) Prognostic value of estrogen receptors in primary breast cancer. Cancer 44: 671–675

9. Hilf R, Feldstein ML, Gibson SL, Savlov ED (1980) The relative importance of estrogen receptor analysis as a prognostic factor for recurrence or response to chemotherapy in women with breast cancer. Cancer 45: 1993–2000

10. Kiang DT, Frenning DH, Goldman AI, Ascensao VF, Kennedy BJ (1978) Estrogen receptors and responses to chemotherapy and hormonal therapy in advanced breast cancer. N Engl J Med 299: 1330–1334

11. Lippman ME, Allegra JC, Thompson EB, Simon R, Barlock A, Green L, Huff KK, Do HMT, Aitken SC, Warren R (1978) The relation between estrogen receptors and response rate to cytotoxic chemotherapy in metastatic breast cancer. N Engl J Med 298: 1223–1228

12. McGuire WL (1978) Hormone receptors: Their role in predicting prognosis and response to endocrine therapy. Semin Oncol 5: 428–433

13. McGuire WL (ed) (1978) Progress in cancer research and therapy. X. Hormones, receptors and breast cancer. Raven, New York

14. Meyer JS, Hixon B (1979) Advanced stage and early relapse of breast carcinomas associated with high thymidine labeling indices. Cancer Res 39: 4042–4047

15. Scatchard G (1949) The attractions of protein for small molecules and ions. Ann NY Acad Sci 51: 600–672

16. Silvestrini R, Daidone MG, Di Fronzo G (1979) Relationship between proliferative activity and estrogen receptors in breast cancer. Cancer 44: 665–670

17. Tubiana M, Pejovic MJ, Renaud A, Contesso G, Chavaudra N, Gioanni J, Malaise EP (1981) Kinetic parameters and the course of the disease in breast cancer. Cancer 47: 937–943

18. Valagussa P, Di Fronzo G, Bignami P, Buzzoni R, Bonadonna G, Veronesi U (1981) Prognostic importance of estrogen receptors to select node-negative patients for adjuvant chemotherapy. In: Jones SE, Salmon SE (eds) Adjuvant therapy of cancer, 3rd edn. Grune and Stratton, New York

Relationship of Stromal Elastosis to Steroid Receptors in Human Breast Carcinoma

J. Jacquemier, R. Lieutaud, and P. M. Martin

Laboratoire d'Anatomie Pathologique, Institut J. Paoli I. Calmettes,
232 Boulevard de Sainte Marguerite, 13273 Marseille, Cedex 9 France

Introduction

In an attempt to improve the selection of patients with advanced breast cancer who can be expected to respond to endocrine therapy, we undertook to examine all correlations between the morphological appearance, of the tumor and steroid receptors. In earlier work we established that the combined presence of progesterone and estrogen receptors (PgR and ER respectively), which reflects hormone dependence better than ER alone, is associated with a certain type of differentiated lesion and a moderate degree of malignancy of neoplastic cells [10, 14, 19].

Elastosis arises from stromal modification accompanying the development of human breast cancer. It has been related to the presence of ER, the menopausal status of patients, and the response to endocrine therapy [2, 5, 6, 8, 14–16, 20]. Consequently to investigate the role of elastosis in human breast cancer, we examined three series of lesions, recording their ER and PgR, their histological differentiation, their histological grade, and finally the age and menopausal status of patients.

Materials and Methods

Populations

Five hundred and three cases of breast cancer were routinely investigated for ER and PgR content and pathological features. Of these 503, 113 were chosen for their eosinophilic stroma and investigated by Weigert's stain. This population was called A [18].

In addition, 40 cases without the morphological appearance of elastosis on usual coloration were investigated for Weigert staining. This population was called B.

Finally, we used Weigert staining to investigate the presence of elastosis in tumors of histological grade III. Lesions positive for both ER and PgR were analyzed separately (population c) in view of the usual low receptor positivity of this class of tumor.

Pathological Features

For each sample, a minimum of three sections along the lesion's two main axes were stained with hematein-eosin-saffran (HES). Histological type and grade (Scarff and Bloom) were recorded as previously described [12, 13].

Recent Results in Cancer Research. Vol. 91
© Springer-Verlag Berlin · Heidelberg 1984

Lesional elastosis was assessed according to a previously published technique [4, 10, 14], as follows: First, the presence of hyalin and eosinophilic deposits in the stroma was investigated, since they are thought to reflect the presence of elastin [4, 10]. Such deposits (HES-positive cases) were seen in 113 of our 503 lesions. Since this procedure does not, in fact, discriminate between elastosis and fibrohyalin and/or fibrinoid deposits that are not elastic fibers, elastosis was assessed on additional slides treated with Weigert's stain, which specifically stains elastin and elastic fibers. With this technique only 91 of the 113 lesions containing eosinophilic deposits were found to show true elastosis. Elastosis was graded as follows: grade 0, no evidence of elastic fibers; grade 1, presence of some thin elastic fibers; grade 2, moderate elastosis; and grade 3, marked evidence of elastosis. Five groups of lesions were considered according to the location of the elastosis: ductal, interstitial, ductal + interstitial, vascular, and vascular + ductal.

Steroid Receptor Analysis

The ER and PgR content of lesions was determined, as previously described [11], by a dextran-coated charcoal adsorption technique in which moxestrol and promegestone are used as radioligands. Results are expressed in femtomoles per milligram of cytosol protein and lesions were considered positive if they were above 10 fmol.

Menopausal status was assessed on the basis of plasma hormone levels and clinical examination (a minimum of 2 years without menstruation was used as the criterion for attainment of menopause). In this particular series, as well as in our general population of patients (more than 2,000 [12, 13], menopause occurred on average at the age of 50 years.

Statistical Analysis

The statistical analysis was based on Student's t-test and the χ^2 test, with Yate's correction for small populations. To investigate the possibility of bias in the composition of the HES-positive population (113 cases), a paired control population (also 113 cases) was randomly chosen from 450 human breast cancer patients not included in the 503 cases of this series, and was used to further validate the statistical analysis. For populations B and C, we used the Fisher exact probability test and the χ^2 test.

Results

Elastosis and Menopausal Status

The distribution of patients according to either their menopausal status or the histological type of lesion was statistically identical with the distribution found in both the overall and in the control populations. The same distribution of menopausal and premenopausal patients was observed in both the Weigert-negative and the Weigert-positive populations (Table 1). Furthermore, the mean number of pregnancies was unrelated to the grade of elastosis (Table 2).

In both premenopausal and menopausal patients, neither the grade of elastosis (Table 2) nor the ductal and interstitial topography of elastosis (Table 3) led to any discrimination among patients. However, vascular elastosis was only encountered in menopausal patients (Table 3).

Table 1. Relationship between elastosis and menopausal status[a]

	Overall population	Control population	Hes-positive population	Weigert's stain	
				Negative	Positive
Premenopausal patients	144 (28.6%)	26 (22.2%)	35 (30.9%)	7 (31.8%)	28 (30.7%)
Menopausal patients	359 (71.8%)	88 (77.8%)	78 (69.1%)	15 (68.2%)	63 (69.3%)
Total	503	113	113	22	91

[a] Results are expressed as numbers of cases and, in parentheses, as percentages of their respective populations

Table 2. Relationship between grade elastosis, menopausal status, and number of pregnancies in population A[a]

	Elastosis, grade			
	0	1	2	3
Premenopausal patients	7 (31.8%)	10 (43.5%)	9 (23.1%)	9 (31.0%)
Menopausal patients	15 (68.2%)	13 (56.5%)	30 (76.9%)	20 (69.0%)
Pregnancies (mean)	2.4	2.6	2.1	3.1

[a] Results are expressed as numbers of cases and, in parentheses, as percentages of their respective populations

Table 3. Relationship between elastosis topography and menopausal status in population A[a]

Topography	Ductal	Interstitial	Ductal and Interstitial	Vascular	Vascular and ductal
Premenopausal patients	7 (30,4%)	11 (34.4%)	10 (30.3%)	–	1 (12.5%)
Menopausal patients	16 (69.6%)	21 (65.6%)	23 (69.7%)	3	7 (87.5%)
Total	23	32	33	3	8

[a] Results are expressed as numbers of cases and, in parentheses, as percentages of their respective populations

Elastosis and Histopathological Differentiation and Prognosis

Elastosis was encountered more often in histologically differentiated lesions ($P < 0.01$). The grade of elastosis was not, however, related to this feature (data not shown) (Table 4).

Table 4. Relationship between elastosis and histological type of lesion[a]

Histological type	Overall population	Control population	Hes-positive population	Weigert's stain	
				Negative	Positive
Well-differentiated	30	5	7	0	7
Polymorphic	250	58	76	11	65
Atypical	156	38	17	6	11
Lobular infiltrate	22	7	8	1	7
Isolated cells	4	1	1	0	1
Ductal	14	2	2	2	0
Medullary	11	1	1	1	0
Colloid	8	1	1	1	0
Total	503	113	113	22	91

[a] Results are expressed as numbers of cases

Table 5. Relationship between elastosis and histological grade of lesion[a]

	GI	GII	GIII	Total
General population	53	228	163	503
	(10,8%)	(45,3%)	(32,4%)	
Population B	7	21	12	40
	(17.5%)	(52.5%)	(30%)	
Rate of elastosis	7	16	7	30
in population B	(100%)	(76.1%)	(58.3%)	

[a] Results are expressed as numbers of cases and, in parentheses, as percentages of their respective populations

In population B, investigated by Weigert staining, the distribution of histological grades was not significantly different from that among the total population of 503 cases (Table 5). The rate of elastosis in population B was 75% (30/40), which is similar to that found by other authors [2, 4, 8, 10]. Elastosis was significantly correlated with histological grade, being more frequent in tumors of grades I and II than in those of grade III ($P < 0.06$).

Elastosis and Steroid Receptors

The presence of elastosis was found to be associated with the presence of steroid receptors (Table 6). In premenopausal patients whose lesions showed signs of elastosis, an increased incidence of both ER and PgR was observed ($P < 0.05$). In these patients, elastosis-positive lesions showed a higher ER content (177 ± 187 fmol) than either the overall population (83 ± 63 fmol) or the control (76 ± 70 fmol) population ($P < 0.01$). Similarly, in menopausal patients there was a relationship between the presence of elastosis and both ER and PgR ($P < 0.02$). In these patients, elastosis-positive lesions apparently had higher ER contents (213 ± 177 fmol) than did elastosis-negative specimens (170 ± 220 fmol), but this relationship was not statistically significant.

Table 6. Relationship between elastosis and steroid receptors for population A[a]

Menopausal status	Receptor status	Overall population	Control population	Hes-positive population	Weigert's stain	
					Negative	Positive
Premeno-	ER+	86	17	25	2	23
pausal	ER−	38	8	10	5	5
patients	PgR+	37	9	7	3	4
	PgR−	87	16	22	20	2
Menopausal	ER+	272	67	57	9	48
patients	ER−	107	21	21	6	15
	PgR+	116	32	34	6	28
	PgR−	263	56	17	7	10

[a] Results are expressed as numbers of cases with (+) or without (−) ER or PgR

Table 7. Elastosis and histological grade III in populations B and C[a]

	Grade III, population B	Grade III, population C
Elastosis positive	7 (58.3%)	12 (80%)
Elastosis negative	5 (41.6%)	3 (20%)
Total	12	15

[a] Results are expressed as numbers of cases and, in parentheses, as percentages of their respective populations

Elastosis and Hormonedependency

In Table 7 we compare the presence of elastosis in patients with grade III tumors from populations B and C. Population C was hormone dependent as shown by the presence of both ER+ and PgR+. Elastosis was more frequent in population C than in population B; however, the difference was not significant ($\chi^2 = 3.33$) in view of the small number of cases.

Discussion

Following works from other authors [11, 17] which showed a good correlation between steroid receptors and morphological epithelial features, our attention has been focused on the stromal changes leading to elastosis in breast carcinomas. Our results indicate (a) that the presence of elastosis is not related to menopausal status and (b) that its topography is not related to the number of pregnancies. The vascular elastosis only encountered in menopausal patients was not considered for the correlations. But the stromal reaction of elastosis may be related to the morphological differentiation of the breast carcinomas. This relationship is supported by in vitro findings showing that the onset of extracellular matrix protein synthesis, including elastin synthesis, is associated with cell differentiation processes [9]. Thus elastosis in lesions could be related to the presence of cells that have retained, at least in part, both their physiological differentiation and their tissular dependence.

Histological grade reflects the degree of malignancy of lesions and is a factor of prognostic significance for the survival of patients [13]. We report here that elastosis is related to lesions of histological grades I and II, i.e., those exhibiting a moderate degree of malignancy. As a tentative explanation for such findings, it has been suggested that the elastic fibers wall in the cells and constitute a mechanical barrier to tumor spread [3]. An increased 5-year survival rate has been reported for patients having elastosis-positive lesions [20], supporting the idea of a relationship between elastosis and lesions of histological grades I and II.

Elastosis is related to the presence of ER and PgR in human breast carcinomas, the statistical relationship depending upon menopausal status and receptor hormone class. In premenopausal women, the relationship between elastosis and ER was found to be more significant than in menopausal patients, whereas the reverse was true for PgR. These results suggest that before the menopause, the frequency of elastosis is lower in cases where ER and PgR are both present. In postmenopausal patients, the frequency of ER is higher than in premenopausal women [12]. Since the combination of ER and PgR probably reflects hormone dependence better than ER alone, some of the ER may, for some reason, be nonfunctional and unable to induce PgR [7, 13]. The combination of elastosis and ER status has been shown to give a better prediction of clinical response to endocrine therapy than either ER or elastosis alone [17].

The above findings strongly suggest that elastosis results from the presence of hormone-dependent neoplastic cells in human breast carcinomas. To confirm this idea we investigated the presence of elastosis in a small population of patients with less differentiated carcinoma who were ER and PgR positive. Our results confirm that elastosis is strongly correlated with hormone dependence in this population, but the population was too small for the results to be of statistical significance.

The underlying mechanism regulating elastosis in human breast cancer remains to be established, but these results suggest that the presence of hormone-dependent cells can be demonstrated both by their biochemical and by their pathological features.

References

1. Adnet JJ, Pinteaux A, Pousse G, Caulet T (1976) Caractérisation du tissu élastique normal et pathologique en microscopie électronique. Pathol Biol (Paris) 24:293–296
2. Azzopardi JG, Path CP, Laurini RN (1974) Elastosis in breast cancer. Cancer 35:174–183
3. Cameron E, Pauling L, Leibowitz B (1979) Ascorbic acid and cancer. A review. Cancer Res 39:663–681
4. Douglas-Davis J (1973) Hyperelastosis, obliteration and fibrous plaques in major ducts of human breast. J Pathol 110:13–26
5. Fisher RR, Gregorio RM, Fisher B (1975) The pathology of invasive breast cancer. Cancer 36:1–85
6. Hornebeck W, Adnet JJ, Robert L (1978) Age dependent variation of elastic and elastase in aorta and human breast cancers. Exp Gerontol 13:293–298
7. Horwitz KB, McGuire WL (1977) Estrogen and progesterone, their relationships in hormone-dependent breast cancer. In: McGuire WL, Raynaud JP, Baulien EE (eds) Progesterone receptors in normal and neoplastic tissues. Raven, New York, pp 102–124

 8. Jackson JG, Orr JW (1957) The ducts of carcinomatous breasts with particular reference to connective tissue changes. J Pathol 74: 265−273
 9. Jones PJ, Scott-Burden T, Gevers W (1979) Glycoprotein, elastin and collagen secretion by rat smooth muscle cells. Proc Natl Acad Sci USA 76: 353−357
10. Lundmark C (1972) Breast cancer and elastosis. Cancer 30: 1195−1201
11. Martinez-Hernandez A, Francis DJ, Silverberg G (1977) Elastosis and other stromal reactions in benign and malignant breast tissue: an ultrastructural study. Cancer 40: 700−706
12. Martin PM, Rolland PH, Jacquemier J, Rolland AM, Toga M (1978) Multiple steroid receptors in human breast cancer I. Technological features. Biomedicine 28: 278−287
13. Martin PM, Rolland PH, Jacquemier J, Rolland AM, Toga M (1979) Multiple steroid receptors in human breast cancer. II. Estrogen and progestin receptors in 672 primary tumors. Cancer Chemother Pharmacol 2: 107−113
14. Martin PM, Rolland PH, Jacquemier J, Rolland AM, Toga M (1979) Multiple steroid receptors in human breast cancer. III. Relationships between steroid receptors and the state of differentiation and the activity of carcinomas throughout the pathologic features. Cancer Chemother Pharmacol 2: 115−120
15. Masters JRW, Sangster K, Hawkins RA, Shivas AA (1976) Elastosis and estrogen receptors in human breast cancer. Br J Cancer 33: 342−343
16. Masters JW, Hawkins RA, Sangster K, Hawkins W, Smith II, Shivas A, Roberts MM, Forrest APM (1978) Estrogen receptors, cellularity, elastosis in human breast cancer. Eur J Cancer 14: 303−307
17. Masters JRW, Millis RR, King RJB, Rubens RD (1979) Elastosis and response to endocrine therapy in human breast cancer. Br J Cancer 39: 356−547
18. Rolland PH, Jacquemier J, Martin PM (1980) Histological differentiation in human breast cancer is related to steroid receptors and stromal elastosis. Cancer Chemother Pharmacol 5: 73−77
19. Shivas AA, Douglas JG (1972) The prognostic significance of elastosis in breast carcinomas. JR Coll Surg Edinb 17: 315−320
20. Tremblay G (1976) Ultrastructure of elastosis in scirrhous carcinoma of the breast. Cancer 37: 307−316

Part III: A Critical Summary

G. Contesso, J. C. Delarue, F. May-Levin, H. Sancho-Garnier, and H. Mouriesse

Institut Gustave-Roussy, 39 Rue Camille Desmoulins, 94805 Villejuif Cedex, France

At present, assay of hormone receptors is a good method of estimating the hormone sensitivity or independence of a patient with breast cancer. However, in certain cases the results should be analyzed circumspectly.

The close connection, which varies in degree, between these assays and the specific clinical and histological characteristics of a tumor has been noted by several teams and allows the determination of groups of patients with a greater or lesser risk of metastases and thus a better treatment plan, adapted to each patient.

As far as the interpretation of assays of certain types of tumors is concerned, in the literature one can find reference to a small but not negligible number (5%−10%) of estrogen receptor negative (ER−) breast tumors which were nevertheless hormone sensitive. Until now, it has been thought possible that this phenomenon is due to faulty storage of a sample or to an incorrect assay having brought about the denaturation of the receptors. The articles in this section have shown that endogenic hormones may be implicated: estradiol either circulating in premenopausal women or synthesized inside the tumor in postmenopausal women.

The paper by S. Saez et al. shows that in premenopausal women:

1. The presence of circulating estrogen is necessary for the stimulation of ER, without these receptors varying according to the hormone cycle. Whether or not ER might be blocked by endogenic estradiol is unknown. Although this idea has been accepted by many authors, it has been disputed by others.

2. The cytosolic progesterone receptors (PgR), on the other hand, vary during the hormone cycle. These results confirm that PgR synthesis is estrogen dependent and that the theoretical hormone resistance of an ER+ PgR− tumor should be regarded with circumspection in the presence of a high concentration of plasmatic progesterone.

Simultaneous assay of cytosolic and nuclear receptors and determination of the concentration of circulating progesterone should allow evaluation of the exact role played by endogenic hormones (we are currently studying this question).

In postmenopausal women, concentrations of plasmatic estradiol are obviously low and the intratumoral biosynthesis of estradiol may then have a certain clinical importance. According to K. Carlström, this biosynthesis takes place mainly by hydrolysis of estrogenic conjugates. Biosynthesis of estradiol may saturate the receptor sites, leading to a low concentration of ER, even with low concentrations of peripheral estrogens.

The connections between hormone receptors and the other characteristics of breast tumors were the subject of several chapters:

Recent Results in Cancer Research. Vol. 91
© Springer-Verlag Berlin · Heidelberg 1984

In a series of 490 patients, Andry and co-workers show that the size of the tumor and the invasion of lymphnodes are both independent of receptor status. However, some histological types, like the tubular and lobular carcinomas and especially tumors of low histological grade (I or II), entail a higher ER concentration.

This observation is confirmed by the study by Silvestrini and co-workers on the labeling index (LI). They found a low LI level, i.e., a low proliferative rate, in ER+ tumors. However, the presence of hormone receptors may reflect not only the biological activity of a tumoral cell but also that of its connective environment; thus the work of Jacquemier and co-workers shows that a close relationship exists between considerable elastotic stromal modification and ER positivity. On the other hand, Contesso and co-workers show (as might have been expected) that hormone receptors are usually totally absent in inflammatory tumors of the human breast, which are characterized by their rapid rate of growth and which are often undifferentiated, having a high histological grade.

The clinical importance of these observations lies in being able to foresee the evolution of the disease and thus being able to prepare a better treatment plan for each patient. With regard to the most common groups of mammary carcinoma (directly operable), many teams have observed that recurrences are more frequent, occur earlier, and have a lower survival rate when no ER are present. As shown by Contesso and co-workers, this also pertains to inflammatory tumors (Pev 2 and 3): patients without ER had a much more serious evolution, the rate of remission being only 5% after 3 years despite treatment.

The above-mentioned studies of hormone receptor assays generally take into account only a single characteristic (such as cell proliferation and elastosis) and can therefore be considered individually. This is not the case with studies concerning prognostic factors. The prognostic value of certain clinical and histological characteristics − e.g., the evolutionary phase, the number of metastatic nodes, and the histological grade − has, in fact, been extensively demonstrated both in Europe and in the United States. Thus when analyzing the role of hormone receptors, all the prognostic factors known from multifactorial analyses, such as that recently carried out by Rosen et al., should be taken into account. An independent role can then be assigned to these receptors and taken into consideration alongside other prognostic factors when planning the individualized treatment of breast cancer.

Part IV. The Course of Disease

Estrogen Receptor Variations in Neoplastic Tissue During the Course of Disease in Patients with Recurrent Breast Cancer*

S. Toma, G. Leclercq, N. Legros, R. J. Sylvester, J. C. Heuson, and R. J. Paridaens

Institut Jules Bordet, Centre des Tumeurs de l'Université Libre de Bruxelles, Service de Médicine, Clinique et Laboratoire de Cancérologie Mammaire, Rue Héger-Bordet 1, 1000 Bruxelles, Belgium

Introduction

In recent years, it has been repeatedly demonstrated that estrogen receptor (ER) assays are useful as a therapeutic guide in the treatment of advanced breast cancer. The validity of this tool in predicting the results of endocrine treatments has been confirmed in our laboratory [1, 2] as well as in many others (review article, ref. [3]). Moreover, we found that among several variables known to have a predictive value, receptor concentration was the one most significantly related to the therapeutic response; the presence or absence of ER was of lesser value [1, 2].

In our experience, receptor concentrations of multiple biopsies taken on the same day from the same patient are quite consistent [4]. A good consistency was also observed in patients who had multiple sequential assays during the course of their disease, when no intervening systemic therapy was given [1]. From these data it was concluded that ER concentration was a characteristic feature of a given patient, and that routine receptor determination on the primary could provide a useful guide to therapy at the time of relapse in previously untreated patients [1]. Little, however, is known about the possible influence of systemic treatments such as hormones or chemotherapy on the ER content in a given patient. Here we intend to report our experience concerning receptor variations during the course of disease in patients with recurrent breast cancer.

Patients and Methods

Patients

The medical records of all patients with breast cancer for whom two or more consecutive ER assays were performed in our laboratory were reviewed. We excluded from the analysis those patients with bilateral breast cancer and those who had received a systemic antineoplastic treatment with hormones and/or chemotherapy before the first assay.

---

* Part of this work was supported by a grant from the Fonds Cancérologique de la Caisse Générale d'Epargne et de Retraite (CGER) de Belgique and by grant number 5R10-CA 11488-11 awarded by the National Cancer Institute, DHEW

ER Assay

All samples subjected to the ER assay were also verified histologically for the presence of neoplastic tissue. All biopsies came from our operating room and were immediately processed to remove blood, necrotic tissue, and adipose tissue, before being stored in liquid nitrogen [5]. ER concentration of the samples was evaluated by measuring the ^{3}H-estradiol-17β binding capacity of their cytosol fraction using a dextran-coated charcoal method previously described [5]. Binding capacity was expressed as femtomoles (10^{-15} mol) per milligram of tissue protein. Evaluation of ER concentration was considered impossible in samples with low protein content (< 1 mg/ml).

Results

General Characteristics of the Samples Analyzed

The samples consisted of primary tumors, local recurrences, or distant soft tissue metastases, except in four cases, in which they were taken from the bone (one patient), the liver (two patients), or the ovary (one patient). Premenopausal patients generally had lower receptor values than postmenopausal patients, but receptor concentrations varied over a wide range in both groups.

Consecutive ER Assays in the Absence of Intercurrent Systemic Treatment

The data pertaining to 44 patients are given in Fig. 1. The symbols designate the results of two consecutive assays in individual patients in the absence of intervening treatment. Two patients underwent three consecutive assays and are thus represented twice on the graph.

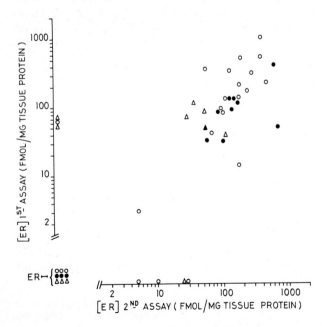

Fig. 1. Estrogen receptor *(ER)* concentrations in consecutive biopsies of neoplastic tissue without intercurrent systemic treatment. The following symbols are used: premenopausal patients, first assay performed on the primary ($\triangle$) or on a metastasis ($\blacktriangle$); postmenopausal patients, first assay performed on the primary ($\bigcirc$) or on a metastasis ($\bullet$)

The details of the statistical analysis have already been published [1, 2], so that only the conclusion will be summarized here.

Taking into consideration the 33 patients in whom the first ER assay was positive (ER+), a significant correlation was found between the two consecutive values ($P = 0.013$). The correlation remained significant in the subset of 26 postmenopausal patients ($P = 0.018$). However, no conclusion could be drawn for the premenopausal patients, the sample size being too small.

Among 13 patients with an initially negative (ER−) assay, nine (69%) remained negative at the second assay whereas only four became ER+. In the latter, ER concentration was always very low, i.e., always below 30 fmol/mg tissue protein.

Finally, the time lapse separating the consecutive assays (range, 15 days to 63 months; median 16 months) did not influence the ER variations.

Effect of Systemic Treatments on the ER Assay (Unpublished Data)

The data pertaining to 42 patients are presented in Fig. 2. Intercurrent treatments were as follows: single endocrine therapy in 12 patients, consisting of oophorectomy in two premenopausal patients and of either estrogens (one patient) or antiestrogens (nine patients) in postmenopausal patients; combination chemotherapy (CMF)[1] in 14 cases, generally administered as an adjuvant treatment after mastectomy; hormonochemotherapy in 16 cases, combining various modalities of endocrine treatment (mainly tamoxifen) with various standard chemotherapy regimens (CMF, AV[2], etc.).

Considering only the first assay performed after systemic therapy, the mean receptor concentration was markedly lower after treatment (71 fmol/mg tissue protein) than before

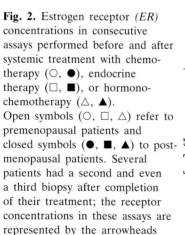

Fig. 2. Estrogen receptor *(ER)* concentrations in consecutive assays performed before and after systemic treatment with chemotherapy (○, ●), endocrine therapy (□, ■), or hormonochemotherapy (△, ▲). Open symbols (○, □, △) refer to premenopausal patients and closed symbols (●, ■, ▲) to postmenopausal patients. Several patients had a second and even a third biopsy after completion of their treatment; the receptor concentrations in these assays are represented by the arrowheads

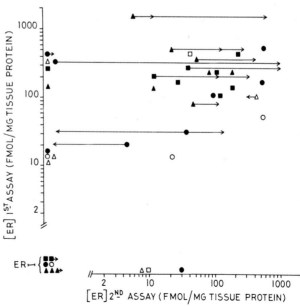

---

1 Cyclophosphamide, methotrexate, fluorouracil
2 Adriamycin, vincristine

Table 1. Mean ER concentration (fmol/mg tissue protein) before and after systemic antineoplastic treatment

	All cases	All drugs stopped since			
		< 3 months	3–12 months	> 12 months	> 24 months
No. of cases	42[a]	16	21	21	10
ER before treatment	195	237	215	229	161
ER after treatment	71[b]	17	143	170	243
Ratio $\left(\frac{\text{after}}{\text{before}} \times 100\right)$	36%	7%	67%	74%	151%

[a] Note that 13 patients underwent more than one receptor assay after systemic treatment
[b] First assay after treatment

(195 fmol). Five cases with high receptor values, above 100 fmol, were even negative at the second assay. Such a phenomenon did not occur in the group of untreated cases.

After completion of treatment, 13 patients underwent more than one receptor assay. Interestingly, as shown by the arrows in Fig. 2, ER values generally tended to rise when the delay after treatment interruption increased. In Table 1, the receptor variations are analyzed in relation to the time elapsed since drug withdrawal. Mean receptor values were low when the assays were performed less than 3 months after the end of treatment. ER concentrations later increased and became very close to their initial values when the delay exceeded 1 year.

The effects of hormonotherapy and chemotherapy have also been analyzed (data not shown in detail). The mean receptor concentration dropped apparently more after hormonotherapy (12 patients; 199 fmol before vs 57 fmol after treatment) or hormonochemotherapy (16 patients; 251 vs 46 fmol) than after chemotherapy alone (14 patients; 128 vs 110 fmol).

Discussion

As stated above, performing routine receptor assays on the primary tumor is useful. Since tumor tissue is not always available at the time of generalization, the information obtained from the assay on the primary can serve as a guide for therapy. This is true when no intercurrent treatment has been given. Our present results indicate that systemic treatment with hormones and/or chemotherapy markedly affects the results of ER assays in patients with advanced breast cancer. Thus, receptor concentrations are frequently lower after treatment, sometimes reaching undetectable levels, especially if treatment has been administered within 3 months of the assay. This effect tends, however, to vanish with time, and ER values in recurrences arising more than 1 year after drug withdrawal are close to those of the initial assay performed before treatment.

How systemic treatment affects the receptor content of tumors is largely unknown and remains a matter for speculation. Tumors might be a mixture of cells with various degrees of hormone sensitivity. Endocrine treatments kill specifically hormone-dependent cells and are thus likely to favor the emergence of receptor-negative clones. This could explain, at least in part, why the receptor concentrations dropped apparently more after endocrine treatments than after chemotherapy alone. As shown elsewhere in this book (Part III;

chapter by G. Andry et al.), the receptor content within a tumor might reflect its degree of differentiation, the latter being influenced by systemic treatments for more or less prolonged periods. In addition, drugs might interact directly with the ER machinery. In this regard, tamoxifen is known to induce a depletion of cytoplasmic receptors by translocating them into the nucleus and by inhibiting their resynthesis (review, ref. [6]). This effect will persist for a long time after discontinuation of treatment since tamoxifen and its principal antiestrogenic metabolite, desmethyltamoxifen, have very long biologic half-lives [7]. It is not known whether tamoxifen-induced receptor depletion would transiently affect the response to other modalities of endocrine therapy.

From a practical point of view, whenever possible and especially after systemic treatment, a biopsy of neoplastic tissue should be carried out before any therapeutic decision is made. The results of an assay performed during treatment or within a few weeks after drug withdrawal should, however, be interpreted with great caution. In this situation, the hormone dependency of the tumor could be underestimated by a falsely low or negative assay.

References

1. Paridaens R, Sylvester RJ, Ferrazzi E, Legros N, Leclercq G, Heuson JC (1980) Clinical significance of the quantitative assessment of estrogen receptors in advanced breast cancer. Cancer 46: 2889–2895
2. Heuson JC, Paridaens R, Ferrazzi E, Legros N, Leclerq G, Sylvester RJ (1981) Contribution of estrogen receptors to the strategy of breast cancer treatment. In: Hollmann KH, de Brux J, Verley JM (eds) New frontiers in mammary pathology. Plenum, New York, pp 267–285
3. Hawkins RA, Roberts MM, Forrest APM (1980) Oestrogen receptors and breast cancer: current status. Br J Surg 67: 153–169
4. Leclercq G, Heuson JC (1976) Estrogen receptors in the spectrum of breast cancer. Curr Probl Cancer 1 (6): 3–34
5. Leclercq G, Heuson JC, Schoenfeld R, Mattheiem WH, Tagnon HJ (1973) Estrogen receptors in human breast cancer. Eur J Cancer 9: 665–673
6. Paridaens RJ, Heuson JC (1979) Steroids, In: Pinedo HM (ed) Cancer chemotherapy. Excerpta Medica, Amsterdam, pp 167–181
7. Patterson JS, Settatree RS, Adam AK, Kemp JV (1980) Serum concentrations of tamoxifen and major metabolite during long-term Nolvadex therapy, correlated with clinical response. In: Mouridsen HT, Palshof T (eds) Breast cancer – experimental and clinical aspects. Pergamon, Oxford, pp 89–92

Prognostic Value of Progesterone Receptors in Primary Breast Cancer

M. F. Pichon, C. Pallud, M. Brunet, and E. Milgrom

Groupe de Recherches sur la Biochimie Endocrinienne et la Reproduction (INSERM U. 135), Faculté de Médecine de Bicêtre, Universite Paris-Sud, 78 rue du Général Leclerc, 94270 Kremlin-Bicêtre, France

Introduction

The presence of estradiol (ER) and progesterone (PgR) receptors in breast tumors determines the likelihood of their hormone dependency. Recently, several studies have shown that, generally, a better clinical evolution is observed when the primitive tumor contains ER, suggesting that steroid receptors might have a prognostic value in early breast cancer.

Almost all the studies on the prognostic value of ER in primary breast cancer report that ER-negative tumors recur earlier than ER-positive tumors. The recurrence rates observed in the two groups are independent of other classical prognostic factors such as age, menopause, and presence and number of invaded lymph nodes [1, 3, 4, 6, 17, 18]. However, the differences between ER-positive and ER-negative tumors in this respect are often small (8% at 30 months follow-up in the study of Saez et al. [16] and 10.5% in the study of Maynard et al. [11]) and require large patient populations to be statistically demonstrated. Indeed, the predictive value of ER status for any one patient is insufficient for it to serve as a basis for therapeutic strategy.

Our results, set out below, show that PgR status is in fact more efficient as a prognostic factor, since clear differences were observed in the evolution of the disease according to PgR presence or absence [cf. 15].

Patients and Methods

Since 1974, PgR has been measured in tumors from all patients with operable breast cancer treated at the Centre René Huguenin. Results were then related to the disease-free interval.

The patient population was composed of 98 women with histologically documented adenocarcinoma of the breast. The mean age of the patients was 60.3 years (range 35–88). The patients were operated on and followed up exclusively at the Centre. Pseudo-inflammatory, bilateral, or multiple cancers were excluded from the study.

Estradiol and progesterone receptor assays were performed on primary tumors using a dextran-coated charcoal technique with 10 fmol/mg cytosol protein as the limit for receptor positivity [14]. Fifty-four tumors were PgR positive and 44 PgR negative.

Recent Results in Cancer Research. Vol. 91
© Springer-Verlag Berlin · Heidelberg 1984

Table 1. Clinical characteristics of the patients

	PgR+ (n = 54)	PgR− (n = 44)	ER+ (n = 94)	ER− (n = 11)
Premenopause	16	11	25	2
Postmenopause[a]	31	26	55	7
With invaded axillary nodes	25	15	36	5
Without invaded axillary nodes	24	24	45	6
Stage of the disease				
I	4	5	9	0
II	36	22	57	6
III	14	17	28	5
Grade of the tumor				
I	4	1	6	0
II	24	13	37	2
III	20	19	34	7

[a] Natural menopauses only

The stage of the disease was determined according to the UICC recommendations, and tumor biopsies were graded by the technique of Scarff, Bloom, and Richardson [2]. Clinical characteristics are summarized in Table 1.

Graphs were derived from the life table analysis by the actuarial method; comparison between groups was by the log rank test, the χ^2 test being used to assess the statistical significance between groups [9, 13].

Results

PgR as a Prognostic Factor in Early Breast Cancer

During a mean follow-up of 25 months, six of 54 patients with PgR-positive tumors presented with recurrences, whereas 17 of 44 in the PgR-negative group did so (Table 2). This difference is significant ($P = 0.04$) (Fig. 1).

Of the 105 patients, nine received adjuvant chemotherapy. Results of statistical analysis are not altered when these patients are excluded.

Further analysis distinguishing between local recurrences and metastatic spread showed that PgR status was not related to both types of evolution. No connection was found between the occurrence of local recurrences and the presence or absence of PgR in the primary tumor: three of seven PgR-positive and four of seven PgR-negative tumors recurred locally ($P = 0.6$).

On the other hand, early metastatic spread was observed among patients with PgR-negative tumors (Fig. 2). During a mean follow-up period of 25 months, 16 patients developed metastases. Among this group, only three of the patients belonged to the PgR-positive group, the other 13 having PgR-negative tumors ($P = 0.02$). Using the log rank test, we estimated that the absence of PgR in a tumor represents a 3.6 times higher risk of metastatic spread.

Table 2. Results of follow-up studies

	PgR+ (n = 54)	PgR− (n = 44)	ER+ (n = 94)	ER− (n = 11)
Deaths	3	8	12	3
Total no. of recurrences[a]	6	16	21	5
Metastases	3	4	7	2
Local recurrences	3	13	15	4

[a] Three patients evidenced both metastases and local recurrences

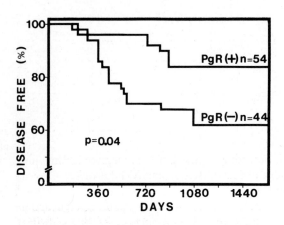

Fig. 1. Disease-free interval and PgR status in primary breast cancer

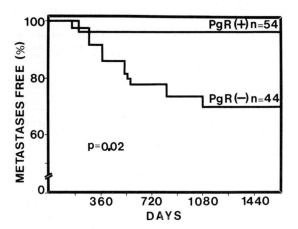

Fig. 2. Occurrence of metastases and PgR in primary tumors

The probability of metastatic spread decreases with increasing concentrations of PgR (Table 3). In the group of 17 patients with a PgR concentration in tumors of more than 200 fmol/mg protein, there were no recurrences during a mean observation time of 23 months.

The difference in the occurrence of metastases according to PgR status in the primary tumor remained significant ($P < 0.05$) when premenopausal and postmenopausal patients were studied separately.

Table 3. PgR concentration in primary tumors and occurrence of metastases

PgR concentration (fmol/mg protein)	No. of patients developing metastases/total no. of patients
0	12/42
1– 9	1/2
10– 99	2/26
100–199	1/11
> 200	0/17

$\chi^2 = 8.1$ $P = 0.08$ χ^2 for trend 5.9 $P = 0.01$

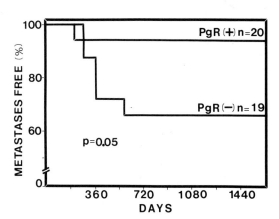

Fig. 3. Occurrence of metastases and PgR in patients with invaded axillary nodes

Fig. 4. Occurrence of metastases and PgR in patients with grade III tumors

Prognostic Value of PgR Among Patients with Invaded Axillary Nodes or Poorly Differentiated Tumors

The presence of neoplastic cells in axillary lymph nodes and the histological grade are well-established prognostic factors in breast cancer. In these patients, the rate of metastatic spread was also found to be related to PgR status of the tumor. In our study, 40 patients were lymph node positive (N+) at the time of surgery (Fig. 3). During a mean follow-up of

18 months, no case of metastases was observed in the PgR-positive group ($n = 25$), whereas five of 15 (33%) in the PgR-negative group evidenced metastases ($P = 0.005$). No significant difference related to PgR status was observed among patients without invaded axillary nodes.

The study of patients according to histological grading showed that PgR presence or absence delineates a different evolution within the grade III group. Indeed, for grade I tumors, corresponding to well-differentiated tumors, no recurrence was observed in our group ($n = 5$). For grade II tumors ($n = 37$), there was no statistically significant difference between PgR-positive and PgR-negative tumors. Thirty-nine tumors were classified as grade III. In this group 23 patients were also N+. In the PgR-positive group two of 20 patients presented with metastases, whereas in the PgR-negative group 6 of 19 did so ($P = 0.05$) (Fig. 4).

Finally, among the patients displaying criteria of bad prognosis, two different types of evolution can be predicted on the basis of PgR presence or absence in the primary tumor.

Conclusion

The prognostic value of steroid receptors in breast cancer is independent of the usual clinical criteria, such as tumor size and node positivity. The synthesis of PgR by target cells is estrogen dependent and is the result of a differentiated process. In breast cancer, ER and PgR are more often present in differentiated tumors as defined by histological grading [10]. In a study of 50 tumors by electron microscopy [7] we also found that PgR presence was associated with the presence of criteria of differentiation. It is generally assumed that differentiated tumors have a relatively slow growth rate (12), and PgR-positive tumors would therefore be expected to evolve at a slower rate.

Since our first report, the prognostic value of PgR in early breast cancer has been investigated by two other groups [8, 16] and similar conclusions regarding the importance of this receptor have been reached. However, long-term studies seem necessary to assess the clinical usefulness of PgR as a prognostic factor, since the behavior of the PgR-positive and PgR-negative tumors over a very long follow-up is not yet known. Indeed, two studies question the long-term prognostic value of ER: Hilf et al. [5] with a maximum of 8 years' follow-up, concluded that ER has no prognostic value in primary breast cancer, while Hanhel et al. [4] showed that patients with ER-positive tumors had a significantly longer disease-free interval and a delayed recurrence time in N+ cases, but also that in this latter group the difference between ER-positive and ER-negative tumors gradually disappeared when follow-up was extended to 5 years after mastectomy. Additional studies are necessary to establish whether PgR-negative tumors display a specific behavior pattern.

References

1. Allegra JC, Lippman ME, Simon R, Thompson EB, Barlock A, Green L, Huff KK, Do HMT, Aitken SC, Warren R (1979) Association between steroid hormone receptor status and disease-free interval in breast cancer. Cancer Treat Rep 63: 1271–1277
2. Bloom HJG, Richardson WW (1957) Histological grading and prognosis in breast cancer. Br J Cancer 2: 359–369

3. Furmanski P, Saunders DE, Brooks SC, Rich MA (1980) The prognostic value of estrogen receptor determinations in patients with primary breast cancer. Cancer 46: 2794–2796
4. Hahnel R, Woodings T, Brian Vivian A (1979) Prognostic value of estrogen receptors in primary breast cancer. Cancer 44: 671–675
5. Hilf R, Feldstein ML, Gibson SL, Savlov ED (1980) The relative importance of estrogen receptor analysis as a prognostic factor for recurrence or response to chemotherapy in women with breast cancer. Cancer 45: 1993–2000
6. Knight WA, Livingston RB, Gregory EJ, McGuire WL (1977) Estrogen receptor as an independent prognostic factor for early recurrence in breast cancer. Cancer Res 37: 4669–4671
7. Le Doussal V, Pallud C, Pichon MF, Brunet M, Gest J (1981) Recepteurs de l'oestradiol et de la progesterone: correlation avec le grading histo-pronostique de Scarff et Bloom et le degré de differentiation cellulaire ultrastructurale. Abstract F-7, 2nd International congress on senology, Barcelona 25–29 May 1981
8. Magdelenat H, Toubeau M, Picco C, Bidron C (1980) Determination des récepteurs d'oestrogènes et de progesterone sur forages-biopsies des tumeurs mammaires. In: Martin PM (ed) Recepteurs hormonaux et pathologie mammaire. Medsi, Paris p 107
9. Mantel N (1966) Evaluation of survival data and two new rank order statistics arising in its consideration. Cancer Chemother Rep 50: 163–170
10. Martin PM, Rolland PH (1980) Differentiation cellulaire des récepteurs de l'oestradiol et de la progesterone dans les tumeurs mammaires humaines. In: Martin PM (ed) Recepteurs hormonaux et pathologie mammaire. Medsi, Paris, p 121
11. Maynard PV, Blamey RW, Elston CW, Haybittle JL, Griffiths K (1978) Estrogen receptor assay in primary breast cancer and early recurrence of the disease. Cancer Res 38: 4292–4295
12. Meyer JS, Hixon B (1979) Advanced stage and early relapse of breast adenocarcinoma associated with high thymidine labelling indices. Cancer Res 39: 4042–4047
13. Peto R, Pike MC, Armitage P, Breslow NE, Cox DR, Howard SV, Mantel N, McPherson K, Peto J, Smith PG (1977) Design and analysis of randomized clinical trials requiring prolonged observation of each patient. II. Analysis and examples. Br J Cancer 35: 1–39
14. Pichon MF, Milgrom E (1977) Characterization and assay of progesterone receptor in human mammary carcinoma. Cancer Res 37: 464–471
15. Pichon MF, Pallud C, Brunet M, Milgrom E (1980) Relationship of presence of progesterone receptors to prognosis in early breast cancer. Cancer Res 40: 3357–3360
16. Saez S, Chouvet N, Israel N, Cheix F, Mayer M (1980) Signification et interêt de l'étude des récepteurs hormonaux dans les tumeurs mammaires humaines. Senologia 5: 155–161
17. Samaan NA, Buzdar AU, Aldinger KA, Schultz PN, Yang KP, Romsdahl MM, Martin R (1981) Estrogen receptor: a prognostic factor in breast cancer. Cancer 47: 554–560
18. Westerberg H, Gustafson SA, Nordenskjold B, Silfwersward C, Wallgren A (1980) Estrogen receptor level and other factors in early recurrence of breast cancer. Int J Cancer 26: 429–433

Estrogen and Progesterone Receptors as Prognostic Factors in Early Breast Cancer*

S. Saez, F. Cheix, and M. Mayer

Centre Leon Berard, 28 Rue Laënnec, 69373 Lyon, Cedex 8, France

Introduction

During the past 10 years, steroid receptors in human breast tumors have been extensively investigated in many laboratories. The initial aim of this clinical research was to help in selecting patients with metastasis for hormonal treatment.

Jensen showed very early that patients whose tumors did not contain estrogen receptors (ER) responded very poorly to hormone therapy [6]. But it was found that reliance on the presence of ER in tumors as a criterion of hormone dependence led to overestimation of the exact number of hormone-dependent cases [10]. Indeed, 60%−70% of tumors are positive for ER content, whereas no more than 30% are clinically hormone dependent.

McGuire pointed out that among the steroids which presumably have an action on breast epithelium (androgens, glucocorticoids, mineralocorticoids), progesterone has a special place. Like estrogen, it is involved in growth processes even if its role is not completely understood. It has a stimulatory effect on experimental tumors when present at high doses [5] but reduces the positive effect of estrogens on tumor appearance and progression [17]. On the other hand, progesterone receptor (PgR) is synthesized under the control of estrogen activity in normal target cells such as endometrial and mammary epithelium [4]. It has therefore been suggested that its maintenance in tumors developed in these organs might be the expression of their capacity to respond to estrogen stimulation. Horwitz and McGuire suggested that PgR determination could help in defining hormone-dependent tumors and in predicting their response to hormone therapy. Further work confirmed this prediction and showed that 80% of tumors which contained both receptors were hormone dependent [9].

In primary tumors, receptor determinations were investigated in relation to the response of patients to initial treatment, independently of their hormone-dependent character. Since ER determinations were developed before those of PgR, the series of patients with the longest follow-ups concern ER only.

Walt [19] and Knight [7] were the first to demonstrate the association between the absence of ER and early recurrence, and this was confirmed by others [2, 3, 9, 11]. The aim of the

* This work was supported in part by the Institut National de la Santé et de la Recherche Médicale (ATP 24-75-47) and CRAT (76-4-490) and the Fédération Française des Centres de Lutte contre le Cancer

present investigation was to analyze long-term follow-up of patients in relation to the presence of ER and to investigate the significance of PgR as another prognostic factor, distinct from hormone dependency.

Materials and Methods

Patients

The distribution of steroid receptors (ER, PgR) was investigated in 310 patients with primary disease.

All patients were treated by modified radical mastectomy. They were evaluated every 3 months for the first year and then every 6 months. They were checked by clinical examination, chest X-ray, radiological bone survey, and liver scan once a year.

The outcome in relation to the tumor ER content is analyzed for a 7-year period. The relationship to PgR data is available in 151 patients followed up for a $3^3/_4$-year period.

Patients were distributed into categories of positive or negative receptor content and their menopausal status was recorded. The stage of the disease was assessed according to the UICC recommendations [18].

The analysis of contingency tables was performed by the χ^2 test with continuity correction. The occurrence of relapses was represented by the actuarial method and comparison between groups was by the log rank test [12].

Steroid Receptor Assays

ER and PgR were measured in tumor samples obtained from primary tumors at the time of initial treatment. Assays were carried out using the dextran-coated charcoal technique with estradiol and R-5020 as tritiated ligands according to the methods previously described [15]. The K_d and receptor content were calculated by the Scatchard method and the results expressed as femtomoles of bound labeled hormone per milligram cytosol protein. The threshold of positivity was 3 and 10 fmol/mg protein for ER and PgR respectively.

Results

The distribution of ER and PgR positive and negative cases in the patients studied here is shown in Table 1. It does not differ from a larger population we have investigated. In both populations the percentage of ER+ tumors is lower in the premenopausal than in the postmenopausal period, whereas the percentage of PgR+ tumors is higher in the premenopausal period. The overall mean of ER positivity is 69%, and that of PgR positivity, 35%.

Clinical parameters such as tumor size and axillary node involvement which define the *extension of the disease* at the time of initial treatment have a well-known prognostic value. For this reason the distribution of receptors has been analyzed in relation to these parameters. Table 1 indicates that the percentage of tumors containing ER or PgR does not vary according to axillary node status.

Table 1. Distribution of the different types of tumor receptor content in relation to menopausal status and degree of extension of the disease, and compared with the type of treatment

	No.	ER+ (%)	ER− (%)	No.	PgR+ (%)	PgR− (%)
Controls						
Total	621	69	36	621	35	65
Premenopause	155	58	42	185	39	61
Postmenopause	436	66	34	436	33	66
Present study						
Total	310	67	32	151	38	61
Premenopause[a]	92	58	42	48	42	58
Postmenopause	195	72	28	90	37	63
Axillary nodes						
N+	172	67	32	89	39	61
N−	112	64	35	62	37	63
N[b]	26	76	23			
Stages						
I	34	62	38	27	52	48
II	137	67	33	83	40	60
III	128	67	33	39	23	77
Adjuvant therapy						
(+)	147	63	36	86	39	61
(−)	155	69	31	65	37	63
Local irradiation						
(+)	154	75	25	40	42	58
(−)	148	58	42	111	37	63

[a] Menopausal status was not known for all patients
[b] Histological examination of palpable axillary nodes. N+ could be underestimated

Classification according to the stage does not show any difference in the percentage of ER+ tumors, but the percentage of PgR+ tumors is significantly lower at the most advanced stages (52%, 40%, and 23% at stages I, II, and III respectively).

Choice of the treatment given to the patients was based only on the size of the tumor and axillary node status. Hence, the distribution of receptor-positive cases is very similar in groups of patients who received adjuvant therapy and in those who did not (Table 1).

Figure 1 represents the length of the disease-free interval of patients in relation to the ER content of their tumors. At 18 months' follow-up, 95% of ER+ cases were disease-free vs 85% of ER− cases. The difference is significant ($P = 0.03$), but the two curves of disease-free interval established over a long period are not significantly different ($P = 0.41$).

A similar pattern of results is observed in the category of patients with invaded axillary nodes (Fig. 2). During the first 3 years only, the rate of recurrence is in favor of the tumors containing ER, but the difference between the ER+ and ER− curves is not significant ($P = 0.07$). In fact, while the presence of ER anticipates a longer disease-free interval within the class with positive axillary node status, it does not predict a higher percentage of

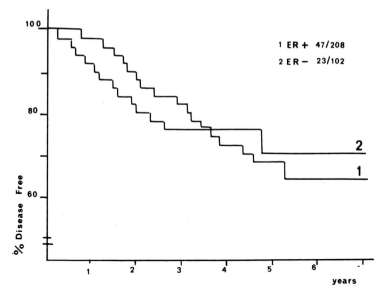

Fig. 1. Disease-free interval in relation to the presence or absence of estradiol receptors in tumors

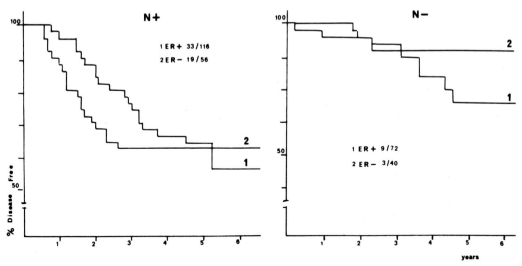

Fig. 2. Disease-free interval in relation to the presence or absence of estradiol receptors in tumors. $N+$, patients with positive axillary nodes; $N-$, patients with negative axillary nodes

cure. In the group with negative axillary nodes, the percentage of relapses is even higher for ER+ than for ER− cases after 3 years' follow-up.

Figure 3 represents the recurrence rate of 151 patients in relation to the PgR content of the tumor. Only one of 58 PgR+ cases relapsed (curve 1) vs 13 of 93 PgR− (curve 2). The difference is significant ($P < 0.05$). Patients whose axillary nodes were not invaded at the time of initial treatment have a low rate of recurrence (three of 62), and the presence or

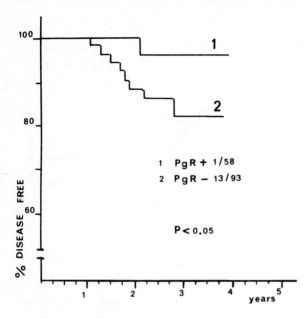

1   PgR + 1/58
2   PgR − 13/93

P < 0.05

Fig. 3. Disease-free interval in relation to the presence or absence of progesterone receptors in tumors

Table 2. Recurrences in the different classes of receptor content

	Total (n)	ER+	ER−	Total (n)	PgR+	PgR−
All patients	310	205	102	151	58	93
Max. follow-up	84 months			45 months		
Recurrences						
Total	70	47/208	23/102	14	1/58	13/93
Premenopause[a]	16	9/54	7/38	4	1/20	3/28
Postmenopause	51	38/148	13/55	7	0/33	7/57
Axillary node status[b]						
(+)		31/116	19/56	11	0/35	11/54
(−)		9/72	3/40	3	1/23	2/39

[a] Menopausal status was not known for all patients
[b] Cases with histological examination of palpable axillary nodes only are not included

absence of PgR does not make any difference (Table 2). As expected, in patients with positive axillary nodes the rate of recurrence was greater. However, there is an important difference between the two subsets in their PgR content (Fig. 4): there was no relapse in the 35 patients of the PgR− group. The difference is significant ($P < 0.001$).

Discussion

Analysis of the total population of 310 patients with primary tumors confirmed the known prognostic value of the extension of the disease at the time of initial treatment. Apparently, subclassification of the patients in relation to the receptor content of the tumor introduces

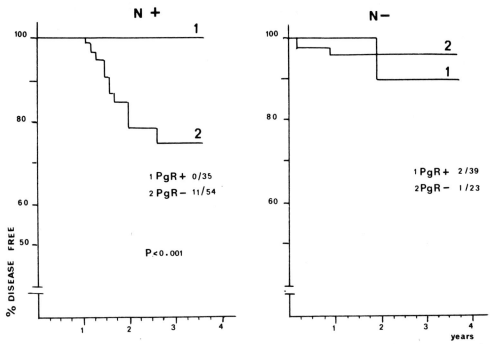

Fig. 4. Disease-free interval in relation to the presence or absence of progesterone receptors in tumors. $N+$, patients with positive axillary nodes; $N-$, patients with negative axillary nodes

another prognostic parameter whose significance is more evident in patients with positive axillary nodes. It is shown that in patients who have the same extension of the disease and undergo the same type of treatment, the length of the disease-free period depends on the receptor content of the tumor.

Since 1976 most studies have shown that ER positivity is associated with a prolonged disease-free interval [19]. Our present results indicate that in the overall patient population the effect of ER status on outcome is more evident during the early period after initial treatment. The better prognosis associated with ER positivity is restricted to the class of patients with invaded axillary nodes.

Very few reports deal with the prognostic value of PgR. According to Allegra et al., it does not influence the disease-free interval [1]. But their receptor data are not quite comparable to those in the present analysis since some were obtained from metastatic lesions in patients who were already under treatment. In an analysis recently published by M. F. Pichon and S. Saez [13, 14, 19], it was found that the PgR assay introduced a more selective criterion than ER. Recent results have confirmed that this receptor could be considered as a marker for estrogen responsiveness. As such it could be an index of more differentiated function and of lower growth rate [8].

According to several lines of data, PgR measurement is preferable to ER quantitative assay. Indeed, PgR positivity is associated with a prolonged disease-free interval, found independently of either the menopausal status, tumor extension to axillary nodes or the type of therapy applied. On the other hand, the absence of PgR may be due to causes other than hormone independence in some physiological circumstances [15]. This could explain unexpected hormone dependence of some rare PgR− tumors.

These present data are nevertheless too preliminary to anticipate the effect of PgR status on survival. Studies on larger populations for longer periods will be necessary to establish the effect of receptor status and type of therapy on long-term outcome. Taking both into consideration should lead to optimal adjustment of adjuvant therapy.

References

1. Allegra JC, Lippman ME, Thompson EB, Simon A, Barlock A, Green L, Huff KK, Do HM, Aitken SC (1979) Distribution, frequency, and quantitative analysis of estrogen, progesterone, androgen, and glucocorticoid receptors in human breast cancer. Cancer Res 39: 1447–1454
2. Dao TL, Nemoto T (1980) Steroid receptors and response to endocrine ablation in women with metastatic cancer of the breast. Cancer 46: 2779–2782
3. Hilf R, Feldstein ML, Gibson SL, Savlon ED (1980) The relative importance of estrogen receptor analysis as a prognostic factor for recurrence or response to chemotherapy in women with breast cancer. Cancer 45: 1993–2000
4. Horwitz K, McGuire WL (1978) Estrogen control of progesterone receptors in human breast cancer. J Biol Chem 253: 2273–2278
5. Huggins L, Grand CC, Brillantes PP (1961) Mammary cancer induced by a single feeding of polynuclear hydrocarbons and its suppression. Nature 189: 204–207
6. Jensen EV, Block GF, Smith S, Kyser K, DeSombre ER (1971) Estrogen receptors and breast cancer response to adrenalectomy. Natl Cancer Inst Monogr 34: 55–70
7. Knight WA, Livingston RB, Gregory EJ, McGuire WL (1977) Estrogen receptor as an independent prognostic factor for early recurrence in breast cancer. Cancer Res 37: 4669–4671
8. Meyer JS, Hixon B (1979) Advanced stage and early relapse of breast adenocarcinoma associated with high thymidine labeling indices. Cancer Res 39: 4042–4047
9. McGuire WL (1980) Steroid hormone receptors in breast cancer treatment strategy. Recent Prog Horm Res 36: 135–156
10. McGuire WL, Pearson OH, Segaloff A (1975) Predicting hormone responsiveness in human breast cancer. In: McGuire WL, Carbone PP, Vollmer EP (eds) Estrogen receptors in human breast cancer. Raven, New York, pp 17–30
11. Nomura Y, Yadagata J, Takenaka K, Tashiro H (1980) Steroid hormone receptors and clinical usefulness in human breast cancer. Cancer 46: 2880–2883
12. Peto R, Pike MC, Armitage P, Breslow NE, Cox DR, Howard SV, Mantel N, McPherson K, Peto J, Smith PG (1977) Design and analysis of randomized clinical trials requiring prolonged observation of each patient. II analysis and exemples. Br J Cancer 35: 1–39
13. Pichon MF, Pallud C, Brunet M, Milgrom E (1980) Relationship of presence of progesterone receptors to prognosis in early breast cancer. Cancer Res 40: 3357–3360
14. Saez S, Chouvet C, Mayer M, Cheix F (1980) Estradiol and progesterone receptor (ER, PGR) as prognostic factors in human primary breast tumors. Proceedings AACR – 553. Cancer Res 21: 139
15. Saez S, Martin PM, Chouvet CD (1978) Estradiol and progesterone receptor in human breast adenocarcinoma in relation to plasma estrogen and progesterone levels. Cancer 38: 3468–3473
16. Skinner LG, Barnes DM, Ribeiro GG (1980) The clinical value of multiple steroid receptor assays in breast cancer management. Cancer 46: 2939–2945
17. Stoll BA (1969) Hormone management in breast cancer. Pittman Medical, London, pp 68–73
18. Union Internationale contre le Cancer (1979) Breast. In: UICC (ed) TNM classification of malignant tumors. pp 47–53
19. Walt AJ, Singhakowinta A, Brooks SC, Cartez A (1976) The surgical implications of estrophile proteins estimations in carcinoma of the breast. Surgery 80: 506–512

Part IV: A Critical Summary

L. Santi

Istituto Nazionale per la Ricerca sul Cancro,
Istituto Scientifico per lo Studio e la Cura dei Tumori,
Istituto di Oncologia Sperimentale e Clinica dell' Università,
Viale Benedetto XV n. 10, 16132 Genova, Italy

Since Jensen [1] described a correlation between response to ablative endocrine therapy in breast cancer patients and estrogen receptor (ER) status, great interest has been shown in assessing the importance of ER and more recently of progesterone receptor (PgR) status in the strategy of breast cancer treatment [2−4]. Attention has been centered mainly on their role in a predictive assay, their value in determining hormone dependence, leading to combined hormonal and cytotoxic treatment of breast cancer, and their possible use as specific carriers of cytotoxic estrogenic or antiestrogenic drugs [5−7].

Various institutes around the world have assayed ER and PgR levels in breast cancer specimens and data on their clinical utilization were studied. Saez et al. demonstrate that the percentage of PgR-positive tumors is lower in the more advanced stages of breast cancer: 52%, 40%, and 23% in stages I, II, and III respectively. By contrast, there is no difference in the percentage of ER present in relation to the staging.

Pichon et al., starting from an analysis of the degree of tumor differentiation, arrive at the conclusion that PgR are present in tumors with higher differentiation. Therefore, if it is true that those tumors which are more differentiated have a slower reproducing time, we can conclude that, within reasonable limits, the presence of PgR in a neoplasm is correlated with less aggressive disease.

As regards the relationship between the disease-free interval and ER, Saez et al. and Pichon et al. demonstrate that after a long period from the time of mastectomy, no difference exists between ER-negative and ER-positive tumors. They do not have sufficient data to draw a conclusion as to whether this is also true of PgR-negative and PgR-positive tumors.

Toma et al. confirm that the information obtained from ER assay during the course of untreated breast cancer is probably a valuable guide for future therapeutic intervention in the metastatic phase, on condition that no intercurrent therapy has been instituted [8]. The interpretation of ER data is less clear in the case of systemic treatment, especially in patients undergoing chemo- and/or hormonotherapy [8−11, 13]. Toma et al. appear to want to confirm that ER data must be interpreted with extreme caution, especially when treatment has been instituted several months before ER assay.

Although radiotherapy apparently has no effect on receptors [11, 14], the available data are insufficient for definite conclusions to be drawn. In summarizing, two question remain: (1) when should the ER and PgR assay be performed and (2) how should they be interpreted?

1. It now seems apparent that ER and PgR evaluation should be performed whenever possible on both primary and metastatic lesions. The determination of PgR and nuclear ER in addition to that of cytoplasmic ER can better delineate whether a tumor is hormone dependent or not [13, 15, 16].

2. *ER*. How ER assays should be interpreted is less clear. Different ways of interpreting ER values may be distinguished as follows:

   a) In postmenopausal untreated patients the ER concentration can be considered a characteristic of the tumor which remains constant throughout the course of the disease. Therefore an ER value from a primary tumor can be utilized at the moment of metastasis, even without an additional ER assay (though this would be preferable), as an indicator of the hormonal dependence of the tumor itself. The situation is less clear in premenopausal patients, where different factors can cause variations in ER values.

   b) ER values from patients who have undergone therapy, especially hormonal therapy, should be interpreted with great caution. There is insufficient data in this area, especially as regards the reliability of ER assays in patients who have undergone recent hormonal therapy. No conclusions can be drawn as to whether chemotherapy affects ER values. Studies have indicated that ER values from postmenopausal women who have undergone radiation therapy can be considered characteristic of the tumor itself.

The above observations have been made on small study groups and cannot be considered conclusive.

PgR. Apparently a better response and a longer disease-free interval are correlated with PgR presence, but at present the prognostic and therapeutic value of PgR is not known with certainty.

ER and PgR data may be of particular value as prognostic indicators and, perhaps, as a guide to the use of adjuvant therapy in patients with breast cancer.

Concluding, the various studies that have been reviewed here show a basic defect inherent in all retrospective studies. On considering, for instance, the studies on ER variations (with and without treatment), it is natural to ask how therapeutic strategy was chosen and if this selection can be a cause of misinterpretation of the results. It is possible that those patients who have undergone a certain therapy may have a less aggressive tumor: patients who have preclinical breast cancer of long duration may not readily accept therapy. Perhaps these cancers have biological characteristics very different from other tumors. This self-selection bias and the insufficient amount of data could be remedied by large randomized controlled trials, which could give a definitive answer to the questions raised above.

Nevertheless, the uncontrolled clinical studies in this chapter have provided a great deal of evidence; this evidence must be interpreted with great care, recognizing the problems and adjusting for them whenever possible.

References

1. Jensen EV, Polley TZ, Smith S, Black GE, Ferguson DI, DeSombre ER (1975) Prediction of hormone dependency in human breast cancer. In: McGuire WL, Carbone PP, Vollmer ED (eds) Estrogen receptors in human breast cancer. Raven, New York, pp 37−56
2. Allegra JC, Lippman ME, Thompson EB, Simon R, Barlock A, Green L, Hoan KK, Do MT, Aitken SC, Warren R (1980) Estrogen receptor status: an important variable in predicting response to endocrine therapy in metastatic breast cancer. Eur J Cancer 323−331

3. Skinner LG, Barnes DM, Ribeiro GG (1980) The clinical value of multiple steroid receptor assays in breast cancer management. Cancer 46: 2939–2945

4. Bloom ND, Tobin EH, Schreibman B, Degenshein GA (1980) The role of progesterone receptors in the management of advanced breast cancer. Cancer 45: 2992–2977

5. Muller ER, Beth ES, Traish A, Wotiz HH (1980) Effect of chemotherapeutic agents on the formation of estrogen receptor complex in human breast tumor breast tumor cytosol. Cancer Res 40: 2941–2942

6. Kiang DT, Frenning DH, Goldman AI, Ascensao VE, Kennedy BJ (1978) Estrogen receptors and response to chemotherapy and hormonal therapy in advanced breast cancer. N Engl J Med 299: 1330–1334

7. Hilf R, Feldstein ML, Scott L, Gibson BS, Savlov ED (1980) The relative importance of estrogen receptor analysis as a prognostic factor for recurrence or response to chemotherapy in women with breast cancer. Cancer 45: 1993–2000

8. Paridaens R, Sylvester RJ, Ferrazzi E, Legros N, Leclerc G, Heuson JC (1980) Clinical significance of the quantitative assessment of estrogen receptors in advanced breast cancer. Cancer 46: 2889–2895

9. Rosen PP, Menendez-Botet CJ, Jerome A, Urban AF, Schwartz MK (1977) Estrogen receptors protein (ERP) in multiple tumor specimens from individual patients with breast cancer. Cancer 39: 2194–2200

10. Allegra JC, Barlock A, Huff KK, Lippman ME (1980) Changes in multiple or sequential estrogen receptor determinations in breast cancer. Cancer 45: 792–794

11. Walt AJ, Singhakowinta A, Brooks SC, Cortez A (1976) The surgical implications of estrophile protein estimations in carcinoma of the breast. Surgery 80: 506–512

12. Nomura Y, Yamagata J, Takenaka K (1980) Steroid hormone receptors and clinical usefulness in human breast cancer. Cancer 46: 2880–2883

13. Waseda N, Kato Y, Imura H, Kurata M (1981) Effects of tamoxifen on estrogen and progesterone receptors in human breast cancer. Cancer Res 41: 1984–1988

14. Burke RE, Mira JG, Datta R, Zava DT, McGuire WL (1978) Estrogen action following irradiation of human breast cancer cells. Cancer Res 38: 2813–2817

15. Garola RE, McGuire WL (1977) An improved assay for nuclear estrogen receptor in experimental and human breast cancer. Cancer Res 37: 3333

16. Silfversward C, Skoog L, Humla S, Gustafsson SA, Nordenskjold B (1979) Intratumoral variation of cytoplasmic and nuclear estrogen receptor concentrations in human mammary carcinoma. Eur J Cancer 16: 39–65

Part V. Treatments

Relationship Between Estrogen Receptors and CMF Adjuvant Chemotherapy*

G. Bonadonna, G. Di Fronzo, G. Tancini, C. Brambilla,
A. Rossi, S. Marchini, and P. Valagussa

Istituto Nazionale per lo Studio e la Cura dei Tumori,
Via Venezian 1, 20133 Milan, Italy

Introduction

The presence of estrogen receptors (ER) has been found to have prognostic significance in patients with resectable breast cancer, regardless of whether axillary nodes are positive or negative [12, 14]. Since adjuvant chemotherapy is now being administered to many patients with histologically positive axillary nodes [9], it could be of practical importance to determine whether ER status can also predict the course of breast cancer in an adjuvant situation. In spite of initial controversial reports [10, 11] several recent retrospective analyses have indicated a lack of significant correlation between tumor ER status and clinical response to cytotoxic chemotherapy. This paper will summarize the clinical experience of the Istituto Tumori of Milan in patients with breast cancer in whom the ER assay was determined before starting polychemotherapy, particularly with CMF.

ER Determination

The ER content was determined on the primary tumor by use of the dextran-coated charcoal method according to the guidelines provided by the EORTC group [7, 8]. The binding parameters (ER concentration or femtomoles per milligram protein and association constant or K_a) were determined through Scatchard analysis. Levels below 5 fmol/mg cytosol protein and $K_2 < 1.5 \times 10^9 \, M^{-1}$ were regarded as negative. No systematic effort was made to verify the ER content through biopsy of recurrent sites in soft tissues.

Advanced Breast Cancer

Table 1 summarizes the response rate according to ER status in patients with advanced breast cancer. Drug treatment included CMF (cyclophosphamide, methotrexate, fluorouracil), AV (adriamycin and vincristine), and CAFP (cyclophosphamide, adriamycin, fluorouracil and prednisone). As detailed in a previous publication [3], irrespective of ER

* This work was supported in part by contract no. N01-CM-33714 with NCI, DCT, NIH, Bethesda, MD, USA

Table 1. Advanced breast cancer: Response to combination chemotherapy according to ER status

	No. of patients	CR + PR (%)	
		Premenopausal	Postmenopausal
Total	85	50	52
ER+	46	58	45
ER−	30	53	53
ER±	9	37	100
		ER+ vs ER−	ER+ vs ER−
		$P = 0.85$	$P = 0.90$

status, complete (CR) and partial (PR) remission occurred in 52% of 85 patients, with no significant difference related to disease presentation (stage $T_{3b}-T_4$, inflammatory carcinoma, disseminated disease). Also, there was no difference between pre- (50%) and postmenopausal (52%) women, and the response rate was comparable to that obtained by us previously [4, 6]. The results failed to provide evidence for a significant difference in response rate according to ER status, and this was also true when a cut-off point of 10 fmol/mg was used. In addition, analysis of median duration of response and the 2-year survival rate were not statistically different between patients with ER-positive tumors and those with ER-negative tumors.

Adjuvant CMF

The analysis of relapse-free (RFS) and total survival rates according to ER status was limited to only a certain percentage of women having operable breast cancer and histologically positive axillary lymph nodes (N+) who were enrolled in our second adjuvant study with CMF [3, 13]. In fact, in 204 women (44.4%) ER assay was not performed (Table 2). Drug therapy consisted in the administration of either 12 or 6 cycles of CMF chemotherapy. In the 4-year analysis patients belonging to the two arms were grouped together since a recent detailed analysis [2] failed to show significant differences in either RFS or total survival rate between the groups treated with 12 or 6 cycles. The comparative 4-year results presented in Table 2 essentially confirmed our previous findings. In fact, the analysis of RFS indicated an absence of significant differences between ER-positive and ER-negative tumors in both pre- and postmenopausal patients. The overall survival rate of premenopausal women with ER-positive tumors was significantly superior to that of women with ER-negative tumors ($P < 0.04$), and this observation supported the evidence against an initial report [11] suggesting that ER-negative tumors could be more responsive to combination chemotherapy. Moreover, the present findings further refute the suggestion that chemotherapy-induced adjuvant castration has a therapeutic role [1].

Sequential Chemotherapy

To test in postmenopausal women less than 65 years of age a form of drug therapy which theoretically could be more effective toward primary cell resistance, a trial utilizing two

Table 2. Actuarial 4-year relapse-free and total survival rates according to ER status following adjuvant CMF

	No. of patients		RFS (%)		Survival (%)	
	Premeno-pausal	Postmeno-pausal	Premeno-pausal	Postmeno-pausal	Premeno-pausal	Postmeno-pausal
Total	324	135	67.2	63.1	78.9	79.8
ER+	138	40	69.8	61.7	80.3	84.4
ER−	33	13	59.4	59.3	70.9	76.5
ER±	21	10	52.9	80.0	70.6	80.0
Unknown	132	72	71.3	65.7	81.0	78.1
			+ vs −	+ vs −	+ vs −	+ vs −
			$P = 0.18$	$P = 0.41$	$P < 0.04$	$P = 0.48$

Table 3. Actuarial 3-year relapse-free and total survival rates in postmenopausal women according to ER status following sequential adjuvant chemotherapy (CMFP → AV)

	No. of patients	RFS (%)	Survival (%)
Total	115	72.2	86.1
ER+	61	75.7	89.6
ER−	20	63.8	82.3
ER±	6	66.7	83.3
Unknown	30	75.0	81.2
		ER+ vs ER−	ER+ vs ER−
		$P = 0.37$	$P = 0.25$

non-cross-resistant regimens (six cycles of CMFP i.e., CMF plus prednisone followed by four cycles of AV) was started in 1977 [2, 5]. In the group of patients in whom the ER assay was performed (85 of 115, or 73.9%), the difference between ER-positive and ER-negative tumors was not significant in the 3-year analysis of RFS and total survival rates (Table 3).

CMF Plus Tamoxifen

This prospective nonrandomized trial utilizing low dose CMF for 12 cycles with concomitant administration of tamoxifen (20 mg/day for 12 months) was started in May 1977 and limited to women older than 65 years or to postmenopausal patients with medical contraindications to treatment with adriamycin. Although the findings are premature, the 3-year analysis yielded a somewhat surprising result, for no significant difference could be detected in either RFS or total survival rate between women with ER-positive and women with ER-negative tumors (Table 4). This could in part be due to the limited number of patients at risk, particularly in the subgroup with ER-negative tumors.

Table 4. Actuarial 3-year relapse-free and total survival rates in postmenopausal women according to ER status following adjuvant CMF plus tamoxifen

	No. of patients	RFS (%)	Survival (%)
Total	93	79.7	90.5
ER+	49	80.0	89.0
ER−	14	92.8	100
ER±	5	75.0	75.0
Unknown	25	76.2	93.3
		ER+ vs ER−	ER+ vs ER−
		$P = 0.80$	$P = 0.26$

Conclusion

The analyses at different follow-up times in our various studies with chemotherapy in advanced as well as in early breast cancer have confirmed that ER status determined prior to the initiation of treatment does not appear useful for predicting response to multiple drug regimens. The lack of significant difference held true both for premenopausal and for postmenopausal patients. Although this should be considered a retrospective analysis and the ER assay was not performed in all patients whose response to chemotherapy could have been evaluated, the consistency of observed findings throughout the studies cannot be merely coincidental. Since our results indicate that in advanced and early breast cancer combination chemotherapy is effective regardless of ER status, there is no reason at present to withhold the administration of effective adjuvant chemotherapy in high-risk patients (i.e., those with positive axillary nodes) in the presence of ER-positive tumors. Whether in this particular subgroup combined chemotherapy-hormone therapy (e.g., CMF plus tamoxifen) would yield superior results compared with chemotherapy alone, remains to be determined through a long-term analysis.

References

1. Bonadonna G, Valagussa P, De Palo G (1981) The results of adjuvant chemotherapy in breast cancer are predominantly due to the hormonal change such therapy induces: Opposed. In: Van Scoy-Mosher MB (ed) Medical oncology: Controversies in cancer treatment. Hall, Boston, pp. 100−109
2. Bonadonna G, Valagussa P, Rossi A, Tancini G, Brambilla C, Marchini S, Veronesi U (1981) Multimodal therapy with CMF in resectable breast cancer with positive axillary nodes. The Milan Institute experience. In: Salmon SE, Jones SE (eds) Adjuvant therapy of cancer III. Grune and Stratton, New York, pp. 435−444
3. Bonadonna G, Valagussa P, Tancini G, Di Fronzo G (1980) Estrogen-receptor status and response to chemotherapy in early and advanced breast cancer. Cancer Chemother Pharmacol 4:37−41
4. Brambilla C, Valagussa P, Bonadonna G (1978) Sequential combination chemotherapy in advanced breast cancer. Cancer Chemother Pharmacol 1:35−39
5. Brambilla C, Valagussa P, Bonadonna G, Veronesi U (1980) Sequential adjuvant chemotherapy in postmenopausal (≤ 65 yr) breast cancer. Proc Am Assoc Cancer Res 21:189 (Abstract 758)

6. De Lena M, Zucali R, Viganotti G, Valagussa P, Bonadonna G (1978) Combined chemotherapy-radiotherapy approach in locally advanced (T_{3b}-T_4) breast cancer. Cancer Chemother Pharmacol 1: 53–59
7. Di Fronzo G, Bertuzzi A, Ronchi E (1978) An improved criterion for the evaluation of estrogen receptor binding data in human breast cancer. Tumori 64: 259–266
8. EORTC Breast Cancer Cooperative Group (1973) Standards for the assessment of estrogen receptors in human breast cancer. Eur J Cancer 9: 379–381
9. Jones SE, Salmon SE (eds) (1981) Adjuvant therapy of cancer III. Grune and Stratton, New York
10. Kiang DT, Frenning DH, Goldman AI, Ascensao VF, Kennedy BJ (1978) Estrogen receptors and response to chemotherapy and hormonal therapy in advanced breast cancer. N Engl J Med 299: 1330–1334
11. Lippman ME, Allegra JC, Thompson EB, Simon R, Barlock A, Green L, Huff KK, Hoan MTD, Aitken SC, Warren R (1978) The relation between estrogen receptors and response rate to cytotoxic chemotherapy in metastatic breast cancer. N Engl J Med 298: 1223–1228
12. National Institute of Health (1979) Steroid receptors in breast cancer. An NIH consensus development conference. Bethesda, Maryland, 27–29 June 1979. Cancer 46 (Suppl): 2759–2962 (1980)
13. Tancini G, Bajetta E, Marchini S, Valagussa P, Bonadonna G, Veronesi U (1979) Preliminary 3-year results of 12 versus 6 cycles of surgical adjuvant CMF in premenopausal breast cancer. Cancer Clin Trials 2: 285–292
14. Valagussa P, Di Fronzo G, Bignami P, Buzzoni R, Bonadonna G, Veronesi U. Prognostic importance of estrogen receptors to select node negative patients for adjuvant chemotherapy. In: Salmon E, Jones SE (eds) Adjuvant therapy of cancer III. Grune and Stratton, New York, pp. 329–333

New Adjuvant Trials for Resectable Breast Cancer at the Istituto Nazionale Tumori of Milan*

G. Bonadonna, P. Bignami, R. Buzzoni, A. Moliterni, P. Valagussa, and U. Veronesi

Istituto Nazionale per lo Studio e la Cura dei Tumori, Via Venezian 1, 20133 Milan, Italy

Introduction

The 5-year results of the CMF adjuvant program carried out in Milan have shown significantly better relapse-free (RFS) and total survival rates in women with positive axillary nodes who were treated with 12 cycles of combination chemotherapy following radical mastectomy than in those treated only with surgery [1, 11]. The 5-year results were subsequently confirmed in the 6-year analysis [2]. In particular:
1. The results were influenced by the extent of axillary involvement as well as by the amount of drugs administered and, for comparative dose levels, the results were not affected by menopausal status.
2. The analysis of RFS failed to detect significant differences between estrogen receptor (ER)-positive and ER-negative tumors, either in pre- or in postmenopausal patients.
3. The comparative 4-year analysis showed that neither the RFS nor the total survival rate varied significantly between the group who received 6 cycles of CMF and that treated with 12 cycles. Most probably, the nadir in surviving tumor cells is reached in the majority of patients in less than 6 cycles, and therefore subsequent cycles (i.e., cycles 7–12) do not reduce the surviving tumor cells by the same fraction as initial cycles. Since cycles 7–12 were providing little or no benefit in the majority of subgroups, even when comparative dose levels were considered, we can conclude that the most important pharmacological factor is the peak level of the drugs rather then their total amount.
4. In the 5-year analysis we failed to detect an increased incidence of second neoplasms compared with the incidence in controls.

Rationale for New Studies

New adjuvant studies utilizing combination chemotherapy were designed with the intent of (a) exploring the efficacy of non-cross-resistant regimens vs CMF; (b) providing constant full drug dosage; (c) testing the efficacy of chemotherapy in node-negative patients with

* This work was supported in part by contract no. N01-CM-07388 with NCI, DCT, NIH, Bethesda, MD, USA

Table 1. New adjuvant trials with chemotherapy being carried out at the Istituto Nazionale Tumori of Milan[a]

ER/nodal status	Adjuvant treatment
Positive and negative/1−3	R ⟨ CMF 12 courses CMF 8 courses → adriamycin 4 courses
Positive and negative/> 3	R ⟨ Adriamycin 4 courses → CMF 8 courses CMF alternated with adriamycin for a total of 12 courses
Negative/negative	R ⟨ No further therapy after surgery CMF 12 courses

[a] Surgery: Simple or modified radical mastectomy (T_{2a}−T_{3a}) or quadrantectomy with axillary dissection (T_{1a})

Table 2. Dose schedule of one course of CMF and adriamycin

Cyclophosphamide	600 mg/m^2 i.v., day 1	
Methotrexate	40 mg/m^2 i.v., day 1	every 3 weeks
Fluorouracil	600 mg/m^2 i.v., day 1	
Adriamycin	75 mg/m^2 i.v., day 1	

To allow a constant full drug dosage, in the presence of myelosuppression on the planned day of drug administration, treatment is delayed until full marrow recovery occurs

ER-negative tumors; and (d) establishing whether less mutilating surgical procedures can affect early and late results.

Table 1 presents an outline of the studies initiated in the fall of 1980. In consideration of the conclusions derived from the NIH Consensus Meeting [15] and our recent favorable results with conservative surgery for T_1 lesions [19], patients are being subjected to less mutilating surgery than in our previous studies. In particular, those whose primary breast cancer is classified as T_{2a} or T_{3a} are subjected to total (simple) mastectomy and complete axillary node dissection. Depending upon the size of the primary tumor and at the discretion of surgeons, modified radical mastectomy with removal of the pectoralis minor can be performed. Patients whose primary tumor is classified as T_1 are subjected to quadrantectomy and complete axillary node dissection. In this group of patients postoperative irradiation to the remaining portions of the breast (50 Gy plus a booster of 10 Gy to the skin surrounding the scar) is started within 2−4 weeks after surgery.

Chemotherapy utilizes a new version of CMF (Table 2). Since the reasons for not being able to administer full dose CMF in many patients was lack of compliance (particularly in elderly women) with respect to oral cyclophosphamide, all drugs are now being administered intravenously. The intervals of 3 weeks between two CMF courses and between two cycles of adriamycin are based on the assumption that longer intervals between two drug doses than those previously applied with CMF can be allowed since the estimated median doubling time of breast cancer cells is 56 days for premenopausal women and 69 days for postmenopausal women [13].

In patients with histologically positive axillary nodes adjuvant chemotherapy is again applied regardless of ER status since previous experience has been that this factor failed to predict significantly the response to chemotherapy, both in advanced disease and in an

Table 3. Breast cancer with negative axillary nodes: percent relapse-free survival related to ER status

	3 years	5 years	P
Total			
ER+	88.7	82.4	0.0005
ER−	67.8	45.2	
Premenopause			
ER+	89.7	85.2	< 0.001
ER−	63.0	38.8	
Postmenopause			
ER+	88.0	81.1	0.07
ER−	76.3	75.3	

adjuvant situation [3, 16]. The administration of non-cross-resistant chemotherapy (CMF and adriamycin) constitutes an attempt to maximize the cell kill of a mixtures of CMF-sensitive and CMF-resistant neoplastic cells. In fact, as suggested by the recent mathematical model of Goldie and Coldman [7], stable genetic alterations arise in tumor cells and result in phenotypic changes in drug sensitivity, and therefore provide a theoretical explanation for CMF-resistant patients. Since the presence of specifically and permanently resistant neoplastic cells is one of the most important causes of chemotherapy failure, sequential or alternating administration of non-cross-resistant regimens could result in a longer RFS and hopefully a higher cure rate than results from continuous administration of a single combination (this has already been observed in Hodgkin's disease [12]). The relative merits of cyclical delivery vs sequential administration will be tested in the very high-risk group, i.e., that having more than three involved axillary nodes, while the potential superiority of sequential chemotherapy vs CMF alone is under evaluation in the subgroup where CMF has produced its best results.

Women with breast cancer operable by conventional procedures and with negative axillary lymph nodes (N−) showed a 10-year relapse-free survival (RFS) rate of about 75% [5, 17]. In the large majority of patients with relapse, the new disease manifestations occur in distant sites, and they are considered to be due to growing micrometastases already present at the time of potentially curative surgery.

In recent years, several attempts have been made to identify the high-risk group with N− breast cancer. Many patients with recurrent disease showed less differentiated tumors, high labeling index, intralymphatic tumor emboli, tumor necrosis and estrogen receptor-negative (ER−) tumors [4, 6, 8−10, 14]. In patients with N−/ER−, the 3-year RFS curve appears almost superimposable to that of N+ patients [4]. The ER status also appears to be an important variable in our recent experience while, for the time being, the significance of other discriminants remains to be fully assessed in large numbers of consecutive patients. In fact, a retrospective analysis has been carried out on 464 consecutive patients operated on for breast cancer between April 1975 and March 1979 at the Istituto Nazionale Tumori of Milan [18]. All patients were histologically N− and none received radiotherapy or chemotherapy. The 3- and 5-year results (median follow-up 36 months) are reported in Table 3. Considering the 5-year RFS and survival results achieved in our Institute with adjuvant CMF in N+ patients [1, 11], the attempt to improve the RFS and survival rates of a high-risk group with N− by utilizing postoperative CMF through a prospective randomized study appears fully justified.

References

1. Bonadonna G, Valagussa P (1981) Dose-response effect of adjuvant chemotherapy in breast cancer. N Engl J Med 304: 10–15
2. Bonadonna G, Valagussa P, Rossi A, Tancini G, Brambilla C, Marchini S, Veronesi U (1981) Multimodal therapy with CMF in resectable breast cancer with positive axillary nodes. The Milan Institute experience. In: Salmon SE, Jones SE (eds) Adjuvant therapy of cancer III. Grune and Stratton, New York, pp. 435–444
3. Bonadonna G, Valagussa P, Tancini G, Di Fronzo G (1980) Estrogen-receptor status and response to chemotherapy in early and advanced breast cancer. Cancer Chemother Pharmacol 4: 37–41
4. Cooke T, George D, Shields R, Maynard P, Griffiths K (1979) Oestrogen receptors and prognosis in early breast cancer. Lancet 1: 995–997
5. Fisher B, Slack N, Katrych D, Wolmark N (1975) Ten-year follow up results of patients with carcinoma of the breast in a cooperative clinical trial evaluating surgical adjuvant chemotherapy. Surg Gynecol Obstet 140: 528–534
6. Fisher ER, Redmond C, Fisher B (1980) Pathological findings from the National Surgical Adjuvant Breast Project (Protocol no. 4) VI. Discriminant for five-year treatment failure. Cancer 46: 908–918
7. Goldie GH, Coldman AJ (1979) A mathematical model for relating the drug sensitivity of tumors to their spontaneous mutation rate. Cancer Treat Rep 63: 1727–1733
8. Knight WA, Livingston RB, Gregory EJ, McGuire WL (1977) Estrogen receptor: an independent prognostic factor for early recurrence in breast cancer. Cancer Res 37: 4669–4671
9. Meyer JS, Rao BR, Stevens SC, White WL (1977) Low incidence of estrogen receptors in breast carcinomas with rapid rates of cellular replication. Cancer 40: 2290–2298
10. Nime FA, Rosen PP, Thaler H, Ashikary R, Urban JA (1977) Prognostic significance of tumor emboli in intramammary lymphatics in patients with mammary carcinoma. Am J Surg Pathol 1: 25–30
11. Rossi A, Bonadonna G, Valagussa P, Veronesi U (1981) Multimodal treatment in operable breast cancer: five-year results of the CMF programme. Br Med J 282: 1427–1431
12. Santoro A, Bonadonna G, Bonfante V, Valagussa P (1982) Alternating non-cross resistant chemotherapy vs MOPP alone in the treatment of advanced Hodgkin's disease. New Engl J Med 306: 770–775
13. Skipper HE (1980) Breast cancer treated by means of mastectomy and mastectomy followed by 12 or 6 cycles of CMF. Southern Research Institute Birmingham, Ala
14. Silvestrini R, Daidone MG, Di Fronzo G (1979) Relationship between proliferative activity and estrogen receptors in breast cancer. Cancer 44: 665–670
15. Special Report (1979) Treatment of primary breast cancer. N Engl J Med 301: 340
16. National Institute of Health (1980) Steroid receptors in breast cancer. An NIH consensus development conference. Bethesda, Maryland, 27–29 Juni, 1979. Cancer (Suppl) 46: 2759–2962
17. Valagussa P, Bonadonna G, Veronesi U (1978) Patterns of relapse and survival following radical mastectomy. Analysis of 716 consecutive patients. Cancer 41: 1170–1178
18. Valagussa P, Di Fronzo G, Bignami P, Buzzoni R, Bonadonna G, Veronesi U (1981) Prognostic importance of estrogen receptors to select node negative patients for adjuvant chemotherapy. In: Salmon, SE, Jones SE (eds) Adjuvant therapy of cancer III. Grune and Stratton, New York, pp. 329–333
19. Veronesi U, Saccozzi R, Del Vecchio M, Banfi A, Clemente M, De Lena M, Gallus G, Greco M, Luini A, Marubini E, Muscolino G, Rilke F, Salvadori B, Zecchini A, Zucali R (1981) Comparing radical mastectomy with quadrantectomy, axillary dissection, and radiotherapy in patients with small cancer of the breast. N Engl J Med 305: 6–11

Effect of Adjuvant Therapy in Primary Breast Cancer in Relation to the Estrogen Receptor Level

A. Wallgren, U. Glas, S. Gustafsson, L. Skoog, N. O. Theve, and B. Nordenskjöld

Stockholm-Gotland Oncologic Center, Karolinska Hospital, S-104 01 Stockholm, Sweden

Introduction

It has repeatedly been shown that the presence of estrogen receptors (ER) in breast cancer tissue is a predictor of the response to endocrine therapy [1−3]; in this respect the quantity of ER is more predictive than simple qualitative classification [2−4]. Little ER in the tumor also predicts an early recurrence of the disease [5, 6]. Consequently adjuvant endocrine manipulations after surgery might be expected to affect short-term recurrence rate only slightly, since the tumors that are the most likely to recur early, i.e., the receptor-poor cancers, are the least likely to be affected by the treatment. In contrast to this expectation, our previous report [7] and that of others [8] have demonstrated that adjuvant tamoxifen therapy results in an increased disease-free survival. We now further detail the results of a prospective trial of tamoxifen treatment for 2 years after surgery. The recurrence rates are correlated to the ER levels in the tumors.

Materials and Methods

Patients

As previously described, after surgery and irrespective of stage or other adjuvant treatment, our postmenopausal women less than 71 years of age were randomly allocated to be treated with tamoxifen (Nolvadex, ICI) 20 mg b.i.d. for 2 years postoperatively or to a control group [7]. Patients with metastatic involvement of the lymph nodes in the surgical

Table 1. Number of eligible patients (a) treated with tamoxifen and (b) in the control group, divided according to other treatment modalities

Treatment group	Total no.	No further treatment (N−)	Radiotherapy (N+)	Chemotherapy (N+)
Tamoxifen	298	175	60	63
Controls	284	172	51	61
Total	582	347	111	124

specimen or whose tumors measured more than 30 mm were also superrandomized to receive 12 courses of polychemotherapy or, alternatively, postoperative radiotherapy as previously detailed [7]. The number of patients in the different treatment groups is given in Table 1.

Compliance

Owing to administrative errors at the beginning of the study, six patients never received tamoxifen. Five patients refused the proposed treatment. So far, 31 patients have interrupted the treatment before 2 years have elapsed because of subjective symptoms and various medical reasons listed in Table 2.

Estrogen Receptors

Estrogen receptor determination of the tumors has been performed in 417 (71.6%) of the patients in the study. Immediately after surgery a piece of the tumor was excised and placed into iced saline and transported to the receptor laboratory at the Karolinska Hospital. The sample was frozen at $-80°$ C and analysis performed within 3 weeks.

After thawing, the specific estradiol binding capacity was determined by isoelectric focusing on polyacrylamide gel as previously described [9]. The amount of receptor was expressed as the binding capacity of estradiol (femtomoles) per microgram of DNA. The distribution of the ER values are given in Fig. 1. For the analysis of recurrence-free survival rates the tumors were divided according to the quartile values of the receptor contents.

Statistical Method

The differences between the two treatment groups in terms of time to the first relapse or to death were tested using the log-rank test. The comparisons were made within each of the three treatment strata (i.e., no further treatment, postoperative chemotherapy, and radiotherapy) to allow for any skewness in distribution.

Table 2. Causes of interruption of tamoxifen treatment

Causes of interruption	No.
Nausea, gastrointestinal disturbance	8
Hot flushes, sweats	4
Thrombosis, thrombophlebitis	4
Sudden death caused by cerebral thrombosis	1
Symptoms of cerebral ischemia	1
Allergy	3
Toxicity of liver	1
Thrombocytopenia	1
Septic infection (concomitant cytotoxic chemotherapy)	1
New cancer	1
Other and unspecified	6
Total	31

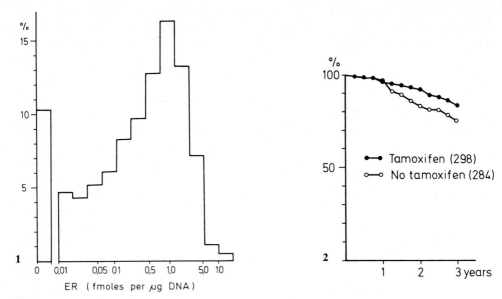

Fig. 1 (*left*). Frequency distribution of ER values in postmenopausal patients

Fig. 2 (*right*). Recurrence-free survival rates in the two patient groups

All patients randomized to either the tamoxifen or the control group were included in the analysis irrespective of whether the treatment was given or not. The mean time for follow-up was 17 months, with a range of 2–49 months.

Results

Recurrence-Free Survival

The recurrence-free survival rates of the patients in the two groups are given in Fig. 2. The rate was significantly better among the tamoxifen-treated patients than in the control group ($\chi^2 = 6.01$, $P = 0.01$).
Figure 3 separately illustrates findings in patients with nodal involvement; in this subgroup tamoxifen again yielded an increased recurrence-free survival rate ($P = 0.01$).

Recurrence-Free Survival and Receptor Level

Figure 4 illustrates that the recurrence-free survival rate was much higher for control patients with more than the median amount of ER. This was true both for patients with and for patients without nodal involvement. The patients were further subdivided into four equally sized groups according to their ER values. The recurrence-free survival rates within these quartile groups are illustrated for control patients and for tamoxifen-treated patients (Fig. 5).

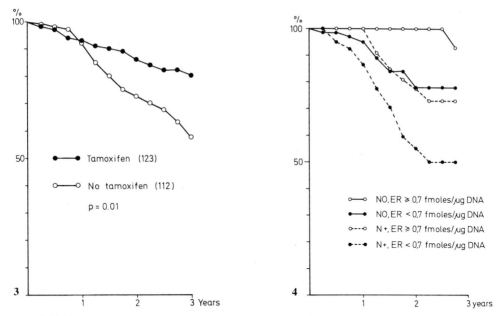

Fig. 3 (*left*). Recurrence-free survival rates in the two patient groups when lymph nodes were involved

Fig. 4 (*right*). Recurrence-free survival rates in the control group according to lymph node involvement and amount of ER

Discussion

This ongoing study shows that adjuvant treatment with the antiestrogen tamoxifen significantly increases the recurrence-free survival rate in postmenopausal women. A long uninterrupted disease-free period after surgery for breast cancer is of great importance. Once the disease has recurred, the woman will always feel less secure, even if the treatment is successful. But on the other hand, prophylactic treatment means unnecessary medication for many women. Even if tamoxifen is well tolerated by most patients, some are troubled by gastrointestinal symptoms and nausea, and younger postmenopausal women often experience hot flushes and sweats that impair the quality of life. Tamoxifen probably increases the danger of thromboembolic disease and is expensive. Therefore before tamoxifen is recommended as a routine adjuvant treatment it should be established beyond doubt that it yields prolonged survival.

The tumoral ER content was found to be a good predictor of early recurrence in patients not treated with tamoxifen, which is in concordance with several other studies [5, 6]. Interestingly, we found that tamoxifen also increased the recurrence-free survival rate in women with receptor-poor tumors. Thus many receptor-poor tumors must have responded to tamoxifen.

Several factors probably contribute to this unexpected finding. The most important is that it is possible to detect a significant reduction in recurrences only in groups of patients with a sufficient recurrence rate, and the receptor-poor tumors do have a high recurrence rate. A second factor is that receptor-poor tumors may in fact respond to tamoxifen although

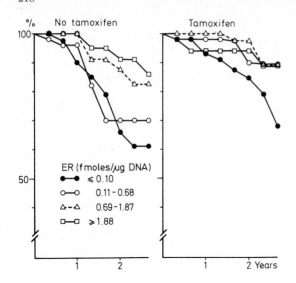

Fig. 5. Recurrence-free survival rates in the two patient groups according to ER levels

experience with metastatic disease tells us that this response is insufficient to classify the patient as a responder [3, 4]. In metastatic disease an objective response probably requires a 90% decrease in cell number. In the adjuvant situation a less pronounced regression or a decreased rate of cell replication [10] may be measurable as a prolonged disease-free interval. A third factor is that the correlation established by many groups between rapid tumor cell replication and low receptor values may partly be an artifact; the experiments by Wilking et al. [11] have demonstrated intratumoral metabolism of estrone sulfate to estradiol which blocks the receptor sites and thereby considerably reduces the levels of unbound receptor. Thus some tumors with rapid replication and low apparent receptor levels may in fact be able to interact with tamoxifen.

Whatever the reason for the effect, the conclusion of the study is that the ER level of a breast cancer does not necessarily predict the response to adjuvant treatment with tamoxifen. This gives a less pessimistic outlook for patients with low tumoral receptor contents than ER negativity usually implies. The early reduction in recurrences in postmenopausal women also gives us hope that tamoxifen will improve survival. The low toxicity compared with cytotoxic chemotherapy and the easy administration would make tamoxifen an excellent agent for "adjuvant" treatment. Further follow-up of our patients and further studies will reveal the place of tamoxifen in the treatment of breast cancer.

References

1. Jensen EV, Block GE, Smith S, Kyser K, Sombre ER (1971) Estrogen receptors and breast cancer response to adrenalectomy. Natl Cancer Inst Monogr 34: 55
2. Heuson JC, Longeval E, Mattheiem WH, Deboel MC, Sylvester RJ, Leclerq G (1977) Significance of quantitative assessment of estrogen receptors for endocrine therapy in advanced breast cancer. Cancer 39: 1971
3. Westerberg H, Nordenskjöld B, Wrange Ö, Gustafsson JÅ, Humla S, Theve NO, Silfverswärd C, Granberg PO (1978) Effect of antiestrogen therapy on human mammary carcinomas with different estrogen receptor contents. Eur J Cancer 14: 619–622

4. Allegra JC, Lippman ME, Thompson EB, Simon R, Barlock A, Green L, Huff KK, Do HMT, Aitken SC, Warren R (1980) Estrogen receptor status: An important variable in predicting response to endocrine therapy in metastatic breast cancer. Eur J Cancer 16: 323−331

5. Knight WA III, Livingston RB, Gregory EJ, McGuire WL (1977) Estrogen receptor as an independent prognostic factor for early recurrence in breast cancer. Cancer Res 37: 4669−4671

6. Westerberg H, Gustafsson SA, Nordenskjöld B, Silfverswärd C, Wallgren A (1980) Estrogen receptor level and other factors in early recurrence of breast cancer. Int J Cancer 26: 429−433

7. Wallgren A, Baral E, Glas U, Kaigas M, Karnström L, Nordenskjöld B, Theve NO, Wilking N, Silfverswärd C (1981) Adjuvant breast cancer treatment with tamoxifen and combination chemotherapy in postmenopausal women. In: Salmon SE, Jones SE (eds) Adjuvant therapy of cancer III. Grune and Stratton, New York

8. Fisher B, Redmond C, Brown A et al. (1981) Treatment of primary breast cancer with chemotherapy and tamoxifen. N Engl J Med 305: 1−6

9. Wrange Ö, Nordenskjöld B, Gustafsson JÅ (1978) Cytosol estradiol receptor in human mammary carcinoma: an assay based on isoelectric focusing in polyacrylamide gel. Anal Biochem 85: 461−474

10. Nordenskjöld B, Löwhagen T, Westerberg H, Zajicek J (1976) ^{3}H-Thymidine incorporation into mammary carcinoma cells obtained by needle aspiration before and during endocrine therapy. Acta Cytol 20: 137−143

11. Wilking N, Carlström K, Gustafsson SA, Sköldefors H, Tollbom Ö (1980) Oestrogen receptors and metabolism of oestrone sulphate in human mammary carcinoma. Eur J Cancer 16: 1339−1344

Part V: A Critical Summary

J. C. Heuson

Institut Jules Bordet, Centre des Tumeurs de l'Université Libre de Bruxelles, Service de Médecine, Clinique et Laboratoire de Cancérologie Mammaire, Rue Héger-Bordet 1, 1000 Bruxelles, Belgium

The three papers presented in this section involve some consideration of the potential usefulness of estrogen receptors (ER) in the planning of adjuvant therapy for breast cancer. Hence the problem is briefly reviewed.

The significance of ER in primary breast cancer is twofold: (a) they have prognostic implications and (b) they provide information on the hormone dependence of the tumor.

The prognostic value of ER in primary breast cancer has been the subject of several publications which have recently been reviewed by Hähnel [1]. According to this author, in a large majority of studies it was found that the presence of ER is associated with a longer disease-free interval. This conclusion was based on almost 2,000 patients. However, in six studies involving 326 patients, no difference in disease-free interval between ER+ and ER− carcinomas was observed. With regard to survival, all published series on the association with ER status agree that patients with ER+ breast carcinomas have an advantage over those with ER− carcinomas. The prognostic value of ER, when it existed, was often independent of the axillary nodal status. The latter finding is of particular interest in regard to the selection of patients for adjuvant trials. Thus, node-negative cases have fair prognosis overall except, although some authors [2, 3] have suggested that there is a subset of ER− tumors where the prospect is about as dire as in node-positive cases. It is tempting to test adjuvant chemotherapy in this subset.

Apart from their prognostic value, ER are most important as a marker of the hormone dependence of breast cancer [4]. Thus, in stage IV cases it was found that the likelihood of a response to endocrine therapy is a direct function of ER concentration [5−7]. It is most likely that similar relationships will be found in the adjuvant treatment of stage I or II patients. Indeed, there are already data consistent with this assumption. Adjuvant tamoxifen either alone or in combination with polychemotherapy has proven especially beneficial in ER+ cases and, in some subsets, only in association with higher receptor levels [8−11].

Should these data be confirmed, ER will be useful for the selection or stratification of patients in adjuvant trials. For collaborative studies, the major issue will then lie in the reproducibility of the assay results. In order to achieve this goal, the organization of an interlaboratory quality control program will be mandatory [12].

References

1. Hähnel R (1982) Steroid receptor status, tumor growth and prognosis. In: Stoll BA (ed) Endocrine relationship in breast cancer. Heinemann Medical, London, p 107
2. Knight WA III, Livingston RB, Gregory EJ, McGuire WL (1977) Estrogen receptor as an independent prognostic factor for early recurrence in breast cancer. Cancer Res 37:4669
3. Bonadonna G, Bignami P, Buzzoni R, Moliterni A, Valagussa P, Veronesi U (1983) New adjuvant trials for resectable breast cancer at the Istituto Nazionale Tumori of Milan. This book, pp 210–213
4. DeSombre ER, Carbone PP, Jensen EV, McGuire WL, Wells SA Jr, Wittliff JL, Lipsett MB (1979) Steroid receptors in breast cancer. N Engl J Med 301:1011
5. Heuson JC, Longeval E, Mattheiem WH, Deboel C, Sylvester RJ, Leclerq G (1977) Significance of quantitative assessment of estrogen receptors for endocrine therapy in advanced breast cancer. Cancer 39:1971
6. Paridaens R, Sylvester RJ, Ferrazzi E, Legros N, Leclercq G, Heuson JC (1980) Clinical significance of the quantitative assessment of estrogen receptors in advanced breast cancer. Cancer 46:2889
7. Osborne CK, Yochmowitz MG, Knight WA III, McGuire WL (1980) The value of estrogen and progesterone receptors in the treatment of breast cancer. Cancer 46:2884
8. Palshof T (1981) Adjuvant endocrine therapy in the management of primary breast cancer. Reviews on Endocrine-Related Cancer (Suppl) 7:65
9. Wallgren A, Baral E, Glas U, Kaigas M, Karnström L, Nordenskjöld B, Theve NO, Wilking N, Silfverswärd C (1981) Adjuvant breast cancer treatment with tamoxifen and combination chemotherapy in post-menopausal women. In: Salmon S, Jones SE (eds) Adjuvant therapy of cancer III. Grune and Stratton, New York, p 345
10. Hubay CA, Pearson OH, Marshall JS, Rhodes RS et al. (1980) Adjuvant chemotherapy, antiestrogen therapy and immunotherapy for stage II breast cancer: 45-month follow-up of a prospective, randomized clinical trial. Cancer 46:2805
11. Fisher B, Redmond C, Brown A, Wolmark N et al. (1981) Treatment of primary breast cancer with chemotherapy and tamoxifen. N Engl J Med 305:1
12. Sarfaty GA, Nash AR, Keightley DD (eds) (1981) Estrogen receptor assay in breast cancer. Laboratory discrepancies and quality assurance. Masson, New York

Endocrine Surgery in Breast Cancer

F. Badellino, G. Canavese, and G. Margarino

Istituto Nazionale per la Ricerca sul caucro, Istituto Scientifico per lo Studio e la Cura dei Tumori,
Istituto di oncologia sperimentale e clinica dell'università,
Viale Benedetto XV n. 10, 16132 Genova, Italy

Introduction

Endocrine cancer therapy began its development only after the availability of synthetic steroids made bilateral adrenalectomy and hypophysectomy possible.

Numerous different therapeutic schedules based on hormonal manipulation have been tried with patients suffering from cancer of the breast, prostate, thyroid, or endometrium. The term "hormone dependence" signifies that pharmacological or surgical suppression of specific endocrine functions can, in a certain number of cases, result in the regression of the primitive tumor and its metastases.

In endocrine therapy of mammary and prostatic cancer, ablative endocrine surgery is of primary importance. The most important procedures include:

1. Castration
   a) Oophorectomy (Beatson 1896)
   b) Orchiectomy (Prostatic carcinoma — Huggins 1941) (Male breast cancer — Farrow and Adair 1942)
2. Adrenalectomy (Huggins and Scott 1945)
3. Hypophysectomy (Welker 1948; J. le Beau 1951)

Oophorectomy

Oophorectomy as endocrine treatment for mammary cancer dates back to 1896, when Sir G. Beatson of Glasgow performed this procedure on three women suffering from breast cancer.

The use of castration in cancer treatment as an adjuvant to mastectomy in the absence of clinically evident metastases, which resulted in an increased disease-free interval but had no effect on mortality [13, 20], has for the most part been abandoned.

Therapeutic oophorectomy in patients with inoperable or disseminated breast cancer has, on the whole, given satisfactory results. In 639 cases reported by Veronesi [32], the overall response to oophorectomy was 29.5%, with an average duration of 16 months. The 5-year survival rate for patients who demonstrated a regression was 19%; 33% of premenopausal patients showed a regression while only 17.9% of women under 35 years of age and 6% of postmenopausal women did so. In a study performed by the New York Memorial Hospital [11], 34.5% of premenopausal women showed regression while no response to castration was seen in women in the first year of menopause. Oophorectomy has rarely been effective in postmenopausal women. Best results have been obtained with metastases of the soft tissues (40%), while bone, pleural, and lung metastases responded in only 26% of patients [6].

Of the patients with positive ER levels, 70% have shown a response to oophorectomy, compared with an extremely small percentage of responders among ER-negative patients, prompting the limitation of castration to patients with ER+ tumors [9, 34].

The result obtained by therapeutic castration can be of great help in predicting the response to subsequent adrenalectomy or hypophysectomy. Castration can be done either by surgical oophorectomy or by irradiation of the ovaries. The surgical procedure offers the advantage of complete and immediate removal of the hormonal influence of ovaries and permits exploration of the abdomen to exclude the possible presence of visceral or parenchymal metastases. When castration has been by irradiation of the ovaries, there is a possibility, especially in young patients, of resumption of the menstrual cycle and, as has occasionally been reported, an eventual pregnancy. The morbidity and mortality for oophorectomy are, in general, very low. Large case studies have reported a mortality rate of 2.5% in 191 cases [31] and 3% in 270 patients operated on [33]. A loss of menstrual-like blood may occur immediately after surgery in patients who have undergone oophorectomy during the luteinic phase. Urinary excretion of estrogens tends to fall to very low levels during the first few days after surgery, but then rises to approximately 50% of the presurgical level. Only estriol seems to remain at very low levels [10].

Orchiectomy

In man castration may be indicated in breast and prostatic cancer. Though the low frequency of breast cancer in males makes any comprehensive study difficult, it is generally accepted that endocrine surgery offers an effective form of therapy at minimal risk.

Adrenalectomy

In 1951, the synthesis and subsequent availability of the 11-deoxycorticoids made bilateral adrenalectomy possible without fear of hypoadrenal crisis [16]. Removal of the ovaries alone does not completely eliminate circulation of the sex steroids. Though there is no direct evidence for the production of estrogen in the adrenal cortex, it is well known that adrenal androstenedione is converted to estrogen in the peripheral tissues. Excision of the adrenal glands causes a net reduction in these hormones. Response to this treatment ranges from 23% to 46%. Average survival in responsive patients is 26 months vs 10 months in nonresponsive subjects [29]. The incidence of regression seems to be greater in subjects who have undergone adrenalectomy without previous hormone therapy [7]. In premenopausal women the response rate is apparently equal for those who have undergone oophorectomy and for those who have undergone both castration and adrenalectomy. Adrenalectomy performed at the moment of relapse of the disease in a patient previously oophorectomized results in longer survival.

From 50% to 60% of ER-positive tumors responded to endocrine ablation, the degree of response being proportional to the quantity of hormone receptors present in the tumor. The presence of both estrogen and progesterone receptors is associated with the highest percentage of response. Patients below 45 years of age show a low response rate (19%) of

Table 1. Treatment schedule of cortisone acetate (Cortone) and hydrocortisone hemisuccinate (Flebocortid) in bilateral adrenalectomy and hypophysectomy patients before and after surgery

---

A) Day before surgery: cortisone (Cortone)
    8:00 a.m. 50 + 50 mg i.m. (left and right gluteus)
    6:00 p.m. 50 + 50 mg i.m. (left and right gluteus)

B) Day of surgery: cortisone and hydrocortisone
    8:00 a.m. 50 mg i.m.
    During surgery: 100 mg i.v. (hydrocortisone)
                                (Flebocortid)
    6:00 p.m. 50 mg i.m.

C) After surgery: cortisone
   1st–2nd day: 50 mg i.m. a.i.d. (every 6 h)
   3rd–4th day: 50 mg i.m. t.i.d. (every 8 h)
   6th–9th day: 50 mg i.m. b.i.d. (every 12 h)
   10th day onward: 25 mg p.o. t.i.d. (every 8 h)

The dose of Cortone, in the absence of blood pressure variation, is gradually reduced to 37.5 mg p.o./day. In the event of adrenal crisis with cortisol deficiency, cortisone dosage can be increased or hydrocortisone can be administered (100–300 mg/day)

short duration [2]. The metastatic sites which respond most markedly to adrenalectomy are those which involve the soft tissues, the bones, and the lungs. Objective relief of bone pain and general improvement in the patient may sometimes be seen in the first few days following surgery.

Adrenalectomy is performed using one of the following surgical approaches:

1. *Transpleuric-diaphragmatic and thoracic-laparotomic approach,* indicated in tumors of the adrenals but rarely used in breast or prostate cancer patients.
2. *Transperitoneal approach,* preferred by some authors since it allows access to the ovaries and the adrenals, with the possibility of removing accessory adrenal tissue. It presents notable difficulties in obese patients and when the liver is enlarged [26].
3. *Extraperitoneal approach.* There are two possibilities: the posterior retroperitoneal method of Young (1936), which allows the relatively rapid removal of both glands without repositioning the patient, and the posterolateral lombotomic approach, which is generally employed in two-step adrenalectomy [26].

Postoperative treatment is extremely critical [6] since adrenalectomy results in the elimination of the glucocorticoids and mineralocorticoids, both of which are indispensable for maintenance of homeostasis. Permanent substitution therapy must be started with cortisone. The most commonly used treatment schedule is that described by Higgins and Bergenstal in 1951 (Table 1) [17]. A variation in the technique which bypasses the need for substitution therapy has been proposed by Dargent et al. [8, 22]. The operation consists of the removal of the ovaries and the right adrenal and then the implantation of a portion of left adrenal in the spleen. In this way a certain quantity of the endocrine secretion passes through the spleen to the liver, where estrogens and androgens would be degraded without denaturation of the corticosteroids. Theoretically this procedure could be considered the ideal method, but the high incidence (approximately 20%) of metastases in the adrenal glands must be kept in mind [30]. In 118 patients who underwent oophoro-adrenalectomy, 41% presented metastases of the ovary and adrenal [4]. The postoperative complications of

Table 2. Complications following bilateral adrenalectomy in 500 consecutive breast cancer patients [A. Fracchia (1967), Surg Gynecol Obstet 125:749]

Type of complication	No. of patients
No complications	301
Pneumothorax	65
Atelectasia, pneumonia	61
Postoperative hemorrhage	19
Cardiovascular insufficiency	16
Electrolyte disturbances	16
Infections	14
Herniated lumbar disc	5
Orthostatic hypotension	3

adrenalectomy are those common to most types of abdominal and extraperitoneal procedures (Table 2). The overall mortality reported by different authors without reference to the methods employed ranges from 2.7% to 16%.

Studies carried out on patients after oophoro-adrenalectomy have not demonstrated complete elimination of the sex steroids, but no relationship has been seen between the persistence of a certain quantity of hormones and treatment failure.

In recent years different compounds have been employed to block the action or synthesis of estrogens. Aminoglutethimide (AG) blocks the conversion of cholesterol to pregnenolone by inhibiting 20-hydroxylation in the adrenal [12, 18, 24]. In extra-adrenal sites it is a potent inhibitor of the metabolization of androstenedione and testosterone to estrogens. AG is usually used in association with dexamethasone or hydrocortisone for their effect on ACTH secretion. Some authors have demonstrated a response to AG similar to that obtained with adrenalectomy [27, 28]. However, it should be remembered that AG is not without side-effects whose severity may at times necessitate suspension of treatment. It is possible that AG plus corticosteroid therapy may replace surgical adrenalectomy in the near future, but presently it should be considered an alternative to adrenalectomy in those patients who represent a high surgical risk, and can be used to predict which patients will respond to surgical adrenalectomy.

It is improbable that another widely tested compound, tamoxifen, will be able to replace endocrine ablation [29].

Hypophysectomy

For more than 25 years hypophysectomy has been successfully used in the treatment of breast cancer (approx. 42% remissions), and it has also been employed with success in patients with prostate and thyroid cancer [3, 19, 21]. Adrenalectomy and hypophysectomy seem to give equivalent results. Hypophysectomy can be performed using various techniques, including surgery, radioisotopes, ultrasound, freezing, and diathermocoagulation.

The surgical approaches to the sella turcica used to perform hypophysectomy can be either extra- or intracranial. The most commonly followed technique is transfrontal craniotomy, and more recently transnasal and transphenoidal hypophysectomy has gained wide acceptance, allowing excision of only the anterior lobe, as is done in cases of diabetic retinopathy [14, 15].

The stereotactic cryohypophysectomy technique described by Rand [25] and the stereotactic radiofrequency procedure of Zervas [35] have shown a 29% success rate in 66 patients. These methods are relatively easy, take little time, and involve few risks.

The first attempt to destroy the hypophysis by radioactive material was made by Northfield (1949), who used radon in the treatment of some forms of acromegaly and Cushing's syndrome. Later Rasmussen et al. (1954) demonstrated that the intrapituitary implantation of ^{90}yttrium pellets resulted in a 2−3 mm thick necrotic area surrounding the single rods of ^{90}Y. This isotope, a pure β emitter with a half-life of approximately 64 h, has remained the most popular radioactive preparation used for this procedure. Up to 10,000 rads can be administered as close as 3 mm from the axial section of the rod. Radioactive material can be implanted intracranially through the diaphragm of the sella turcica (Rasmussen 1954), via the nasal transethmoid-sphenoidal route (Bauer 1956) and via the nasal transsphenoidal route (Greening and Stevenson 1957, Dogliotti and Ruffo 1958) [26]. The needle is directed toward the floor of the sella turcica, its ascent being continuously checked on a scope, using an image intensifying apparatus.

Other radioactive isotopes have been used, including radon (^{222}Rn), phosphorus (^{32}P), and gold (^{198}Au).

Surgical hypophysectomy gives a higher response rate than the radiobiological technique. The average duration of objective regressions is 18 months with the surgical technique, compared with about 12 months with the methods using radioactive material. After surgical hypophysectomy responsive patients have a greater survival rate than nonresponsive patients. Postmenopausal patients have shown a greater response. The metastatic sites that respond more often are those located in the lymph nodes, bone, pleura, and skin [5].

Postoperative complications are particulary severe. About 20% of the patients present permanent diabetes insipidus, 30% have olfactory disturbances, 20% suffer from rhinorrhea and meningism, and a small percentage show lesions of the cranial nerves and optic pathway. Hypoadrenalism appears immediately after surgical hypophysectomy and requires substitution treatment similar to that given after adrenalectomy. Manifestation of decreased thyroid function appears more slowly, necessitating treatment when serum thyroxin levels drop. The diabetes insipidus which appears in the first few days following surgery, together with marked polyuria, can be corrected with hypophyseal extracts administered either intramuscularly or by nasal inhalation.

Postoperative mortality ranges from 6% to 10%; in one study utilization of the transsphenoïdal technique gave a mortality of 1% [24].

In a study conducted on 93 patients who underwent destruction of the hypophysis by ^{80}Y and ^{32}P, no signs of hypothyroidism serious enough to require treatment were observed [1].

In patients who have undergone hypophysectomy with radioactive isotopes, hypoadrenalism appears more slowly; the mortality for this procedure is no greater than 1%−2%.

Inactivation of the hypophysis is a useful therapeutic method in patients with advanced breast cancer, especially when other forms of therapy are no longer capable of controlling the evolution of the disease (Tables 3, 4).

Encouraging results have been obtained in experiments using antiprolactin and antiestrogen compounds.

Table 3. Regressions after surgical hypophysectomy in breast cancer patients

Authors	No. of cases	Regressions	
		n	*%*
Kennedy et al. (1956)	28	18	64
Luft et al. (1958)	54	27	50
Jessiman et al. (1959)	45	27	60
Pearson and Ray (1960)	333	144	43
Boesen et al. (1961)	92	42	46
Peck and Olson (1963)	44	16	36

Table 4. Regressions after radiobiological hypophysectomy with ^{90}Y in breast cancer patients

Authors	No. of cases	Regressions	
		n	*%*
Forrest et al. (1959)	28	9	32
Moseley et al. (1959)	42	11	26
Evans et al. (1959)	31	8	26
Juret et al. (1964)	150	56	37
Notter and Melander (1966)	100	32	32

Conclusions

Removal of the ovaries and the adrenal glands gives beneficial results in breast cancer therapy if performed following precise indication. It is obvious that the hormonal receptor levels are of essential importance, but other clinical and biological parameters must be considered as being of equal importance. These include the menopausal status of the patient (no later than 5 years postmenopause), the metastatic sites involved, and the disease-free interval (at least 2 years). Another valid criterion in menstruating women is an increase in metastatic pains at the time of ovulation. Remission obtained with previous hormonal or ablation therapy should also be taken into account. These signs, combined with positive hormonal receptor levels, can almost guarantee a positive response.

References

1. Badellino F (1976) Results of pituitary ablation by ^{90}Y and ^{32}P interstitial implants in breast carcinoma. In: Eharyulu KKN, Sudarsanam A (eds) Hormones and cancer. Stratton Medical, New York, p 233
2. Brown PW, Terz JJ, King R, Lawrence W Jr (1975) Bilateral adrenalectomy for metastatic breast carcinoma. Arch Surg 110: 77
3. Bucalossi P, Veronesi U, Cascinelli N, Buraggi G, Miserocchi E, Monfardini S (1976) Pituitary ablation with ^{90}Y implant in advanced thyroid cancer. Cancer 20: 724

4. Caldarola L, Badellino F, Molinatti GM (1971) Ovariectomie avec surrénalectomie bilatérale pour cancer du sein en stade avancé (A propos de 118 cas). Presse Med 79: 1743

5. Caldarola L, Badellino F, Santoro L, Lesca F, Reali F, Ferrero B (1973) Resultati a distanza in 73 ipofisectomie radiobiologiche per cancri mammari inoperabili e/o metastatizzati. Gaz Med Ital 132: 276

6. Catania VC, Paolucci R (1977) Indicazioni, risultati e prospettive della terapia endocrino-chirurgica. In: Casa (ed) I tumori della mammella. Ambrosiana, Milano, p 289

7. Dao TL, Nemoto T, Bross IDJ (1967) A controlled, randomized comparative study of early and late adrenalectomy in women with advanced mammary cancer. In: Forrest APM, Kunklers PB (eds) Prognostic factors in breast cancer. Livingstone, Edinburgh, p 177

8. Dargent M, Mayer M (1959) La transplantation surreno-splenique dans le traitment du cancer du sein en phase avancée. A propos de 24 cas. Mem Acad Chir 85: 112

9. De Sombre ER, Carbone PP, Jensen EV, Lipsett MB, McGuire WL, Wells SA, Witliff JL (1979) Steroid receptors in breast cancer. An NIH consensus development conference, 27−29 June, 1979

10. Diczfalusy E, Notterg G, Edsmyr F, Westman A (1959) Estrogen excretion in breast cancer patients before and after ovarian irradiation and oophorectomy. J Clin Endocrinol 19: 1230

11. Fracchia AA, Farrow JH, De Palo AJ, Conolly DT, Huvos AG (1969) Castration for primary inoperable or recurrent breast carcinoma. Surg Gynecol Obstet 128: 1226

12. Gower DB (1974) Modifiers of steroid-hormone metabolism. A review of their chemistry, biochemistry and clinical applications. J Steroid Biochem 5: 501

13. Hayward S (1970) Hormones and human breast cancer. Springer, Berlin Heidelberg New York (Recent results in cancer research, vol 24)

14. Hardy J (1967) Hypophysectomie trans-sphenoidale. In: Dargent M, Romieu CL (eds) Major endocrine surgery for treatment of the cancer of the breast in advanced stages. Simep, Lyon, p 97

15. Hardy J, Ciric IS (1968) Selective anterior hypophysectomy in the treatment of diabetic retinopathy: a transphenoidal microsurgical technique. JAMA 203: 73

16. Huggins C, Scott WW (1945) Bilateral adrenalectomy in prostatic cancer. Ann Surg 122: 1031

17. Huggins C, Bergenstal DM (1952) Inhibition of human mammary and prostatic cancers by adrenalectomy. Cancer Res 12: 134

18. Hughes SWM, Burley DM (1970) Aminoglutethimide. A "side effect" turned to therapeutic advantage. Postgrad Med J 46: 409

19. Juret P (1966) Endocrine surgery in human cancers. Thomas, Springfield

20. Kennedy BJ, Mielke PW Jr, Fortuny IE (1960) Therapeutic castration versus prophylactic castration and breast cancer. Surg Gynecol Obstet 118: 524

21. Luft R, Olivecrona H (1975) Hypophysectomy in management of neoplastic disease. Bull NY Acad Med 33: 5

22. Mayer M, Dargent M, Pommatau E, Leaz S (1967) Resultats de la transplantation surrenosplenique associée à la surrenalectomie droite et à l'ovariectomie. In: Dargent M, Romieu Cl (eds) Major endocrine surgery for the treatment of cancer of the breast in advances staged. Simep Lyon, p 67

23. Pearson OH, Ray BS (1960) Hypophysectomy in the treatment of advanced cancer. Am J Surg 99: 544

24. Philbert M, Laudaut MH, Bricaire LH (1966) Etude clinique et biologique d'un inibiteur de l'hormonosynthèse corticosurrénale: l'aminoglutethimide. Ann Endocrinol 29: 189

25. Rand RW, Dashe AM, Paglia DE, Conway LW, Solomon DH (1964) Stereotactic cryohypophysectomy. JAMA 189: 255

26. Ruffo A, Badellino F, Rossotto P et al. (1960) Il trattamento endocrino-chirurgico dei tumori maligni. Omnia Therapeutica, vol XI, genn.-marzo

27. Santen RJ, Lipton A, Kendall J (1974) Successful medical adrenalectomy with aminoglutethimide. Role of altered drug metabolism. JAMA 230: 1661

28. Santen RJ, Wells SA Jr (1980) The use of aminoglutethimide in the treatment of patients with metastatic carcinoma of the breast. Cancer 46: 1066
29. Schweitzer RJ (1980) Oophorectomy-adrenalectomy. Cancer 46: 1061
30. Sirtori C, Pizzetti F, Catania VC (1958) Studio istologico e istochimico dei surreni e delle ovaie in pazienti portatrici di carcinoma mammario. Tumori 44: 263
31. Treves N, Finkbeiner JA (1958) An evaluation of therapeutic surgical castration in the treatment of metastatic recurrent and primary inoperable mammary carcinoma in women. An analysis of 191 patients. Cancer 11: 421
32. Veronesi U, Pizzocaro G (1962) Oophorectomy for advanced carcinoma of the breast. Surg Gynecol Obstet 115: 443
33. Veronesi U, Pizzocaro G (1966) L'ovariectomia nella terapia del carcinoma avanzato della mammella. Tumori 52: 465
34. Weick JK, Cooperman AM (1978) Ovarian suppression and breast cancer. Surg Clin North Am 58: 795
35. Zervas NT (1969) Stereotaxic radiofrequency surgery of the normal and abnormal pituitary gland. N Engl J Med 280: 429

Treatment of Advanced Breast Cancer with Tamoxifen

C. Rose and H. T. Mouridsen

Department of Oncology I, Finsen Institute,
49 Strandboulevarden, 2100 Copenhagen, Denmark

Introduction

The overall response rate in advanced breast cancer patients treated with endocrine therapies is in the range of 30% [1, 2]. In recent years it has been demonstrated that response to various forms of endocrine treatment can be predicted in approximately 60% of cases provided that the patient's tumor tissue contains the estrogen receptor (ER) protein [3]. This response rate is in the same range as that obtained with cytotoxic therapy [1, 2]. Furthermore, a response to endocrine therapy seems to predict that a response to subsequent cytotoxic treatment will be of longer duration and lead to prolonged survival [4, 5]. Another aspect of endocrine therapy is that new remissions can be achieved when using subsequent endocrine therapies [6−11]. Therefore, taking into account the fact that treatment of patients with metastatic disease is, at best, palliative, it appears that there is a sound clinical rationale behind the use of the relatively nontoxic endocrine treatment modalities.

The various forms of endocrine treatment in advanced breast cancer can be divided into four groups according to their mode of biological action (Table 1). The rationale for the use of the ablative procedures oophorectomy, adrenalectomy, and hypophysectomy [12−16] is that hormones promote the growth of some mammary tumor cells. Thus, a decrease in the concentration of these hormones is assumed to induce tumor regression. The concentration of adrenal steroid hormones can be diminished by treatment with aminoglutethimide (AG), which inhibits production of these hormones [17−20]. Furthermore, the peripheral aromatization of androstenedione to estrone [21] is inhibited by AG.

The mode of action underlying the paradoxical effect of pharmacological doses of steroid hormones such as estrogens, androgens, progestins, and glucocorticoids on tumor growth is largely unknown [22−26]. Owing to the pronounced side-effects of treatment with these steroids, competitive treatment with antihormones such as the nonsteroidal antiestrogenic compound tamoxifen (TAM) has been evaluated [27]. The primary step in its action is the competition with estradiol for binding to the cytoplasmic ER which renders the tumor cells insensitive to circulating levels of estrogens [28−30]. At the chromatin level the mechanism of action of TAM is complex [31, 32], and ultimately it leads to both a partial block of the cell cycle in the early G_1-phase [33] and an increase in the concentration of the progesterone receptor protein in the tumor cells [34, 35]. Furthermore, recent studies have shown [36, 37] that TAM binds to high-affinity, saturable sites that appear to be different from the ER-binding sites.

Recent Results in Cancer Research. Vol. 91
© Springer-Verlag Berlin · Heidelberg 1984

Table 1. Endocrine therapy of breast cancer

Ablative:	Oophorectomy
	Adrenalectomy
	Hypophysectomy
Inhibitive:	Aminoglutethimide
	Δ^1-Testololactone
	Bromocriptine
	L-dopa
Additive:	Estrogen
	Progestin
	Androgen
	Glucocorticoid
Competitive:	Antiestrogen
	Antiandrogen

This review will present the therapeutic results achieved with tamoxifen in treatment of advanced breast cancer when used as a single agent or in combination with other treatment modalities. For reviews concerning the biochemical, biological, and pharmacological properties of TAM, the reader is referred to the comprehensive works by Furr et al. [38] and Patterson [39].

Patient Population

The clinical trials reviewed here met the following conditions:
1. More than 20 patients randomized in each treatment arm within the trial
2. Statements of criteria for response (compatible with UICC criteria)
3. Information about relevant data such as side-effects and dominant site of disease

Criteria of Response

With few exceptions of minor importance, responses were classified according to the UICC criteria [40].
Some authors did not distinguish between complete (CR) and partial remission (PR), and other investigators did not give the exact numbers of no change (NC) and progressive disease (PD). The majority of the authors calculated the mean or median duration of response, while only a few reported the time to treatment failure (TTF) [10, 41–43], and the survival time [11, 41, 42, 44, 45].

Clinical Results

Tamoxifen Used as a Single Agent

Recently, the efficacy of TAM in various trials encompassing 1,269 patients with advanced breast cancer was reviewed [27]. Most of the patients were from nonrandomized trials.

Table 2. Results of treatment with tamoxifen irrespective of previous systemic treatment

References	No. of patients evaluable	Treatment results				CR + PR		Response duration[a] (mean or median)
		PD	NC	PR	CR	No.	%	
47	68	30	12	–	–	26	38	–
49	29	–	–	–	–	9	31	38 w
43	68	14	31	17	6	23	33	171 d
44	30	18	2	–	–	10	33	11 m
10	37	20	6	–	–	11	30	14.4 + m
50	36	9	18	–	–	9	25	10 m
51	32	9	8	10	5	15	47	10–20+ m
52	24	9	5	7	3	10	42	13 m
11	60	31	11	–	–	18	30	15 m
55	45	18	7	16	4	20	44	10 m
53	65	20	20	14	11	25	39	11+ m
41	52	26	18	8	0	8	15	230 d
57	23	12	6	–	–	5	22	–
Total	569	204/530	144/541	–	–	189/569		
Percent		39	27			34		
95% C.L.[b] (%)		35–44	23–31			30–39		

[a] d, days; w, weeks; m, months
[b] 95% C.L. = 95% confidence limits

Irrespective of previous systemic treatment, the response rate ranged from 16% to 52%, with an average of 32%. In the present review the responses in 569 patients randomized to treatment with TAM alone are summarized in Table 2. The response rates range from 15% to 52%, with an average of 34% (95% C.L. = 30%–39%). The rates for PD and NC were also comparable in both the former and the present patient populations. Table 2 includes three studies which the two reviews have in common [41, 47, 53].

Dosage

In spite of the extensive use of TAM in the treatment of advanced breast cancer, the optimal dose has yet to be established. Doses in the range of 20–40 mg daily are currently recommended and have been used in the majority of the clinical trials. At this dose level the steady-state blood values are obtained within 12–16 weeks, and blood concentrations known to be associated with a response are reached after 6 weeks [46]. Using many different dose levels (Table 3) with a relatively small number of patients at each level (half of the patients were also treated with androgens), Tormey et al. [41] did not find a significantly different therapeutic effect at the highest TAM doses compared with the low doses. Higher blood concentrations at the higher dose levels could conceivably lead to a more rapid response. However, in the present study no significant difference in median time to first response was observed. Ward [47] compared 20 mg and 40 mg per day and failed to find any advantages in using the higher dose.

Table 3. Randomized trials comparing different dose levels of tamoxifen

References	Dose of tamoxifen	Response rate (CR+PR/N)	%	95% C.L. (%)	Time to first response
41	< 12 mg/m^2 b.i.d.	10/37	27	(14−44)	34 d
	12−32 mg/m^2 b.i.d.	8/45	18	(8−32)	63 d
	> 32 mg/m^2 b.i.d	11/26	42	(23−63)	56 d
47	10 mg b.i.d.	12/33	36	(20−55)	−
	20 mg b.i.d.	14/35	40	(24−58)	−

Tamoxifen Compared with Other Endocrine Therapies

The efficacy of treatment with tamoxifen compared with other endocrine therapy modalities has been subject to many investigations. A prospective comparison between oophorectomy and treatment with TAM in premenopausal patients with advanced breast cancer has yet to be done. Data from two phase II trials indicate that the rate of response is approximately 30% [62, 63].

In a study including 26 patients, all of whom had responded to prior oophorectomy or additive hormone treatment, Kiang et al. [48] found that the rate and duration of response to TAM was similar to that obtained by major ablative procedures such as hypophysectomy and adrenalectomy. The response rate to pharmacological doses of sex steroid hormones is approximately 30%−40% (Table 4). Three studies [43, 44, 49] comparing treatment with pharmacological doses of estrogens and treatment with TAM failed to demonstrate differences in the overall response rates and durations of remission. In all three studies the side-effects were both more frequent and more serious in the patients treated with estrogens.

Although the difference was not statistically significant, Westerberg [10] reported a higher remission rate (30%) in patients receiving tamoxifen than in those treated with fluoxymesterone (19%). Survival was significantly longer in the tamoxifen-treated group. Toxicities were mild and comparable in the two groups except for the symptoms of virilization, which occurred only in the androgen-treated group.

No difference in response rates or durations of remission were demonstrated in either of two studies comparing treatment with TAM and treatment with medroxyprogesterone acetate (MPA) given either orally [50] or intramuscularly [51].

Two studies have compared the efficacy of inhibitive treatment with the enzyme antagonist AG combined with a glucocorticoid and treatment with TAM [11, 52]. Both studies indicate that the two treatment modalities are equally effective with respect to overall rate and duration of response, but objective responses in bone metastasis are achieved more often with AG than with TAM (18/44 = 41% vs 9/47 = 19%). Side-effects were more frequent and pronounced in the AG-treated group, and prompted discontinuation of the therapy in some patients.

In conclusion, the overall treatment results with TAM are as good as those obtained with other endocrine therapies. In addition, the side-effects of TAM seem minor. However, in none of these studies comparing TAM with other endocrine therapies were sufficient numbers of patients included to allow analysis for subsets of patients who might gain greater benefit from one or other of the treatments.

Table 4. Randomized trials comparing tamoxifen with other endocrine therapies

References	Treatment (dose)	Response rate (CR + PR/N)	%	95% C.L. (%)	Duration of response (median or mean)	Time to treatment failure (median)	Survival (median)
49	TAM (10 mg × 3)	9/29	31	(15–51)	38 w	–	–
	DES (5 mg × 3)	6/27	22	(9–42)	32.5 w	–	–
43	TAM (10 mg × 2)	23/68	34	(22–47)	238 d	171 d	–
	DES (5 mg × 3)	30/74	41	(29–53)	393 d	142 d	–
44	TAM (20 mg × 2)	10/30	33	(17–53)	11 m	–	25 m
	EE_2 (0.5–15 mg/d)	9/29	31	(15–51)	12 m	–	31 m
10	TAM (20 mg × 2)	11/37	30	(16–47)	14.4+ m	8.5 m	–
	FLU (10 mg × 2)	8/42	19	(9–34)	10.6+ m	5 m	–
50	TAM (20–30 mg/d)	9/36	25	(12–42)	10 m	–	–
	MPA (400–1,000 mg p.o./d)	10/40	25	(13–41)	7 m	–	–
51	TAM (10 mg × 2)	15/32	47	(29–65)	CR 21+ m PR 10 m	–	–
	MPA (1,000 mg d 1–30 1,000 mg/w)	14/26	54	(33–73)	CR 17+ m PR 7 m	–	–
52	TAM (20 mg × 2)	10/24	42	(22–63)	13 m	–	–
	AG + H (1,000 + 40 mg/d)	10/21	48	(26–70)	10 m	–	–
11	TAM (10 mg × 2)	18/60	30	(19–43)	15 m	–	24+ m
	AG + H (1,000 + 60 mg/d)	17/57	30	(18–43)	15 m	–	19 m

TAM, tamoxifen; *DES*, diethylstilbestrol; EE_2, ethinyl estradiol; *MPA*, medroxyprogesterone acetate; *AG*, aminoglutethimide; *FLU*, fluoxymesterone; *H*, hydrocortisone

Table 5. Response of tamoxifen related to ER status

References	Responders (CR + PR)/total	
	ER-positive	ER-negative
43	5/11	–
44	7/13	0/7
51	6/9	–
49	7/18	0/5
55	7/11	2/9
53	6/12	1/9
41	7/23	0/7
Total	45/97 (46%)	3/37 (8%)

Table 6. Response to second-line endocrine therapy in relation to response to previous therapy with tamoxifen

References	2nd-line drug	Non-cross-resistance CR+PR/NR	%	95% C.L. (%)	Cross-sensitivity CR+PR/R	%	95% C.L. (%)
49	DES	1/19	5	(0−26)	2/5	40	(5− 85)
43	DES	4/22	18	(5−40)	5/11	46	(17− 77)
10	FLU	1/10	10	(0−45)	–	–	–
51	MPA	2/6	33	(4−78)	4/4	100	(40−100)
11	AG + H	5/34	15	(5−31)	4/6	67	(22− 96)

CR + PR, response to second-line therapy; *R*, responders to first-line therapy; *NR*, nonresponders to first-line therapy; *DES*, diethylstilbestrol; *FLU*, fluoxymesterone; *MPA,* medroxyprogesterone acetate; *AG* aminoglutethimide; *H*, hydrocortisone

Response of Tamoxifen Related to Estrogen Receptor Status

Only seven studies have correlated the response to TAM with the presence of ER. In all of these studies only small subsets of the total groups of patients were analyzed for ER, and the different investigators used different techniques and cut-off limits. The results are summarized in Table 5. In the ER-positive group 46% of the patients experienced a response, in contrast to only 8% in the ER-negative group. These results correlate well with the figures previously found [27]. The rather low remission rate in the ER-positive group may be due to the fact that the TAM treatment was second- or third-line therapy in most cases.

Tamoxifen as a Single Agent Compared with Combinations of Tamoxifen with Other Endocrine Therapies

The available data analyzing the response to second-line endocrine therapy in relation to response to previous therapy with tamoxifen are summarized in Table 6. The numbers of

Table 7. Randomized trials comparing tamoxifen with tamoxifen in combination with other endocrine therapies

References	Treatment (dose)	Response rate (CR + PR/N)	%	95% C.L. (%)	Duration of response (mean or median)	Time to treatment failure (median)	Survival (median)
53	TAM (10 mg × 3)	25/65	39	(27–51)	11+ m	–	–
	TAM DES (1 mg × 3)	21/57	37	(25–51)	9+ m	–	–
41	TAM (2–100 mg/m² × 2)	8/52	15	(7–28)	230 d	64 d	329 d
	TAM FLU (7 mg/m² × 2)	21/56	37	(25–52)	212 d	180 d	380 d
55	TAM (10 mg × 3)	20/45	44	(30–60)	CR 10 m / PR 9 m	–	–
	TAM MPA (100 mg/d)	14/55	26	(15–39)	CR 9 m / PR 12+ m	–	–
56	TAM (10 mg × 2)		33	–	–	–	–
	TAM AG+H (750+20 mg/d) Danazol (100 mg × 3)		55	–	–	–	–
57	TAM (20 mg × 2) Placebo	5/23	22	(8–44)	–	–	–
	TAM Bromocriptin (2.5 mg × 4)	4/20	20	(6–44)	–	–	–

TAM, tamoxifen; *DES*, diethylstilbestrol; *FLU*, fluoxymesterone; *MPA*, medroxyprogesterone acetate; *AG*, aminoglutethimide; *H*, hydrocortisone

patients are small, and the data should, therefore, be interpreted with caution. There appears to be partial cross-sensitivity and a lack of complete cross-resistance between treatment with TAM and the other endocrine therapies. These clinical experiences indicate that the different endocrine therapies may not share the same ultimate modes of action and provide a rationale for the simultaneous application of different endocrine therapies. The data of randomized trials comparing TAM and combinations of TAM with other endocrine treatments are summarized in Table 7. One trial [53] analyzed the efficacy of TAM in combination with diethylstilbestrol (DES). It appears that the addition of DES to TAM improved neither the rate nor the duration of response. The dose of DES (3 mg/daily) was lower than that often used in the treatment of advanced disease. But, according to Carter et al. [54], the therapeutic gain is minimal when the dose is increased from 1.5 mg to 1,500 mg per day. Tormey et al. [41] compared TAM with TAM plus the androgen fluoxymesterone, using doses of TAM ranging from 2 mg/m^2 to 100 mg/m^2 twice daily. The observed difference in response rate, 15% vs 38%, is significant, as is the difference in median time to treatment failure. However, the durations of response and the median survival times did not differ significantly. In another study [55], TAM was compared with a combination of TAM and MPA. The response rate was lower in the group treated with MPA + TAM than in the group treated with TAM alone, but this difference was not significant. The MPA dose was 100 mg/daily given orally. Although this dose may have been too low, the dose-response relationship of oral treatment with MPA has not yet been properly analyzed.

Preliminary data from a trial including a total of 140 patients followed up for at least 3 months [56], where TAM alone was compared with a combination of TAM, AG + H (hydrocortisone) and the synthetic androgen danazol, reveal a response rate of 55% for the combination and 33% for TAM alone.

Finally, no advantage of combining TAM with the prolactin-inhibiting drug bromocriptine has been demonstrated to date [57].

Tamoxifen in Combination with Cytotoxic Therapy

The concept of tumor heterogeneity provides a rationale for combining endocrine and cytotoxic chemotherapy, and the different modes of action of endocrine therapies and cytotoxic drugs should theoretically lead to higher rates of response with the combined treatments. To date six randomized studies of treatment of postmenopausal women with cytotoxic agents in combination with TAM have been published (Table 8).

Cocconi et al. [45] analyzed 133 evaluable patients and found a response rate of 74% and 51% in favor of the combination. No real difference was found in duration of remission and survival. The EORTC cooperative group [58] randomized 215 patients to the same therapeutic regimens. The results confirm the superiority of CMF + TAM regarding response rates (72% vs 46%). The median time to treatment failure (70 weeks vs 40 weeks) was significantly longer in the combined treatment group. However, the therapeutic benefit was limited to patients more than 60 years of age and to patients with metastases in bones and viscera. Tormey et al. [42] tested the efficacy of dibromodulcitol (D) plus adriamycin (A) alone or in combination with TAM in 122 patients eligible for study after exposure to previous chemotherapy and/or ablative endocrine treatment. Although utilizing a second-line regimen, response rates of 36% and 55% respectively were achieved. The median duration of response, overall median time to treatment failure, and the median time of survival were in favor of the combined treatment. When comparing these results

Table 8. Randomized trials of cytotoxic therapy in combination with tamoxifen

References	Treatment (dose)	Response rate (CR + PR/N)	%	95% C.L. (%)	Duration of response (mean or median)	Time to treatment failure (median)	Survival (median)
42	DA	16/55	29	(18−43)	160 d	110 d	270 d
	DA	34/67	51	(38−63)	280 d	170 d	340 d
	TAM (20 mg/d)						
59	CFVe	35/64	55	(42−67)	–	–	–
	CFVe	46/69	67	(54−78)	–	–	–
	TAM (20 mg/d)						
45	CMF	36/71	51	(39−63)	47 w	–	118 w
	CMF	46/62	74	(62−85)	51 w	–	84 w
	TAM (10 mg × 2)						
60	CMFV/AC	8/20	40	(19−64)	–	–	–
	CMFV/AC	15/20	75	(51−91)	–	–	–
	TAM (10 mg × 2)						
58	CMF	47/103	46	(37−57)	–	40 w	–
	CMF	81/112	72	(64−82)	–	70 w	–
	TAM (20 mg × 2)						
61	CAF → CMF	46/54	85	(73−93)	–	–	–
	CAF → CMF	50/58	86	(75−94)	–	–	–
	TAM (20 mg/d)						

TAM, tamoxifen; *D*, dibromodulcitol; *A*, adriamycin; *C*, cyclophosphamide; *F*, 5-fluorouracil; *M*, methotrexate; *Ve*, velbe; *V*, vincristine

with those from the EORTC study, it is noteworthy that DA-TAM was found to be superior to DA both in patients older than 56 years of age and in those less than 46 years of age. However, a group of perimenopausal patients did not benefit from the combined treatment.

In two other studies [59, 60] the trend of a higher rate of remission observed in the chemohormonal treatment regimen seems to be confirmed. However, in one study [61] the addition of TAM to sequential treatment with CAF for ten cycles followed by CMF did not improve the remarkably high remission rate of 85% obtained with the chemotherapy regimen alone.

Conclusions

Treatment of advanced breast cancer with TAM has proved to be an alternative to other endocrine treatment modalities. The response rate is approximately 35% irrespective of previous treatment and ER status. These response rates are similar to those obtained with other endocrine therapies in postmenopausal patients. Toxicity to tamoxifen is milder and less frequent than is the case with estrogens, androgens, and AG. Furthermore, a substantial percentage of patients can obtain a second response to additive or inhibitive endocrine treatment following relapse or progression while on treatment with TAM. Knowledge of the correct dose level and drug scheduling of TAM is still limited and should be further analyzed in comparative studies. Based upon the data available today, it seems that the simultaneous administration of TAM and other endocrine therapies is not significantly superior to treatment with TAM alone. This question may be answered within the next few years when a number of ongoing randomized trials are completed.

Since endocrine therapy acts mainly by decreasing the growth rate of the hormone-sensitive tumor cells, it could be that simple additional endocrine and cytotoxic treatments would be antagonistic. There is, however, clinical evidence for the superiority of combined chemohormonal therapy compared with chemotherapy alone. Thus, in five out of six randomized trials the addition of TAM to various regimens of cytotoxic therapies improved the response rate and in two of the studies [42, 58] also improved the time to treatment failure.

In conclusion, TAM is as effective as other endocrine therapies in the treatment of advanced breast cancer in postmenopausal patients, whereas its role in the treatment of premenopausal patients remains to be defined. Its placement in combined treatment modalities is still under investigation, but limited data suggest a therapeutic benefit of its addition to cytotoxic therapy.

References

1. Henderson IC, Canellos GP (1980) Cancer of the breast. N Engl J med 302: 17
2. Henderson IC, Canellos GP (1980) Cancer of the breast. N Engl J med 302: 78
3. McGuire WL, Pearson OH, Segalof A (1975) Predicting hormone responsivenes in human breast cancer. In: McGuire WL, Carbone PP, Vollmer EP (eds) Estrogen receptors in human breast cancer. Raven, New York, p 17
4. Legha SS, Buzdar AU, Smith TL, Swenerton KD, Hortobagyi GN, Blumenschein GR (1980) Response to hormonal therapy as a prognostic factor for metastatic breast cancer treated with combination chemotherapy. Cancer 46: 438

5. Manni A, Trujillo JE, Pearson OH (1980) Sequential use of endocrine therapy and chemotherapy for metastatic breast cancer: effects on survival. Cancer Treat Rep 64:111
6. Pearson OH, Ray DS (1959) A comparison of the results of adrenalectomy and hypophysectomy in carcinoma of the breast. In: Raven RW (ed) Cancer hormone therapy, vol 6. Butterworth, London, p 335
7. Manni A, Trujillo JE, Marshall JS, Brodkey J, Pearson OH (1979) Antihormone treatment of stage IV breast cancer. Cancer 43:444
8. Manni A, Pearson OH, Brodkey J, Marshall JS (1979) Transsphenoidal hypophysectomy in breast cancer. Cancer 44:2330
9. Manni A, Arafah BM, Pearson OH (1981) Androgen-induced remissions after antiestrogen and hypophysectomy in stage IV breast cancer. Cancer 48:2507
10. Westerberg H (1980) Tamoxifen and fluoxymesterone in advanced breast cancer: a controlled clinical trial. Cancer Treat Rep 64:117
11. Smith IE, Harris AL, Morgan M, Ford HT, Gazet J-C, Harmer CL, White H, Parsons CA, Villardo A, Walsh G, McKinna JA (1981) Tamoxifen versus aminoglutethimide in advanced breast carcinoma: a randomized cross-over trial. Br Med J 283:1432
12. Dao TL (1972) Ablation therapy for hormone-dependent tumours. Annu Rev Med 23:1
13. Robin PE, Dalton GA (1977) The role of major endocrine ablation. In: Stoll BA (ed) Breast cancer management-early and late. Chicago Year Book, Chicago, p 147
14. Hayward J (1970) Hormones and human breast cancer. Springer, Berlin Heidelberg New York, pp 10, 33 (Recent results in cancer research, vol 24)
15. Dao TL (1978) The value of adrenalectomy in patients with metastatic breast cancer. Surg Clin North Am 58:801
16. Hayward JL, Atkins HJB, Falconer MA et al. (1970) Clinical trials comparing transfrontal hypophysectomy with adrenalectomy and with transethmoidal hypophysectomy. In: Joslin CAF, Gleave EN (eds) The clinical management of advanced breast cancer. Alpha Omega, Cardiff, p 50
17. Griffiths CT, Hall TC, Saba Z, Barlow JJ, Nevinny HB (1973) Preliminary trial of aminoglutethimide in breast cancer. Cancer 32:31
18. Samojlik E, Santen RJ (1978) Adrenal suppression with aminoglutethimide. III. Comparison of plasma Δ^4- and Δ^5-steroids in postmenopausal women treated for breast carcinoma. J Clin Endocrinol Metab 47:717
19. Samojlik E, Veldhuis JD, Wells SA, Santen RJ (1980) Preservation of androgen secretion during estrogen suppresion with aminoglutethimide in the treatment of metastatic carcinoma. J Clin Invest 65:602
20. Santen RJ, Worgul TJ, Samojlik E, Interrante A, Boucher AE, Lipton A, Harvey HA, White DS, Smart E, Cox C, Wells SA (1981) A randomized trial comparing surgical adrenalectomy with aminoglutethimide plus hydrocortisone in women with advanced breast cancer. N Engl J Med 305:545
21. Santen RJ, Santner S, Davis B, Veldhuis J, Samojlik E, Ruby E (1978) Aminoglutethimide inhibits extraglandular estrogen production in postmenopausal women with breast carcinoma. J Clin Endocrinol Metab 47:1257
22. Lippman M, Bolan G, Hoff K (1976) The effects of estrogens and antiestrogens on hormone-responsive human breast cancer in long-term tissue culture. Cancer Res 36:4595
23. Zava DT, McGuire WL (1978) Human breast cancer: androgen action mediated by estrogen receptor. Science 199:787
24. Nicholson RL, Davies P, Griffiths K (1978) Interaction of androgens with oestradiol-17β receptor proteins in DMBA-induced mammary tumours — a possible oncolytic mechanism. Eur J Cancer 14:439
25. Løber J, Rose C, Salimtschik M, Mouridsen HT (1981) Treatment of advanced breast cancer with progestins. Acta Obstet Gynecol Scand [Suppl] 101:39
26. Santen RJ, Samojlik E (1979) Medical adrenalectomy for treatment of metastatic breast carcinoma. In: McGuire WL (ed) Breast cancer: advances in research and treatment, vol 3. Plenum, New York, p 79

27. Mouridsen HT, Palshof T, Patterson J, Battersby L (1978) Tamoxifen in advanced breast cancer. Cancer treat Rev 5: 131
28. Nicholson RI, Davies P, Griffiths K (1977) Effects of oestradiol-17β and tamoxifen on nuclear oestradiol-17β receptors in DMBA-induced rat mammary tumours. Eur J Cancer 13: 201
29. Jordan VC, Dix CJ, Naylor KE, Prestwich G, Rowsby L (1978) Nonsteroidal antiestrogens: their biological effects and potential mechanism of action. J Toxicol Environ Health 4: 363
30. Koseki Y, Zava DT, Chamness GC, McGuire WL (1977) Estrogen receptor translocation and replenishment by the anti-estrogen tamoxifen. Endocrinology 101: 1104
31. Rochefort H, Borgma JL (1981) Differences between oestrogen receptor activation by oestrogen and anti-oestrogen. Nature 292: 257
32. Ip MM, Milholland RJ, Rosen F, Kim U (1981) Dichotomus effects of tamoxifen on a transplantable rat mammary tumour. Cancer Res 41: 984
33. Butler WB, Kelsey WH (1981) Effect of the antiestrogen tamoxifen on synchronized cultures of MCF-7 cells. 17th Annual meeting Am Soc Clin Oncology, Abstr 35
34. Horwitz KB, Kosekiy, McGuire WL (1978) Estrogen control of progesterone receptor in human breast cancer: Role of estrodiol and antiestrogen. Endocrinology 103: 1742
35. Namer M, Lalanne C, Baulieu E-E (1980) Increase of progesterone receptor by tamoxifen as a hormonal challenge test in breast cancer. Cancer Res 40: 1750
36. Sutherland RL, Murphy LC (1980) The binding of tamoxifen to human mammary carcinoma cytosol. Eur J Cancer 46: 1141
37. Sutherland RL, Murphy LC, Foo MS, Green MD, Whybourne AM, Krozowski ZS (1980) High-affinity anti-oestrogen binding site distinct from the oestrogen receptor. Nature 288: 273
38. Furr DJ, Patterson JS, Richardson DN, Slater SR, Wakeling AE (1979) Tamoxifen. In: Goldberg ME (ed) Pharmacological and biochemical properties of drug substances, vol 2. APA, Washington, p 355
39. Patterson JS (1981) Clinical aspects and development of antioestrogen therapy: A review of the endocrine effects of tamoxifen in animals and man. J Endocrinol 89: 67
40. Hayward JL, Carbone PP, Heuson J-C, Kumaoka S, Segaloff A, Rubens RD (1977) Assesment of response to therapy in advanced breast cancer. Cancer 39: 1289
41. Tormey DC, Lippman MF, Edwards BE, Cassidy J (to be published) Evaluation of tamoxifen doses with and without fluoxymesterone in advanced breast cancer
42. Tormey DC, Falkson G, Crowley J, Falkson HC, Voelkel J, Davies TE (1982) Dibromodulcitol and adriamycin $\pm$ tamoxifen in advanced breast cancer. Cancer Clin Trials 5: 33
43. Ingle JN, Ahmann DL, Green SJ, Edmondson JH, Bisel HF, Kvols LK, Nichols WC, Creagan ET, Hahn RG, Rubin J, Frytak S (1981) Randomized clinical trial of diethylstilbestrol versus tamoxifen in postmenopausal women with advanced breast cancer. N Engl J Med 304: 16
44. Beex L, Pieters G, Smals A, Koenders A, Benraad T, Kloppenborg P (1981) Tamoxifen versus ethinyl estradiol in the treatment of postmenopausal women with advanced breast cancer. Cancer Treat Rep 65: 179
45. Cocconi G, Lisi BD, Boni C, Mori P (1981) Chemotherapy vs combination of chemotherapy and endocrine therapy in advanced breast cancer. A prospective randomized study. UICO conf clin oncol breast cancer, Abstr. 03−0141
46. Fabian C, Sternson L, El-Serafi M, Cain L, Harne E (1981) Clinical pharmacology of tamoxifen in patients with breast cancer: correlation with clinical data. Cancer 48: 876
47. Ward HWC (1973) Anti-oestrogen therapy for breast cancer: A trial of tamoxifen at two-dose levels. Br Med J 1: 13
48. Kiang DT, Frenning DH, Vosika GJ, Kennedy BJ (1980) Comparison of tamoxifen and hypophysectomy in breast cancer treatment. Cancer 45: 1322
49. Stewart HJ, Forrest APM, Gunn JM, Hamilton T, Langlands AO, McFadyen IJ, Roberts MM (1980) The tamoxifen trial − A doubleblind comparison with stilbestrol in postmenopausal women with advanced breast cancer. Eur J Cancer [Suppl] 1: 83
50. Luporini G, Beratta G, Tabiadon D, Tedeschi L, Rossi A (1981) Comparison between oral medroxyprogesterone acetate (MPA) and tamoxifen (TMX) in advanced breast carcinoma. 17th Annual meeting Am Soc Clin Oncology, Abstr C-398

51. Mattsson W (1980) A phase III trial of treatment with tamoxifen versus treatment with high-dose medroxyprogesterone-acetate in advanced postmenopausal breast cancer. In: Iacobelli S, Marco AD (eds) Role of medroxyprogesterone in endocrine-related tumours. Raven, New York, p 65

52. Lipton A, Harvey HA, Santen RJ, Worgul T, Boucher A, White D (1981) Randomized trial of aminoglutethimide versus tamoxifen in metastatic breast cancer. 17th Annual meeting Am Soc Clin Oncology, Abstr. C-437

53. Mouridsen HT, Salimtschik M, Dombernowsky P, Gelshøj K, Palshof T, Rørth M, Daehnfeldt JL, Rose C (1980) Therapeutic effect of tamoxifen versus combined tamoxifen and diethylstilbestrol in advanced breast cancer in postmenopausal women. Eur J Cancer [Suppl] 1:107

54. Carter AC, Sedransk N, Kelley RM, Ansfield FJ, Rawdin RG, Talley RW, Potter NR (1977) Diethylstilbestrol: Recommended dosages for different categories of breast cancer patients. JAMA 237:2079

55. Mouridsen HT, Ellemann K, Mattsson W, Palshof T, Daehnfeldt JL, Rose C (1979) Therapeutic effect of tamoxifen versus tamoxifen combined with medroxyprogesterone acetate in advanced breast cancer in postmenopausal women. Cancer Treat Rep 63:171

56. Powles TJ (1981) Multiple endocrine therapy with tamoxifen, aminoglutethimide and danazol for treatment of patients with metastatic breast cancer. UICC conf clin oncology, Abstr 03-0106

57. Settatree RS, Butt WR, London DR, Holme GM, Morrison JM (1979) Tamoxifen and bromocriptine combination in advanced breast cancer. Advances in medical oncology. Research and education, vol 12. Pergamon, New York, p 806(5)

58. Mouridsen HT, Palshof T, Engelsman E, Sylvester R (1980) CMF versus CMF + tamoxifen in advanced breast cancer in postmenopausal women. An EORTC trial. Int Congress Senology

59. Galmarini F, Santos R, Brunu R, Casas O, Chiesa J, Bertacchini C, D'Auria A, Domingoez E (1981) Tamoxifen + CIVEFU vs CIVEFU in advanced breast cancer. UICC conf oncology, Abstr 03-0359

60. Boccardo F, Rubagotti A, Sertoli MR, Rosso R (1981) Randomized trial of chemo-hormone therapy in advanced breast cancer. 17th Annual meeting Am Soc Clin Oncology, Abstr. C397

61. Arraztora J, Ramirez G (1981) Chemotherapy with and without hormonal manipulation in the treatment of advanced breast cancer. 17th Annual meeting Am Soc Clin Oncology, Abstr C-401

62. Pritchard KI, Thomson DB, Meakin JW, Myers RE, Sutherland DJA, Mobbs VG, Campbell J (1981) The role of tamoxifen in premenopausal women with metastatic carcinoma of the breast: an update. 17th Annual meeting Am Soc Clin Oncology, Abstr C-405

63. Wada T, Koyama H, Terasawa T (1981) Effect of tamoxifen in premenopausal Japanese women with advanced breast cancer. Cancer Treat Rep 65:728

Therapeutic Activity of Medroxyprogesterone Acetate in Metastatic Breast Cancer: A Correlation Between Estrogen Receptors and Various Dosages

M. De Lena, S. Villa, and G. Di Fronzo

Ospedale oncologico, Via Scipione l'Africano 191, 70100 Bari, Italy

Introduction

It has been known for a relatively long time that progestogens, and especially medroxyprogesterone acetate (MPA), induce objective regression of the neoplasia in women with metastatic breast cancer. Some authors have recently reported [1, 7−9] that the response to MPA may be increased by employing high daily dosages. On this basis, we tested different dosages of MPA in patients who had become resistant to combined chemotherapy. Furthermore, we correlated the response of the patient with estrogen receptor status of the tumor.

Patients and Methods

Medroxyprogesterone acetate was administered at different dosages in 73 women with metastatic breast cancer during a period of several years (June 1976 to January 1981). All patients had previously been treated with different types of combined chemotherapy [usually CMF and adriamycin + vincristine (AV)]; only four women had undergone endocrine manipulation, i.e., oophorectomy (two) or tamoxifen administration (two). The age of the patients averaged 54 years (ranging from 29 to 74), whereby 63 were postmenopausal and 10 premenopausal.

In 50 ER+ women (68%), the dominant sites of the lesion were bone (28 cases), soft tissue (18), and viscera (four). Twenty-seven patients (17 ER+, 5 ER−, and 5 ER borderline) received 100 mg MPA three times a week per os; 37 (27 ER+, 8 ER−, and 2 ER borderline) were put on 500 mg/day i.m. for 30 days; and nine patients (6 ER+ and 3 ER−) were treated with 1,000 mg/day i.m. for 40 days.

Before initiating MPA therapy, the following parameters were controlled: life expectancy of at least 6 weeks, performance statuts of 50 or more (Karnofsky scale) blood count, liver chemistry, serum calcium, renal function, and precise determination of the physical and radiographic aspects of the indicator lesion. The patients were then physically evaluated at intervals of 1−2 months, and blood tests, X-rays, and scans were carried out when neccesary.

We considered the response as complete (CR) when the metastatic lesions were no longer present and osteolytic metastasis had recalcified for at least 1 month. Furthermore, response was defined as partial (PR) when a decrease of more than 50% in the product of the two largest perpendicular diameters in all measurable lesions or partial recalcification of osteolytic metastasis (without any change in the osteoblastic lesions) was found for a minimum of 1 month. The disease was considered as stabilized (SD) when there was a decrease of 25%−50% in one measurable lesion without regression at another metastatic site. Finally, progression of the disease (PD) was defined as in increase of 25% or more in the initial lesion irrespective of the presence of concomitant regression at other tumor sites, new lesions, or progression of the osteolytic metastasis.

In all women, ER determination was carried out on the primary tumor; in only two cases was it also evaluated in skin metastasis, resulting in one unmodified finding (positive in both biopsies) and one modified finding (positive in the primary tumor and negative in the metastatic lesion).

Estrogen Receptor Assay

The frozen (−80° C) tissue samples, trimmed of fat and debris, were dipped in liquid nitrogen and pulverized in a Micro-dismembrator. The powdered tissue obtained was then vigorously homogenized in 6 vol of ice-cold TEN buffer (tris-HCl pH 7.4 at 4° C, 1 mM EDTA and 3 mM NaN$_3$). The homogenate was centrifuged at 100,000 g at 2° C in a Heraeus W 60/44 A1 rotor for 60 min. After centrifugation, the layer of floating lipids was carefully removed and the clear cytoplasmatic extract (cytosol) recovered and used immediately for estrogen binding activity assay with the dextran-coated charcoal technique (DCC). The cytosol protein contents were determined by the Bio-Rad assay according to Bradford [2] by using a standard protein solution that contained 5.0% human serum albumin and 3.0% human γ-globulin for the calibration curve.

Aliquots of cytosol (200 μl) were incubated in ice-cold 12 × 75 mm glass tubes with 100 μl of tritiated 17β-estradiol (^{3}H-E$_2$) (85−110 Ci/mM) solution at decreasing concentrations (7.5 − 0.375), in the presence (aspecific binding) or absence (total binding) of 100-fold molar excess of unlabeled binding competitor diethylstilbestrol (DES). After 16−18 h of incubation at 0°−4° C, 500 μl of DCC suspension [0.5% (w/v) Norit-A charcoal, 0.05% (w/v) dextran T-70 in TEN buffer] was added to each test tube and then vigorously vortexed. The charcoal was then sedimented out after 15 min by centrifugation at 2,000 g at 4° C for 10 min. Aliquots of the clear supernatant were pipetted into polyethelene vials for the determination of the bound radioactivity content in a Packard 3255 Tri-Carb Spectrometer; quench correction was obtained with the external standardization method. Five milliliters of a prepared cocktail (Emulsifier Scintillator) were added to each sample. The results were analyzed as previously described [5] and plotted for Scatchard analysis [10].

Results

Table 1 illustrates the response to MPA treatment in ER+ patients. No difference in the percentage of objective response (CR + PR) was observed between the group treated with MPA three times a week (100 mg per os) and the group treated for 30 consecutive days (500 mg/day i.m.). In fact, the results were 24% and 22%, respectively. On the other hand, the number of women treated for 40 days (1,000 mg/day i.m.) was too small (only six patients) to draw any definite conclusions; nevertheless, it should be noted that no objective response was observed in these cases. In total, 10 (20%) objective responses and

Table 1. Correlation between different dosages of MPA and response in ER+ patients

MPA dosage (mg)	No. of patients	Type of response				CR + PR	
		CR	PR	SD	PD	No.	%
100 × 3/week	17	1	3	3	10	4	24
500 × 30 days i.m.	27	2	4	9	12	6	22
1,000 × 40 days i.m.	6	–	–	3	3	–	–
Total	50	3	7	15	25	10	20

Table 2. Response to MPA according to dominant site and to individual metastatic site of disease in ER+ patients

	No. of patients	Type of response				CR + PR	
		CR	PR	SD	PD	No.	%
Dominant site							
Soft tissue	18	3	4	3	8	7	39
Bone	28	–	2	11	15	2	7
Viscera	4	–	1	1	2	1	25
Metastatic site							
Breast	12	1	3	3	5	4	33
Skin	18	6	1	5	6	7	39
Nodes	17	2	3	7	5	5	29
Bone	30	–	3	11	16	3	10
Liver	3	–	–	–	3	–	–
Lung	6	–	1	–	5	1	17
Pleura	2	–	–	–	2	–	–
Mediastinum	1	–	–	1	–	–	–

15 (30%) stabilizations of the disease were observed for the 50 women who were ER+. On the other hand, no objective regression was found in the women (23) considered as ER− or presenting borderline lesions; the disease stabilized in only four cases (3 ER− and 1 borderline).

Table 2 shows how the various sites of metastasis reacted to therapy: soft tissue 39%, bone 7%, and viscera 20%. The objective response was evaluated for the individual organs of metastasis. Breast (33%), skin (39%), and nodal lesions (29%) accounted for the highest incidence of CR + PR, whereas only partial recalcification of bone metastasis was observed in three of 30 (10%) patients. One partial response was noted for the pulmonary lesions, while no response was found for hepatic, pleural, or mediastinal sites.

In those women presenting a disease-free interval of less than 2 years, objective response was higher (28%) than in those who were disease-free for more than 2 years (14%), but as this study population was not very numerous (36 and 14 cases, respectively) this difference cannot be considered statistically significant. Three of the seven ER+ premenopausal women presented objective responses (43%), whereas the response was more marked in

Table 3. Correlation between age, groups, and response in ER+ patients

Age groups (years)	No. of patients	Type of response				CR + PR	
		CR	PR	SD	PD	No.	%
29–30	2	–	–	1	1	–	–
40–49	16	–	1	5	10	1	6
50–59	15	1	2	5	7	3	20
59 +	17	2	4	4	7	6	35
Total	50	3	7	15	25	10	20

postmenopausal patients, and it was interesting to note that the women in menopause for more than 5 years responded better to MPA therapy than did those women who had been in menopause for less than 5 years (33% and 16%, respectively). In fact, upon analyzing all data and correlating the response rate to the various age groups, it was found that the regression rate increased in correspondence with the increase in age (Table 3).

The median duration of response to MPA was 7 months (3–16+). Treatment was well tolerated, and MPA was never suspended because of toxic side-effects.

Discussion

In view of the results we obtained previously with cytotoxic chemotherapy, we would like to point out the following:

1. The percentage of ER+ women (68%) was higher in our series than in most series reported in the literature.
2. In ER– or borderline patients, no complete or partial response was observed.
3. Response was not MPA dosage-dependent in ER+ women: in fact, when the dosage was 100 mg three times a week per os, objective regression occurred in 24% of the cases, whereas at the dosage of 500 mg/day i.m. for 30 days the figure was 22%. This percentage of regressions confirms our previous data obtained with high dosages of MPA in patients in whom ER was not determined [3].
4. The regression rate seemed to be age dependent.
5. Soft tissue was more responsive (39%) to MPA therapy than was bone (7%) or viscera (20%).
6. The average duration of response was 7 months, concording with the results obtained by other authors [6].
7. Similar to previous results obtained with endocrine therapy other than MPA [4], ER positivity did not correlate to a high percentage of objective responses.

References

1. Amadori D, Ravaioli A, Barbanti F (1977) The use of medroxyprogesterone acetate in high doses in palliative treatment of advanced mammary carcinoma (clinical experience with 44 cases). Minerva Med 68: 3967–3980
2. Bradford MM (1976) A rapid and sensitive method for the quantitation of microgram quantities of protein utilizing the principle of protein-dye binding. Anal Biochem 72: 248–259

3. De Lena M, Brambilla C, Volagussa P, Bonadonna G (1979) High dose medroxyprogesterone acetate in breast cancer resistant to endocrine and cytotoxic therapy. Cancer Chemother Pharmacol 2: 175–180

4. De Lena M, Brambilla C, Jirillo A (1980) Tamoxifen efficacy in advanced breast cancer previously treated with endocrine and cytotoxic therapy. Tumori 66: 339–348

5. Di Fronzo G, Bertuzzi A, Ronchi E (1968) An improved criterion for the evaluation of estrogen receptor binding data in human breast cancer. Tumori 64: 259–266

6. Ganzina F (1979) High dose medroxyprogesterone acetate (MPA) treatment in advanced breast cancer. A review. Tumori 65: 563–585

7. Pannuti F, Martoni A, Lenaz CR, Piana E, Manni P (1978) A possible new approach to the treatment of metastatic breast cancer: Massive dose of medroxyprogesterone acetate. Cancer Treat Rep 62: 499–504

8. Pannuti F, Martoni A, Di Marco AR, Piana E, Saccani F, Becchi G, Mattioli G, Barbanti F, Marra GA, Persiani W, Cacciari L, Spagnuolo F, Polenzana D, Rocchetta G (1979) Prospective, randomized clinical trial of two different high dosages of medroxyprogesterone acetate (MPA) in the treatment of metastatic breast cancer. J Cancer 15: 593–601

9. Robustelli Della Cuna G, Calciati A, Bernando Strada MR, Bumma C, Campio L (1978) High dose medroxyprogesterone acetate (MPA) treatment in metastatic carcinoma of the breast: a due response evolution. Tumori 64: 143–150

10. Scatchard G (1949) The attraction of protein for small molecules and ions. Ann NY Acad Sci 51: 660–672

Estrogen Receptor Status and the Clinical Response to a Combination of Aminoglutethimide and Cortisol in Advanced Breast Cancer*

R. Paridaens, G. Leclercq, and J. C. Heuson

Institut Jules Bordet, Centre des Tumeurs de l'Université Libre de Bruxelles,
Service de Médecine, Clinique et Laboratoire de Cancérologie mammaire,
Rue Héger Bordet 1, 1000 Brussels, Belgium

Introduction

Griffiths et al. [1] have shown that when aminoglutethimide, a nonsteroidal nonhormonal compound formerly used as an anticonvulsant, is given together with replacement corticoids, it produces remissions in postmenopausal patients with advanced breast cancer. The remarkable effectiveness of this association has recently been confirmed [2−6]. The therapeutic results appear similar to those achieved with transsphenoidal hypophysectomy [7] or surgical adrenalectomy [8, 9]. Since our initial report in 1980 of a phase II trial conducted at the Institut Jules Bordet [5], our clinical experience with this combination has expanded considerably. Here we intend to report on our entire experience, paying particular attention to the relationship between the pattern of therapeutic response and the quantitative estrogen receptor (ER) assay.

Patients and Methods

Selection of Patients

The criteria of eligibility for the phase II trial of aminoglutethimide in combination with cortisol have been described previously [5]. Briefly, all patients were postmenopausal and had histologically proven advanced breast cancer with progressive disease and measurable or evaluable lesions. Patients with either a second malignancy, a poor general condition (Karnofsky < 50%), CNS metastatic involvement, or rapidly progressive visceral metastases were excluded.

Treatment and Criteria of Response

Our therapeutic regimen was as follows: Aminoglutethimide was given orally at a daily dose of 1 g in four divided doses. At a later stage of our trial, we started with 500 mg daily

* Part of this work was supported by a grant from the Fonds Cancérologique de la Caisse Générale d'Epargne et de Retraite de Belgique. We wish to thank Dr. J. M. Tyberghein (Ciba-Geigy) for supplying aminoglutethimide

and then increased the dose slowly, since we became aware that this regimen improved tolerance. Hydrocortisone was given according to the schedule described by Santen [10]: 10 mg at 8 a.m. and 5 p.m. and 20 mg at bedtime. All patients were treated for a minimum of 3 months unless there was evidence of rapid progression. Treatment was maintained in responders and in patients with no change until evidence of progressive disease appeared. All cases were reviewed by two clinicians (RP and JCH) in order to assess the response according to the criteria defined by the UICC [11].

ER Assay

All samples assayed for ER were histologically examined for the presence of tumor tissue. They consisted of local recurrences or distant soft tissue metastases. All biopsy specimens came from our operating room and were immediately processed to remove blood, necrotic tissue, and adipose tissue before being stored in liquid nitrogen [12]. ER concentration of the samples was evaluated by measuring the ^{3}H-estradiol-17β binding capacity of their cytosol fraction using a dextran-coated charcoal method previously described [12]. Binding capacity was expressed as femtomoles (10^{-15} mol) per milligram of tissue protein. Samples with low protein content (< 1 mg/ml) were considered nonevaluable for the receptor assay.

Relationship Between ER Assays and Therapeutic Response

Since hormones or chemotherapy could significantly affect the results of ER assays, as described elsewhere in this book, we only acknowledged as evaluable those patients who did not receive any of these drugs during the time between the ER assay and the onset of treatment with aminoglutethimide. Patients with systemic antineoplastic treatment prior to ER determination were taken into consideration only if 2 months or more had elapsed since all drugs had been withdrawn.

Results

Of the 54 eligible patients included in the study, three were found to be nonevaluable owing to either lack of measurable lesions (one patient) or death by neoplastic progression within 1 month of initiation of treatment (two patients). Seven patients refused further treatment because of intolerance consisting of somnolence and/or skin rashes. This occurred especially in the initial stage of our trial when we started the full dose of 1 g aminoglutethimide from the first day of treatment.

The main characteristics of the 44 evaluable patients were as follows: (a) median age 64 years (range 37−85); (b) median performance status 80% (Karnofsky index, range 60%−100%); and (c) involved sites were soft tissues in 66%, bones in 59% and viscera in 43%, the latter being mainly the lung and pleura.

As shown in Table 1, there were 17 objective remissions, of which three were complete, representing a 39% response rate. At present, the median duration of remission exceeds 11 months. There was a higher percentage of responses among the nine patients with soft tissue metastases only (56%) than among the 16 patients with bone as the predominant metastatic site (31%) or the 19 patients with visceral involvement (37%).

Table 1. Therapeutic response to aminoglutethimide plus hydrocortisone in 44 evaluable patients

Response			Median duration of treatment		Deaths	
Type	No.	%	Months	Range	No.	%
Complete	3	7	11+	9+ to 24+ ⎫	2	12
Partial	14	32	12	2+ to 22 ⎬		
No change	8	18	7	5+ to 11+ ⎫		
Mixed	2	4		9 and 23 ⎬	9	53
Progression	17	39	3	1 to 8 ⎭		

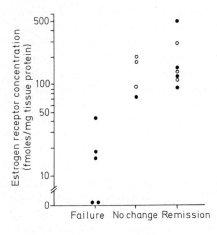

Fig. 1. Estrogen receptor concentration and response to aminoglutethimide. The *open circles* (O) refer to previously untreated cases and the *closed circles* (●) to patients who had prior systemic treatment

The relationship between ER assays and clinical response to treatment could be studied in 16 cases. The results are presented in Fig. 1. All seven patients who responded had high receptor concentrations in their metastases, with a mean value of 197 fmol/mg tissue protein (range 93–499). Four of these patients had been previously treated with hormones (two) or chemotherapy (two). All five patients who failed to respond had received prior systemic treatment with hormones (one), chemotherapy (one), or both (three). Two of these patients had no detectable receptors in their metastases and the remainder had low concentrations, the mean ER concentration in this group being 15.4 fmol (range 0–42). Interestingly, the intermediate category of patients with no change had higher receptor concentrations than cases of failure, the mean value being 129.5 fmol (range 71–186).

Discussion

Aminoglutethimide at the usual dose of 1 g per day given together with near-physiological replacement doses of either cortisone (50 mg/day) or hydrocortisone (40 mg/day) is attracting increasing interest as a treatment of advanced breast cancer in postmenopausal patients. This combination, often referred to as "medical adrenalectomy", blocks adrenal steroidogenesis and thereby decreases the circulating levels of estrogens by an extent similar to that achieved using surgical adrenalectomy [6]. Additional antineoplastic action of aminoglutethimide could evolve from its demonstrated inhibitory effect on the enzyme aromatase, which converts androgens into estrogens in peripheral tissue or within the neoplastic tissue itself [13]. The 39% response rate found in this trial falls within the range reported in the literature [1−6].

It is now generally accepted that estrogen receptors are a good biological marker of hormone dependency in advanced breast cancer. Thus, objective response to endocrine treatments is obtained in only 10% of ER-negative tumors, but in 50%−60% of ER-positive tumors. This holds true for various modalities of treatment, including endocrine ablative surgical procedures (oophorectomy, adrenalectomy, hypophysectomy) and hormone administration (estrogens or antiestrogens, androgens) [14]. Our results in the present study are consistent with our previous observation that the rate of response to endocrine treatments is positively correlated with ER concentration in the neoplastic tissue [15]. Thus, ER-negative cases as well as cases with low ER values, say below 50 fmol, did not respond to medical adrenalectomy. In marked contrast, of the 11 patients with higher receptor concentrations, a high percentage (64%) had a remission. Moreover, within this group, all nonresponding patients had stabilization of their disease for periods exceeding 5 months. In fact, the latter patients had receptor concentrations comparable to those observed in remissions, since their ranges of variation overlap widely. Similar observations were recently made by Lawrence et al. [16], who reported increasing proportions of remissions and stabilizations parallel with increasing ER concentrations.

In conclusion, medical adrenalectomy represents an effective treatment for advanced breast cancer in postmenopausal patients. The efficacy of this therapeutic regimen compares favorably with the results of conventional modalities of endocrine treatment such as surgical adrenalectomy or tamoxifen. A useful selection of patients who are likely to respond to aminoglutethimide could be made by examining ER concentration in metastases. Since a previous systemic treatment can significantly affect the ER concentration in a given patient, it is recommended that whenever possible ER assay be performed just before a therapeutic decision is taken.

References

1. Griffiths CT, Hall TC, Saba Z, Barlow JJ, Nevinny HB (1973) Preliminary trial of aminoglutethimide in breast cancer. Cancer 32: 31−37
2. Santen RJ, Lipton A, Kendall J (1974) Successful medical adrenalectomy with aminoglutethimide. JAMA 230: 1661−1665
3. Gale KE, Sheehe PR, Gould LV, Rohner R (1976) Treatment of advanced breast cancer with aminoglutethimide: an 8 year experience. Clin Res 24: 376 A
4. Smith IE, Fitzharris BM, McKinna JA, Fahmy DR, Nash AG, Neville AM, Gazet JC, Ford HT, Powles TJ (1978) Aminoglutethimide in treatment of metastatic breast carcinoma. Lancet 2: 646−649
5. Paridaens R, Van Haelen C, Heuson JC (1980) Medical adrenalectomy with aminoglutethimide cortisol in the treatment of metastatic breast carcinoma. In: Mouridsen HT, Palshof T (eds) Breast cancer − Experimental and clinical aspects. Pergamon, Oxford, pp 103−106
6. Santen RJ, Wells SA (1980) The use of aminoglutethimide in the treatment of patients with metastatic carcinoma of the breast. Cancer 46: 1066−1074
7. Harvey HA, Santen RJ, Osterman J, Samojlik E, White DS, Lipton A (1979) A comparative trial of transsphenoidal hypophysectomy and estrogen suppression with aminoglutethimide in advanced breast cancer. Cancer 43: 2207−2214

8. Newsome HH, Brown PW, Terz JJ, Lawrence W Jr (1977) Medical and surgical adrenalectomy in patients with advanced breast carcinoma. Cancer 39: 542–546

9. Santen RJ, Worgul T, Veldhuis J, Interrante A, Feil P, Beltz W, Lipton A, Harvey H, Cox C, Wells S (1980) Randomized controlled trial of medical adrenalectomy with aminoglutethimide and surgical adrenalectomy. Proc Am Soc Clin Oncol 21: 410

10. Santen RJ, Samojlik E, Lipton A, Harvey A, Ruby EB, Wells SA, Kendall J (1977) Kinetic, hormonal and clinical studies with aminoglutethimide in breast cancer. Cancer 39: 2948–2958

11. Hayward JL, Carbone PP, Heuson JC, Kumaoka S, Segaloff A, Rubens RD (1977) Assessment of response to therapy in advanced breast cancer. Cancer 39: 1289–1294

12. Leclercq G, Heuson JC, Schoenfeld R, Mattheiem WH, Tagnon HJ (1973) Estrogen receptors in human breast cancer. Eur J Cancer 9: 665–673

13. Santen RJ, Veldhuis JD, Samojlik E, Lipton A, Harvey H, Wells SA (1979) Mechanism of action of aminoglutethimide in breast cancer. Lancet 1: 44–45

14. Hawkins RA, Roberts MM, Forrest APM (1980) Oestrogen receptors and breast cancer: current status. Br J Surg 67: 153–169

15. Paridaens R, Sylvester RJ, Ferrazzi E, Legros N, Leclercq G, Heuson JC (1980) Clinical significance of the quantitative assessment of estrogen receptors in advanced breast cancer. Cancer 46: 2889–2895

16. Lawrence BV, Lipton A, Harvey HA, Santen RJ, Wells SA, Cox CE, White DS, Smart E (1980) Influence of estrogen receptor status on response of metastatic breast cancer to aminoglutethimide therapy. Cancer 45: 786–791

Steroid Receptors in Megestrol Acetate Therapy

J. Alexieva-Figusch, F. A. G. Teulings, W. C. J. Hop,
J. Blonk-van der Wijst, and H. A. van Gilse*

Department of Internal Medicine, Rotterdamsch Radio-Therapeutisch Instituut,
Groene Hilledijk 301, 3075 EA Rotterdam, The Netherlands

Introduction

The role of megestrol acetate (17α-acetoxy-6-methyl-pregna-4,6-diene-3,20-dione), a synthetic progestin derived from hydroxyprogesterone, in the treatment of advanced breast cancer has long been established: generally, remission can be achieved in ca. 30% of postmenopausal patients [1–3, 12, 13, 16, 18, 19]. It is difficult to define the physiological and pharmacological effects of progesterone and synthetic progestins, since virtually none of them are due exclusively to these hormones. Nevertheless, while estrogens and androgens have mainly growth-stimulating effects, the action of progestins is directed more towards modification and differentiation [14]. Megestrol acetate has been studied in both man and animals and seems to have antiestrogenic, antiandrogenic, and glucocorticoid-like properties [4–8, 10, 15] (Fig. 1). There is little information correlating the effect of megestrol acetate treatment and receptor content in human tumor tissue. Morgan reported response to megestrol acetate in seven of 16 patients with ER+ and in two of five patients with ER− [13]. In our previous study on steroid receptors in megestrol acetate-induced regression of human breast cancer [17], it was demonstrated that megestrol and medroxyprogesterone acetates are strong competitors for steroids which bind specifically to androgen, glucocorticoid, and progesterone receptors, indicating that these progestins

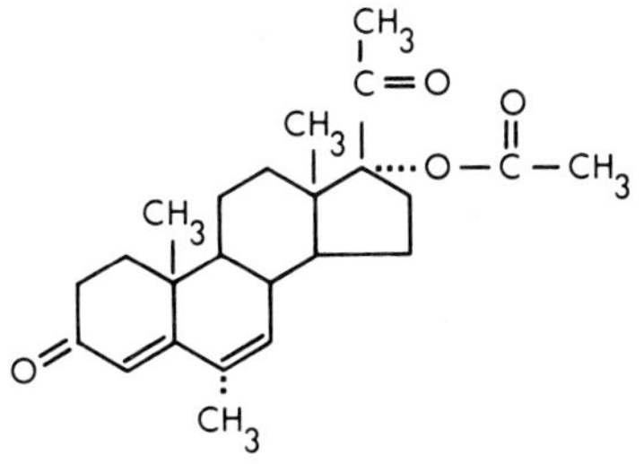

Fig. 1. Megestrol acetate   17 α – acetoxy – 6 – methyl – pregna – 4,6 – diene – 3,20 – dione

* The authors wish to thank Mr. M. S. Henkelman and Mr. H. Portengen for performing the receptor analysis, and Mrs. A. Sugiarsi, Mr. P. van Assendelft, and Mrs. J. L. Wike-Hooley for their assistance

are able to bind to these receptors with high affinity. In contrast, they do not compete with estradiol for estrogen receptor binding. Regressions were significantly associated with tumors containing large amounts of androgen receptors, tumors which also generally contain estrogen receptors.

The possibility that megestrol acetate acts on breast cancer via the progesterone receptor mechanism with subsequent increase in estradiol 17β-dehydrogenase could not be confirmed, although the presence of estradiol 17β-dehydrogenase in human breast cancer has been demonstrated [11].

The present study correlates steroid receptors to response in primary and metastatic breast tumor tissues of 60 postmenopausal patients treated with megestrol acetate.

Materials and Methods

One or more steroid receptors were assessed in 22 primary and 38 metastatic breast cancer specimens. Estrogen receptor was determined in 59 patients, androgen in 32, glucocorticoid in 34, and progesterone in 45. Tumors were classified as receptor negative if they contained less than 10 fmol/mg protein. The receptor assay methods used have been reported previously [17].

Some characteristics of the patients in this study are shown in Table 1. At the start of treatment all patients received megestrol acetate for progressive disease as objectively demonstrated by appropriate clinical and biochemical investigation. After 6 weeks of

Table 1. Characteristics of the 60 patients whose tumors were assayed for steroid hormone receptors

Mean age in years (range)	60
	(32−86)
Menopause age	
1−5 years	25
> 5 years	35
Disease-free interval	
0 months	10
1−12 months	14
13−24 months	19
25−36 months	7
> 36 months	10
Previous hormonal therapy	21
No previous hormonal therapy	39
Dominant sites	
Soft tissue	28
Bones	21
Viscera	11
Response to megestrol acetate therapy	
Remission	20 (33%)
Stable disease	24 (40%)
Progression	16 (27%)

treatment, response was assessed according to EORTC criteria [9]. The clinicians who evaluated response were unaware of the receptor contents of the tumors.

Megestrol acetate (Niagestin 15) was given in daily oral doses varying from 120 to 180 mg in four equal fractions. The drug was continued until the disease progressed.

Results

In our series of 60 patients treated with megestrol acetate, we found the following: estrogen receptor positivity in 64%, progesterone receptor positivity in 56%, glucocorticoid and androgen receptor positivity in 53% and 56% respectively. With increasing amounts of estrogen receptor there was a corresponding increase in the quantities of the other receptors.

Figure 2 gives estrogen receptor data according to response to treatment. Neither the presence of the receptor nor its amount was demonstrably related to the outcome of treatment. However, the duration of remission in patients with estrogen receptor-positive tumors was significantly longer (log-rank test: $P < 0.01$) than in those who lacked estrogen receptor (Fig. 3).

Figure 4 gives data on androgen, glucocorticoid, and progesterone receptors in relation to treatment outcome. A statistically significant higher amount of androgen receptor was noted in the group with remission as compared with the group with stable or progressive disease (Wilcoxon test: $P < 0.05$). No correlation between response to treatment and the amount of glucocorticoid or progesterone receptor was demonstrated. Remission in the group of patients with androgen receptor exceeding 30 fmol/mg protein was 60% (six of 10), while in the group with androgen receptor below that limit the figure was 23% (five of

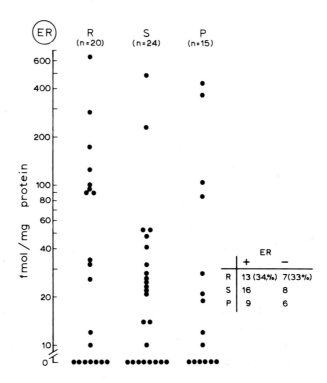

Fig. 2. Response to megestrol acetate treatment according to estrogen receptor values. *R,* remission; *S,* stable; *P,* progression; *ER,* estrogen receptor

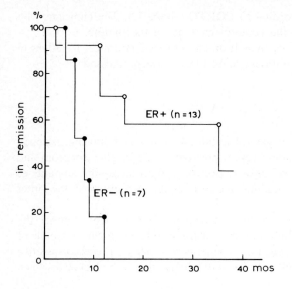

Fig. 3. Acturial percentages of patients in remission according to presence of estrogen receptor *(ER)*

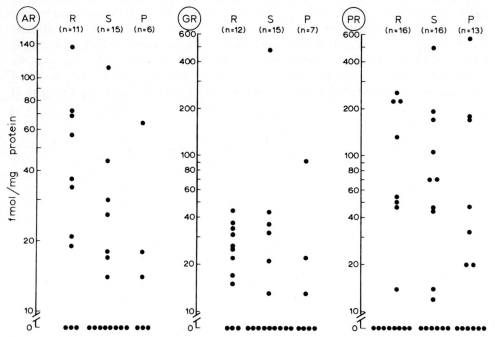

Fig. 4. Response to megestrol acetate therapy according to androgen *(AR)*, glucocorticoid *(GR)*, and progesterone *(PR)* receptor values. R, remission; S, stable; P, progression

22). Moreover, the duration of remission in the group with a high androgen receptor level (> 30 fmol/mg protein) was significantly (log-rank test: $P = 0.05$) longer than that in the group with a low value (< 30 fmol/mg protein) (Fig. 5). The results given in this section did not appreciably differ between patients according to whether receptors were evaluated in primary or in metastatic tumor.

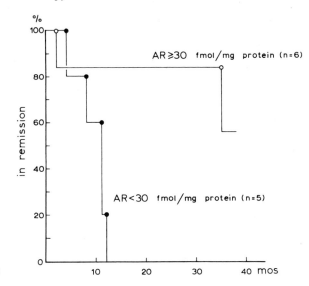

Fig. 5. Actuarial percentages of patients in remission according to amount of androgen receptor *(AR)*

Discussion

Steroid hormone receptors are found in a variety of cancers, including human breast cancer. For megestrol acetate therapy it seems that only the androgen receptor may be useful as an indicator of response. Moreover, this study strongly suggests that a satisfactory remission (i.e., of long duration) may be expected in cases with a large amount of androgen receptor. None of the other receptors appear to predict the probability of remission to megestrol acetate.

The fact that long remissions are associated with estrogen receptor-positive tumors might be explained by the correlation between amounts of androgen and estrogen in breast tumors. All tumors high in androgen receptor were also estrogen receptor positive. However, the number of patients studied is too small to assess fully the additional value of estrogen receptor once the androgen receptor level is known.

References

1. Alexieva-Figusch J, Van Gilse HA, Hop WCJ, Phoa CH, Blonk-v d Wijst J, Treurniet RE (1980) Progestin therapy in advanced breast cancer: Megestrol acetate — An evaluation of 160 treated cases. Cancer 46: 2369—2372
2. Ansfield FJ, Davis HL Jr, Ellerby RA, Ramirez G (1974) A clinical trial of megestrol acetate in advanced breast cancer. Cancer 33: 907—910
3. Ansfield FJ, Davis HL Jr, Ramirez G, Davis TE, Borden EC, Johnson RO, Bryan GT (1976) Further clinical studies with megestrol acetate in advanced breast cancer. Cancer 38: 53—55
4. Briggs MH, Briggs M (1973) Glucocorticoid properties of progestogens. Steroids 22: 555—559
5. Cooper JM, Jones HEH, Kellie AE (1973) The metabolism of megestrol acetate (17α-acetoxy-6-methylpregna-4,6-diene-3,20-dione) in the rabbit. Steroids 22: 255—275
6. Cooper JM, Kellie AE (1968) The metabolism of megestrol acetate (17α-acetoxy-6-methylpregna-4,6-diene-3,20-dione) in women. Steroids 11: 133—148

7. David A, Edwards K, Fellowes KP, Plummer JM (1963) Anti-ovulatory and other biological properties of megestrol acetate. 17α-acetoxy-6 methyl pregna 4:6-diene-3:20-dione (B.D.H. 1298). J Reprod Fertil 5: 331−346

8. Gupta C, Bullock LP, Bardin CW (1978) Further studies on the androgenic, anti-androgenic, and synandrogenic actions of progestins. Endocrinology 120: 736−744

9. Hayward JL, Carbone PP, Heuson JC, Kumaoka S, Segaloff A, Rubens RD (1977) Assessment of response to therapy in advanced breast cancer. Eur J Cancer 13: 89−94

10. Lee AE, Williams PC (1964) Oestrogen antagonists: assay by inhibition of vaginal cornification. J Endocrinol 28: 199−203

11. Lübbert H, Pollow K (1978) Correlation between the 17β-hydroxysteroid dehydrogenase activity and the estradiol and progesterone receptor concentrations of normal and neoplastic mammary tissue. J Mol Med 3: 175−183

12. Morgan LR (1979) Tamoxifen versus megesterol acetate in breast cancer. Cancer Treat Rep 63: 1218 (Abstr 380)

13. Morgan LR, Donley PJ (1981) Tamoxifen versus megestrol acetate in breast cancer. In: Anti-hormones and breast cancer. Reviews on Endocrine-Related Cancer [Suppl] 9: 301−310

14. Neumann F (1978) The physiological action of progesterone and the pharmacological effects of progestogens − a short review. Postgrad Med J 54: 11−24

15. Salander H, Tisell LE (1976) Effects of megestrol on oestradiol induced growth of the prostatic lobes and the seminal vesicles in castrated rats. Acta Endocrinol (Kbh) 82: 213−224

16. Stoll BA (1967) Progestin therapy of breast cancer: Comparison of agents. Br Med J 3: 338−341

17. Teulings FAG, Van Gilse HA, Henkelman MS, Portengen H, Alexieva-Figusch J (1980) Estrogen, androgen, glucocorticoid, and progesterone receptors in progestin-induced regression of human breast cancer. Cancer Res 40: 2557−2561

18. Weeth JB (1974) Large dose progestin palliation. Valuable in solid tumor patients. Proc Am Assoc Cancer Res 15: 726 (Abstr)

19. Weeth JB (1975) Megestrol palliation of breast cancer. Proc Am Assoc Cancer Res 16: 38 (Abstr)

Protocols Based on Steroid Receptors: Great Britain

R. D. Rubens*

Breast Cancer Unit, Guy's Hospital,
London SE1 Medical Oncology Clinic, 9RT, United Kingdom

Introduction

The clinical relevance of steroid receptors to operable, locally advanced and disseminated breast cancer is being studied at centres in Great Britain. Protocols have investigated the use of receptors as guides to response to treatment and prognosis and also the relationship of receptors to other prognostic variables.

Early Breast Cancer

Prognosis

The early results from two studies on women with breast cancer treated by mastectomy have suggested that the prognosis, in terms of both disease-free interval and survival, is improved when tumours are positive for oestrogen receptors (ER) [1, 3]. A larger long-term study at Guy's Hospital and the Imperial Cancer Research Fund's laboratories, in which a thousand patients so far have been accrued for a mean follow-up time of 3.5 years, may, in due course, verify these early results. In this study, analyses of relative independence and interdependence of many other variables including histological characteristics, nodal involvement, serum and urinary hormone profiles and other putative markers of prognosis will also be made.

Adjuvant Systemic Therapy

In a multicentre trial, the use of tamoxifen as adjuvant systemic therapy in operable breast cancer is being studied. In each of the 39 contributing centres, a uniform surgical procedure has been followed, either mastectomy with axillary clearance or mastectomy with node sampling followed by radiotherapy. Accrual to this trial of over one thousand patients has

* I am grateful to Dr. J. F. Stewart for helping in the preparation of this chapter and to the following for providing me with information: Prof. M. Baum (King's College Hospital, London), Prof. R.W. Blamey (University of Nottingham), Dr. R. C. Coombes (Royal Marsden Hospital, Sutton), and Mr. W. D. George (University of Liverpool)

now been stopped. Eligible patients have been premenopausal women with positive axillary lymph nodes and postmenopausal patients with positive or negative axillary nodes. Patients were randomised to receive either no systemic therapy or tamoxifen 10 mg twice daily for 2 years after operation. Oestrogen receptors have been measured in approximately 450 patients (six laboratories have submitted results from 25 centres). This is making possible a study of interlaboratory variation in receptor assays and also a quality control assessment. In due course, the results of the trial in terms of postoperative disease-free interval and overall survival will be interpreted in relation to steroid receptor status.

In 1977, groups at Guy's Hospital, London, and the University of South Manchester amalgamated trials of adjuvant chemotherapy which had begun in 1975 and 1976 respectively. These trials are evaluating the use of adjuvant chemotherapy with either L-phenylalanine mustard or cyclophosphamide, methotrexate and 5-fluorouracil (CMF) in patients with involved nodes after mastectomy with axillary clearance. The trials, which were established to repeat those of the National Surgical Adjuvant Breast Project in the USA and the Istituto Nationale Tumori in Milan, will be analysed in relation to the ER status of tumours as well as other prognostic variables such as menopausal status and extent of axillary involvement.

Locally Advanced Breast Cancer

Although information has become available on the prognostic importance of steroid receptors in operable breast cancer and disseminated disease, there is little in relation to locally advanced breast cancer (stage III). At Guy's Hospital, 60 patients with locally advanced breast cancer on whom ER information was available have been studied [10]. There were no differences in other prognostic variables, responses to treatment or survival between patients with ER-positive (ER+) or ER-negative (ER−) tumours. These results do not suggest that ER status is a prognostic factor in primary locally advanced breast cancer. A number of centres in Great Britain are participating in EORTC protocol 10792. In this trial the value of chemotherapy and/or endocrine therapy as an adjunct to radiotherapy in the treatment of locally advanced disease is being studied. The results of this trial will be interpreted in relation to ER status as well as other prognostic variables.

Disseminated Breast Cancer

Distribution of Metastatic Disease

Observations that visceral metastases from breast cancer respond less often to endocrine treatment than those in bone and soft tissues stimulated a study of the relationship of ER status to the pattern of metastatic disease [12]. In an analysis of 278 patients, it was found that metastases in bones occurred significantly more commonly in patients with ER+ tumours, whilst those with ER− tumours had a significantly higher incidence of metastases in the brain and liver; soft tissue and lung metastases did not appear to be influenced by receptor status. Furthermore, patients with ER+ tumours had a significantly longer survival after first relapse. The essential difference was whether a tumour was positive or negative for receptors, with 5 fmol/mg of cytosol protein as the cut-off point, rather than the absolute amount of receptor present.

Endocrine Treatment

A study sponsored by the British Breast Group and reported in 1978 supported the view that ER status was of value in predicting the response of advanced breast cancer to endocrine therapy [6]. These results were reaffirmed subsequently in a larger series of 191 patient from Guy's Hospital in which the response rate to endocrine treatment was 46 of 136 (34%) in ER+ patients compared with five of 55 (9%) in ER− patients ($P < 0.01$) [7]. It is noteworthy that the five responders with ER− tumours were treated with either androgens or tamoxifen; there were no responses to ovarian ablation, oestrogens, progestogens, corticosteroids or hypophysectomy in patients with ER− tumours. In a small series from the Royal Marsden Hospital, it has been found that there is a marked reduction in ER content in sequential biopsies of tumour tissue during the course of endocrine treatment (Coombes RC, 1981, personal communication).

Further studies at Guy's Hospital and the Imperial Cancer Research Fund laboratories have investigated the predictive value of progesterone receptors (PgR) and preliminary analysis showed that patients with tumours positive for both ER and PgR possibly have an 80% chance of response to endocrine treatment [4]. The results are now being analysed in a series of 148 patients and will be reported shortly. In this series, responses have occurred in patients with tumours of phenotype ER+ PgR− or ER− PgR+, but are most frequent for phenotype ER+ PgR+; ER− PgR− tumours are unlikely to respond.

The presence of elastosis in primary breast tumours also gives an indication of their sensitivity to endocrine treatment [5]. While there is some association between elastosis and receptor status, a combination of these indices gives an improved prediction of the responsiveness of breast cancer to endocrine treatment; ER+ tumours with no elastosis present are unlikely to respond.

A prospective controlled clinical trial at Guy's Hospital has been assessing the contribution of prednisolone to primary endocrine therapy (ovarian ablation in premenopausal patients, tamoxifen in postmenopausal patients). In this trial, the lack of responsiveness of ER− tumours to endocrine therapy has again been confirmed. The preliminary results have indicated that the addition of prednisolone to primary endocrine therapy improves significantly the response rate in patients with tumours which are ER+ or when receptor status is unknown [9].

Cytotoxic Chemotherapy

A retrospective analysis has indicated that the response of advanced breast cancer to cytotoxic chemotherapy is not related to ER status. However, ER+ tumours seem to grow more slowly than ER− tumours, and the response to chemotherapy tends to be longer for ER+ tumours [8]. These data and those in other reports studying the relevance of receptor status to cytotoxic chemotherapy have depended on receptor information obtained on either primary breast tumours or metastatic disease before the commencement of endocrine treatment. Because it is possible that the receptor status of tumours could be changed by prior endocrine treatment, a prospective study has now been undertaken to determine whether the response to cytotoxic chemotherapy is related to receptor status obtaining immediately before chemotherapy is started. Preliminary results again suggest that even under these circumstances, receptor status is not a determinant of response to chemotherapy [11]. An inverse relationship between ER level and thymidine labelling indices of tumours has been found, and the relevance of this to response to cytotoxic chemotherapy is currently being evaluated at the University of Liverpool [2].

Summary

Steroid receptors appear to have prognostic significance in operable and disseminated breast cancer, but not in primary locally advanced disease. Information on receptor status gives some indication of the pattern of metastatic disease. Absence of ER and PgR detect effectively patients who will not benefit from endocrine therapy and the presence of both receptors indicates the patients most likely to respond. Patients with ER+ PgR− or ER− PgR+ tumours have an intermediate frequency of response to endocrine treatment. Receptor status is not a determinant of response to cytotoxic treatment.

References

1. Blamey RW, Bishop HM, Blake JRS, Doyle PJ, Elston CW, Haybittle JL, Nicholson RI, Griffiths K (1980) Relationship between primary breast tumor receptor status and patient survival. Cancer 46: 2765−2769
2. Cooke T, George WD, Griffiths K (1980) Possible tests for selection of adjuvant systemic therapy in early cancer of the breast. Br J Surg 67: 747−750
3. Cooke T, George D, Shields R, Maynard P, Griffiths K (1979) Oestrogen receptors and prognosis in early breast cancer. Lancet 1: 995−997
4. King RJB, Hayward JL, Masters JRW, Millis RR, Rubens RD (1980) Steroid receptor assays as prognostic aids in the treatment of breast cancer. In: Whittliff JL, Dapunt O (eds) Steroid receptors and hormone dependent neoplasia. Masson, New York, pp 249−256
5. Masters JRW, Millis RR, King RJB, Rubens RD (1979) Elastosis and response to endocrine therapy in human breast cancer. Br J Cancer 39: 536−539
6. Roberts MM, Rubens RD, King RJB, Hawkins RA, Millis RR, Hayward JL, Forrest APM (1978) Oestrogen receptors and the response to endocrine therapy in advanced breast cancer. Br J Cancer 38: 431−436
7. Rubens RD, Hayward JL (1980) Estrogen receptors and response to endocrine therapy and cytotoxic chemotherapy in advanced breast cancer. Cancer 46: 2922−2924
8. Rubens RD, King RJB, Sexton S, Minton MJ, Hayward JL (1980) Oestrogen receptors and response to cytotoxic chemotherapy in advanced breast cancer. Cancer Chemother Pharmcol 4: 43−45
9. Rubens RD, Stewart JF, King RJB, Minton MJ, Sparrow GEA, Knight RK (1981) Primary endocrine therapy + prednisolone in advanced breast cancer. Proceedings of AACR and ASCO 22: 436
10. Stewart JF, King RJB, Rubens RD (1981) Estrogen receptors (ER) and prognosis in primary locally advanced breast cancer. Proceedings of AACR and ASCO 22: 148
11. Stewart JF, King RJB, Rubens RD (1981) Oestrogen receptor status of breast cancer immediately before chemotherapy and response to treatment. Br J Cancer 44: 287
12. Stewart JF, King RJB, Sexton S, Millis RR, Rubens RD, Hayward JL (1981) Oestrogen receptors, sites of metastatic disease and survival in recurrent breast cancer. Eur J Cancer 17: 449−435

Currently Active Protocols in the EORTC* Breast Cancer Cooperative Group

H. T. Mouridsen, T. Palshof, W. Mattheiem,
R. J. Sylvester, N. Rotmensz, and R. J. Paridaens

Department of Oncology I, Finsen Institute,
49 Strandboulevarden, 2100 Copenhagen, Denmark

Introduction

Since Jensen's initial work in 1971 [1], many reports have confirmed the utility of estrogen receptor assays for predicting the results of endocrine treatments in advanced breast cancer (review article [2]). These assays, which can be performed either on the primary tumor or on metastases, are deemed to provide the clinician with a tool for measuring the degree of hormone dependence of the tumor. Accordingly, they could be used to select the most appropriate treatment either as palliation in advanced disease or as a prophylaxis against recurrence in stage II cases. We intend to review briefly the currently active protocols in the EORTC Breast Cancer Cooperative Group. We will focus in more detail on those which include endocrine therapy. The possible role of receptor assays in the design of these trials will be analyzed.

Active Protocols for Primary Breast Cancer

The two protocols, summarized in Table 1, concern patients presenting without evidence of distant metastases. In both trials, steroid hormone receptor values will be retrospectively analyzed after completion of the study with regard to their alleged prognostic value. The results of these assays, however, are not taken into account for stratification of the patients when they are included in the trials.

The first protocol (EORTC 10801) concerns operable cases and compares radical mastectomy with conservative surgery completed by radiotherapy. Six cycles of adjuvant chemotherapy with the CMF regimen (cyclophosphamide 100 mg/m^2 p.o. days 1–14; methotrexate 40 mg/m^2 i.v. days 1, 8; fluorouracil 500 mg/m^2 i.v. days 1, 8) are given at 4-week intervals to patients with metastatic involvement of axillary nodes. This schema was chosen on the basis of the Group's experience in a previous trial (EORTC 10761), preliminary results of which will be published in the near future.

Endocrine therapy, which is not included in the former protocol, intervenes as part of the treatment in trial EORTC 10792. This four-arm study is reserved for locally advanced inoperable cases and aims to assess the usefulness of adding endocrine therapy or chemotherapy or both to radiotherapy. The latter modality, considered here as the

---

* European Organization for Research on Treatment of Cancer

Table 1. EORTC Breast Cancer Cooperative Group: Active protocols for primary breast cancer

Protocol number	Stage	Regimen	Study coordinator	Date of activation
10801	I–II	R< Radical mastectomy[a] / Conservative surgery[a]	J. A. van Dongen (Antoni Van Leeuwenhoek Institute, Amsterdam, The Netherlands)	May 1980
10792	III	R< Radiotherapy / Radiotherapy + endocrine therapy / Radiotherapy + chemotherapy / Radiotherapy + endocrine therapy + chemotherapy	J. L. Hayward and R. D. Rubens (Guy's Hospital, London, England)	December 1979

R = Randomized trial
[a] Adjuvant CMF in node-positive cases

reference treatment, is given by a supervoltage technique to the breast and regional nodes, followed by a booster dose to sites of initially palpable disease. Endocrine therapy in premenopausal patients consists of ovarian irradiation plus prednisolone (7.5 mg daily), this drug being continued for 5 years; postmenopausal patients receive tamoxifen (20 mg daily) for a similar period. Chemotherapy consists of 12 cycles of CMF, these drugs being administered in a similar manner as in trial EORTC 10801, i.e., cyclophosphamide 100 mg/m^2 p.o. days 1–14; methotrexate 30 mg/m^2 i.v. days 1, 8; fluorouracil 600 mg/m^2 i.v. days 1, 8.

Active Protocols for Advanced (Stage IV) Disease

Six protocols are now running, their designs being summarized in Table 2. Two of them (EORTC 10807 and EORTC 10808) are used as first-line treatment whereas the other trials intervene at a later stage as second- or third-line treatments. Both protocols EORTC 10802 and EORTC 10807 involve endocrine therapy and are described below.
Trial EORTC 10802 is a pure endocrine phase III study comparing two dosages of medroxyprogesterone acetate (MPA, 300 mg vs 900 mg p.o. daily) in order to investigate the dose-response relationships in view of the recent claims that large doses might dramatically improve therapeutic results [3–5] even in end-stage, heavily pretreated cases. The results will be retrospectively related to the plasma concentrations of MPA and to steroid hormone receptor levels in neoplastic tissue. Such an analysis might be of importance owing to the observation by Teulings et al. [6] that the response to another progestational agent, i.e., megestrol acetate, was more strongly related to androgen receptors than to estrogen or progesterone receptors.

Table 2. EORTC Breast Cancer Cooperative Group: Active protocols for advanced (stage IV) breast cancer

Protocol number	Regimen	Study coordinator(s)	Date of activation
10802	Ⓡ Medroxyprogesterone 300 mg p.o. daily / Medroxyprogesterone 900 mg p.o. daily	H. T. Mouridsen (Finsen Institute, Copenhagen, Denmark)	September 1980
10803	Phase II trial. *CIS*-Platinum 100 mg/m^2 day 1 + vindesine 2 mg/m^2 day 1, 8 q 4 weeks	R. Paridaens (J. Bordet Institute, Brussels, Belgium)	December 1980
10804	Phase II trial. 9-Hydroxy-2 N-methylellipticinium 150 mg/m^2 day 1, 8 q 4 weeks	A. Clarysse (St. Jan Institute, Brugge, Belgium) and A. T. van Oosterom (A. Z. Leiden, The Netherlands)	January 1981
10805	Ⓡ Carminomycin 20 mg/m^2 day 1 q 3 weeks / Adriamycin 75 mg/m^2 i.v. day 1 q 3 weeks	H. T. Mouridsen (Bispebjerg Hospital, Copenhagen, Denmark)	January 1981
10807	Phase II trial. Oophorectomy (premenopausal patients only) + Aminoglutethimide 1 g daily + Hydrocortisone 40 mg daily + Ethinylestradiol 50 mg day 1 q 3 weeks + FAC (see text) day 2 q 3 weeks	R. Paridaens (J. Bordet Institute, Brussels, Belgium)	June 1981
10808	Ⓡ "Classical CMF" q 4 weeks (cyclophosphamide 100 mg/m^2 p.o. day 1–14 methotrexate 40 mg/m^2 i.v. day 1, 8 fluorouracil 600 mg/m^2 i.v. day 1, 8 "New CMF" q 3 weeks (cyclophosphamide 600 mg/m^2 i.v. day 1 methotrexate 40 mg/m^2 i.v. day 1 fluorouracil 600 mg/m^2 i.v. day 1	E. Engelsman (A. Van Leeuwenhoek, Amsterdam, The Netherlands)	June 1981

Ⓡ = randomized trial

Protocol EORTC 10807 is a phase II study of a new regimen of hormonochemotherapy reserved for previously untreated cases. Many empirical associations of standard chemotherapy regimens with oophorectomy in premenopausal patients or steroid hormones or antagonists in postmenopausal patients have been described [7−12]. They generally achieve higher response rates and longer relapse-free periods than the same modalities used singly or in sequence. Improvement of survival, however, seems modest or nil, especially in highly hormone-dependent cases [13], indicating a lack of true synergism between conventional endocrine treatments and cycle active cytotoxic drugs. The originality of the present trial is that it aims to develop a synergistic combination of a deep and prolonged estrogenic suppression achieved by aminoglutethimide plus hydrocortisone (preceded by oophorectomy in premenopausal patients) and cyclic chemotherapy with the FAC regimen (fluorouracil 500 mg/m^2, adriamycin 50 mg/m^2, cyclophosphamide 500 mg/m^2) repeated at 3-week intervals. The latter is preceded by the administration of a single dose of an estrogen (ethinylestradiol 50 μg), which according to results of experimental studies may sensitize estrogen receptor-positive (ER+) cancer cells to the killing effect of cytotoxic drugs [14, 15]. The statistical evaluation of the efficacy of this regimen is based upon the condition that the required lowest limit of therapeutic activity is a 30% complete response rate, at least in ER+ cases. If such a favorable result is obtained, the biologic concept of estrogenic recruitment as an amplifier for chemotherapy will be tested in a randomized phase III trial comparing the present hormono-chemotherapeutic regimen with either ethinylestradiol or placebo given before FAC.

Discussion

Alongside all the new cytotoxic drugs, conventional endocrine treatments retain a privileged place in the treatment of breast cancer. The present review of the EORTC Breast Group's currently active clinical trials shows, however, that estrogen receptor assays, which are the best markers of hormone dependence, are not used as a prospective tool for therapeutic decision. This is particularly obvious when the first treatment has to be initiated for adjuvant or palliative purposes. The great difficulties in the comparison of receptor assays performed in different institutions may explain this fact (see Part II). Another reason is that up to 80% of breast cancers contain detectable amounts of estrogen receptor and are thus likely to benefit, although in varying degrees for each patient, from endocrine treatments [16, 17]. The inclusion of hormonotherapy as part of a multimodal strategy seems justified almost in every case in order to achieve better immediate therapeutic results.

Within each institution of the group, steroid receptor assays performed locally provide the clinician with a useful tool for choosing the appropriate second-line treatment for patients in relapse. Thus, unnecessary hormonal manipulations can be avoided in receptor-poor or receptor-negative cases, which could be included earlier in phase I or phase II trials of new cytotoxic compounds or combinations.

The EORTC Breast Cancer Cooperative Group welcomes all institutions interested in participating in the above-listed clinical trials. Protocols and information can be obtained upon request by writing to Dr. R. Paridaens, Department of Medicine, Rue Héger-Bordet 1, 1000 Brussels, Belgium (telephone 02/538.57.90 − telex 22773).

References

1. Jensen EV, Block GE, Smith S, Kyser K, de Sombre ER (1981) Estrogen receptors and breast cancer response to adrenalectomy. Natl Cancer Inst Monogr 34: 55–70
2. Hawkins RA, Roberts MM, Forrest APM (1980) Oestrogen receptors and breast cancer: current status. Br J Surg 67: 153–169
3. Robustelli Della Cuna G, Calciati A, Strada B, Bumma C, Campio L (1978) High dose medroxyprogesterone acetate (MPA) treatment in metastatic carcinoma of the breast: a dose-response evaluation. Tumori 64: 143–149
4. Pannuti F, Martoni A, Lenaz GR, Piana E, Nanni P (1978) A possible new approach to the treatment of metastatic breast cancer: massive doses of medroxyprogesterone acetate. Cancer Treat Rep 62: 499–504
5. De Lena M, Brambilla C, Valagussa P, Bonadonna G (1979) High-dose medroxyprogesterone acetate in breast cancer resistant to endocrine and cytotoxic therapy. Cancer Chemother Pharmacol 2: 175–180
6. Teulings FA, Van Gilse HA, Henkelman MS, Portengen H, Alexieva-Figusch J (1980) Estrogen, androgen, glucocorticoid and progesterone receptors in progestin-induced regression of human breast cancer. Cancer Res 40: 2557–2561
7. Ahmann DL, O'Connell MJ, Hahn RG, Bisel HF, Lee RA, Edmonson JH (1977) An evaluation of early or delayed adjuvant chemotherapy in premenopausal patients with advanced breast cancer undergoing oophorectomy. N Engl J Med 297: 356–360
8. Brunner KW, Sonntag RW, Alberto P, Senn HJ, Martz G, Obrecht P, Maurice P (1977) Combined chemo- and hormonal therapy in advanced breast cancer. Cancer 39: 2923–2933
9. Falkson G, Falkson HC, Glidewell O, Weinberg V, Leone L, Holland JF (1979) Improved remission rates and remission duration in young women with metastatic breast cancer following combined oophorectomy and chemotherapy. Cancer 43: 2215–2222
10. Robustelli Della Cuna G, Strada B (1980) High dose medroxyprogesterone acetate (HD-MPA) combined with chemotherapy for metastatic breast carcinoma. In: Iacobelli S, di Marco A (eds) Role of medroxyprogesterone in endocrine related tumors. Raven, New York, pp 1–11
11. Heuson JC, Sylvester R, Engelsman E (1980) Alternating cyclical hormonal-cytotoxic combination chemotherapy in postmenopausal patients with breast cancer. An EORTC trial. In: Mouridsen HT, Palshof T (eds) Breast cancer – experimental and clinical aspects. Pergamon, Oxford, pp 113–117
12. Mouridsen HT, Palshof T, Engelsman E, Sylvester RJ (1980) CMF versus CMF plus tamoxifen in advanced breast cancer in postmenopausal women. An EORTC trial. In: Mouridsen HT, Palshof T (eds) Breast cancer – experimental and clinical aspects. Pergamon, Oxford, pp 119–123
13. Glick JH, Creech RH, Torri S, Holroyde C, Brodovsky H, Catalano RB, Varano M (1980) Tamoxifen plus sequential CMF chemotherapy versus tamoxifen alone in postmenopausal patients with advanced breast cancer: a randomized trial. Cancer 45: 735–741
14. Stormshak F, Leake R, Wertz N, Gorski J (1976) Stimulatory and inhibitory effects of estrogen on uterine DNA synthesis. Endocrinology 99: 1501–1511
15. Weichselbaum RR, Hellman S, Piro AJ, Nove JJ, Little JB (1978) Proliferation kinetics of a human breast cancer cell line in vitro following treatment with 17β-estradiol and 1-β-D-arabinofuranosylcytosine. Cancer Res 38: 2339–2342
16. Leclercq G, Heuson JC (1976) Estrogen receptors in the spectrum of breast cancer. Curr Probl Cancer 1 (6)
17. Paridaens R, Sylvester RJ, Ferrazzi E, Legros N, Leclercq G, Heuson JC (1980) Clinical significance of the quantitative assessment of estrogen receptors in advanced breast cancer. Cancer 46: 2889–2895

The Place of Hormone Receptors in the Elaboration of a Therapeutic stategy Against Breast Cancer

P. Pouillart, P. M. Martin, and H. Magdelénat

Section Médicale et Hospitalière, Institut Curie, 26 Rue d'Ulm, 75231 Paris, France

Introduction

When considering the place of hormone receptors in a therapeutic strategy against breast cancer, one must be take into account not only our knowledge of the molecular physiology of hormone-dependent tumors or of their clinical aspects but also the numerous questions concerning these receptors which are still unanswered. These various aspects are dealt with below.

A cell may be termed hormone dependent when there exists an ensemble of intracellular phenomena which depend on the interaction of receptors and specific ligands (whether steroids or not) and evidently mark an intermodulation of the different receptors, implicating a modulation of protein synthesis. Thus, the interaction of estradiol with its specific receptor (ER) indicates a supplementary synthesis of this receptor [2] and the synthesis of the progesterone receptor (PgR) [7].

The PgR is, then, the control of the functional activity of ER. The interaction of progesterone with PgR inhibits the synthesis of ER [2] and PgR [17]. The action of tamoxifen (Tam) on a hormone-competent cell leads to a decrease in the rate of ER synthesis and an increase in that of PgR [21]. Here, PgR still appeared to be the preferred molecular marker of hormonal competence.

It appears that in breast tumors, the presence of PgR is strongly correlated to the degree of cellular differentiation [15], ER being more weakly correlated. PgR seems, then, to be the marker of cellular differentiation. But at a practical level, this information loses its value owing to the cellular heterogeneity of the tumoral population.

It is well known that only 30% of patients with breast cancer respond to hormonal treatment. However, this increases to 60% if ER positivity exists [8], and nearly 80% if both ER and PgR are present [18]. PgR appears to be the better parameter for the prediction of hormonal dependence. Finally, and most importantly, from the results of recent studies [5, 22] it seems that the steroid receptors have a prognostic value independent of the other known parameters. The prognostic value of PgR is even greater than that of ER [12]. In postmenopausal patients, combined hormonal therapy and chemotherapy for the treatment of disseminated breast cancer is far superior to the use of chemotherapy alone, especially in the presence of hormone receptors.

Of the above known facts, three fundamental ideas should be emphasized:

1. That ER and PgR have prognostic significance.

2. That the hormonal dependence of a tumor is correlated with the average amount of receptors.
3. That the tumoral population is heterogeneous, being constituted of both hormone-dependent (HR+) cells and non-hormone-dependent (HR−) cells.

Elaboration of Therapeutic Protocols

The corollary of point 1 above is that therapeutic protocols should vary according to whether hormone receptors are present. Judging by a study of therapeutic protocols for breast cancer that include hormonal therapy [1], this does not yet appear to be the case: in only 12 protocols did the presence of ER influence treatment (protocols 1.0002, 1.0009, 1.0010, 1.0013, 1.0015, 1.0016, 1.0017, 1.0021, 1.0034, 1.0049, 1.0066, and 1.0075) and in only two was PgR positivity taken into account (protocols 1.0060 and 1.0097).

But if it actually seems difficult not to take into consideration the prognostic value of the steroid receptors, it is appropriate at all times to relate the importance of this parameter to the clinical situation.

Advanced Breast Cancer

Other parameters such as serum levels of LDH and albumin, number of metastatic sites initially present, and previous chemotherapy possess a prognostic significance at least as great as the level of receptors. These parameters (independent from one another), which indicate tumoral extension, host reaction, tumoral aggression, tumoral volume, and the therapeutic history of the patient, all permit the identification of at least three different groups of patients for which probability of survival, rate of response, and tolerance to treatment are significantly different.

A recent study (personal clinical trial) shows that in group III patients (essentially characterized by raised LDH levels), who have a very poor prognosis, hormonal therapy has very little effect on HR+ tumors, and the protocols of conventional chemotherapy are accompanied by significant toxicity while again being basically ineffective. In the particular case of inflammatory breast cancer, the prognostic significance of PgR actually disappears completely. There thus appear to be numerous arguments in favor of the elaboration of more complex strategies which take into consideration the diversity of the disease − the biological diversity of the tumor, the great diversity of the host's reaction, etc.

Table 1 lists those parameters shown to have prognostic significance when analyzed according to the method of Cox in a recent personal study.

Table 1. Prognostic factors in disseminated breast cancer

Prognostic parameter	Level of significance
1 − LDH	0.001
2 − LDH + anterior chemotherapy	0.05
3 − LDH + anterior chemotherapy + RP	0.06
4 − LDH + anterior chemotherapy + RP + no. of metastases	0.06

Early Breast Cancer

Numerous trials of adjuvant treatment have now been carried out on patients with breast cancer. At the time of the first controlled trials, the retained indications took into consideration only the prognostic parameters accepted for stages committed to local treatment: that is the size of the tumor and the axillary node invasion. The first two fundamental trials [3, 6] confirmed the prognostic significance of the initial clinical and histological parameters and illustrated the particular significance of age and hormonal status. Thus we have the first elements of a classification:
1. Degree of lymph node invasion.
   a) Absence of node invasion.
   b) Invasion of one to three nodes.
   c) Invasion of more than three nodes.
2. Size of the tumor (the significance of this parameter often appeared to be less).
3. Two age groups
   a) Under 50 years.
   b) Over 50 years.

Two additional parameters that could also be taken into account are:
1. Period of genital activity.
2. Period of menopause.

This classification is important since it appears that the cytotoxic chemotherapy proposed in these first trials affects neither the rate of metastatic relapse nor the rate of short- or long-term survival. Other trials have shown that heavier combinations [28] or those including adriamycin [4] do in fact possess a certain efficacy. Likewise, the analysis of Bonadonna [3] showed that in postmenopausal patients, a significant efficacy appeared when the drug regimen could be brought to completion. However, it was a very small percentage of patients who were thus treated, and even then the efficacy of the combination was inferior to that in the population of young patients.

The systematization of hormone receptor assays introduces a supplementary fundamental notion: Determination of the level of receptors allows one to establish precise indications for adjuvant hormonal therapy, and in addition is of major prognostic significance, attenuating the recognized significance of axillary node invasion. Studies reveal a very pronounced predominance of positive or raised levels of ER in postmenopausal patients. This may explain in part the insufficiencies of the previous adjuvant chemotherapy, and in any case clearly indicates a specific therapeutical modality.

Among the parameters capable of explaining at least partially a bad prognosis, the tumoral doubling time is one of the most standard.

It is known that the histological grade in three classes recovers in part this kinetic notion. Likewise, HR− tumors have a kinetic progression which is more rapid than HR+ tumors [20]. This characteristic is elsewhere amplified before menopause.

Thus this notion of tumoral kinetic progression can be represented by two parameters which partially overlap:
1. Level of hormone receptors.
2. Histological grade.

These observations lead us to propose a different therapeutic strategy according to the parameters initially present. If it is still too early to allot to each parameter a coefficient of significance which rationalizes completely the initial stratification, it is legitimate to propose more specific trials according to the simple scheme shown in Table 2.

Table 2
Premenopause

Group I (high risk)	Group II	Group II'
SBR III	SBR I or II	SBR I or II
HR−	HR+	HR+
Age < 35 years	1−3 nodes	> 3 nodes

Postmenopause

Group III	Group IV
HR+	HR−
SBR I, II, or III	SBR I, II, or III

Several trials are currently taking place and rest on this approach [23] (protocol 2).
In short, information concerning hormone receptor status and in particular that of PgR appears necessary prior to organizing the therapeutic protocols. The main problem becomes, then, access to this information. The conventional methods permit one to determine without ambiguity the levels of ER and PgR in surgical samples (mastectomy, lumpectomy), but it has been necessary to develop a specific methodological approach for cases where surgery is not used. With rigorous control of the quality of sample (measure of the tumoral cellularity) and of the methodological parameters, it is possible to obtain a valid estimation of the levels of intratumoral receptors by means of (a) drill biopsy of the primitive tumor or of a small metastatic nodule or (b) needle aspiration [13, 19, 25]. Since these "micromethods" usually permit determination of only one receptor (ER *or* PgR), priority should be given to assay of PgR, being the more efficient marker of the two. In order to avoid an underestimation of PgR levels in such limited samples, one may amplify the levels by prior administration of tamoxifen (20 mg/day for 7 days before assay), this amplification being specific to the hormone-competent cell (PgR+) [21]. Finally, methods permitting simultaneous measurement of several receptors in these small samples have been proposed [14]. Thus, complete quantitative information can be obtained in all cases of breast cancer, whether they are treated surgically or not.

Optimization of Hormonal Therapy

The second fact worthy of emphasis (the hormonal dependence of a tumor is correlated with the average receptor level and is expressed by the intermodulation of the receptors) raises a problem with regard to optimization of hormonal therapy: Are the intracellular receptors really the target for hormonal therapy, or are they merely the markers of the efficiency of the hormonal treatment? Or even, does the intermodulation of the receptors have any direct relation to therapeutic efficiency? (Receptor status would then have prognostic significance independent of treatment.)
The hypothesis that the receptors are the target of hormonal therapy and consequently are also the markers of the efficiency of treatment leads to a search for the best hormonal therapy. Maximum efficiency of treatment will be attained when the receptor levels are highest. It is appropriate, therefore, to search for those therapeutic combinations which

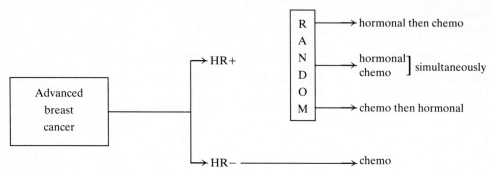

Fig. 1. Protocol 1: Advanced breast cancer

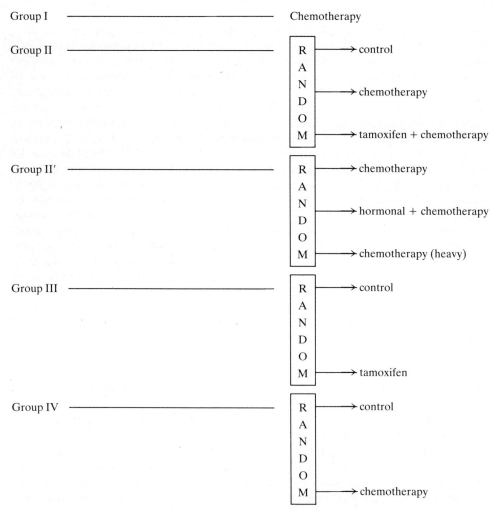

Fig. 2. Protocol 2: Early breast cancer. Adjuvant chemotherapy or hormonal therapy in early breast cancer (see Table 2)

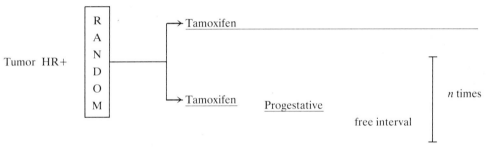

Fig. 3. Protocol 3: Sequential hormonal therapy — study project involving randomized trials to compare the effect of tamoxifen with that of a tamoxifen-synthetic progestin sequence

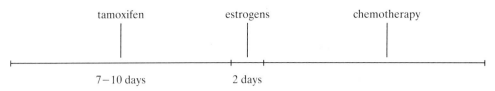

Fig. 4. Protocol 4: Potentiation of the effect of chemotherapy on HR+ cells

maximize the receptor levels (this is the rational basis of sequential hormonal therapy) and to avoid those which lead to a prolonged lowering of these levels (chemotherapy may have such an effect). These considerations provide theoretical justification for the protocols of sequential hormonal therapy [24] (protocol 3). Tamoxifen augments PgR levels [21], which can then be "mobilized" by a progestational agent, whose nature still remains to be optimized. The hormonal sequence can be resumed after a free interval (whose duration and utilization remain to be defined) in order to permit a reinduction of the estrogen receptors which were lowered during the preceding cycle. This theoretical justification, perhaps a little simplistic, remains to be demonstrated. For this purpose one must be able to measure the variations in receptor level (ER and PgR) during the course of treatment; this could be done by repeated measurements at different times using the micromethods of simultaneous dosages of ER and PgR (at the end of each cycle and at intervals of 7–10 days during the free interval). Should this hypothesis be confirmed, it would be possible to envisage that the measurement of the ER and PgR levels will allow an individualized optimization of the different phases of treatment.

Optimization of the Combination of Hormonal Therapy and Chemotherapy

The third fundamental fact concerns the heterogeneity of the cellular population inside the tumor, constituted qualitatively of HR+ cells and HR− cells. Moreover, the individual concentration of receptors varies from one HR+ cell to another (or at least from one tumoral zone to another) [26]. In the actual state of the methodologies of the receptor assays, the character or hormone dependence is only the resultant of the heterogeneous distribution of the cellular populations. The existence of cellular heterogeneity raises the problem of which combination of hormonal therapy and chemotherapy should be employed. If the medical treatment of HR− tumors amounts only to chemotherapy, three combinations of cytotoxic chemotherapy and hormonal therapy can be envisaged for HR+ tumors (protocol 1):

1. Simultaneous administration [10, 23].
2. Hormonal therapy followed by chemotherapy [27].
3. Chemotherapy followed by hormonal therapy.

The decision rests on theoretical considerations relating to the inhibitory effect of efficient cytotoxic chemotherapy on protein synthesis and the selective sensitivity of HR+ and HR− cellular clones to chemotherapy. If chemotherapy exerts an inhibitory effect (even if it is temporary) on the ensemble of the function of cellular metabolic regulation, including protein synthesis, which is functionally dependent on the receptors, hormonal therapy cannot exercise its full effect. If this is indeed the case, simultaneous chemotherapy and hormonal therapy would be contraindicated: hormonal therapy would be of benefit only if it were administered before, or, at least, at a distance from, chemotherapy. Surveillance of the PgR level after 7−10 days of simultaneous treatment with tamoxifen (which alone ought to induce an increase in PgR) and chemotherapy will rapidly resolve this question.

The hypothesis postulating different sensitivity of HR+ and HR− clones during chemotherapy must equally be taken into account. If it was confirmed without ambiguity that in vivo the HR− cells have a kinetic proliferation which is more rapid than that of HR+ cells, chemotherapy ought to affect selectively result in a selective efficiency on the HR+ population. Few convincing arguments in favor of the hypothesis have been presented up till now, and contradictory results have been reported [9, 11], although the apparent discrepancies rest on methodological differences.

One can, however, imagine that the effect of chemotherapy on the HR+ cells could be potentiated by placing these cells in cycle, thanks to an "estrogenic flash" of 24−48 h after 7 days treatment with tamoxifen, followed by immediate administration of chemotherapy (protocol 4). The problem of the cellular selection by hormonal therapy and chemotherapy will only be solved when we acquire precise knowledge of the evolution of the subpopulation of HR+ and HR− cells under hormonal therapy and chemotherapy.

Efforts are currently being made [16], and must be pursued, to improve the sensitivity and specificity of the methods of visualization and of quantification of the population of HR+ and HR− cells on histological sections or on fine-needle aspirates.

The use of specific autofluorescent ligands should allow, if one uses it in an image-intensifying device, replacement of autoradiography, which is poorly adapted for medical practice. Monoclonal antireceptor antibodies will probably have a place in determining the cellular heterogeneity of a tumor, both before and during the treatment.

Conclusion

Hormonal therapy, generally associated with chemotherapy, occupies an important place in the therapeutic strategy against breast cancer for two reasons:

1. Greater efficiency of the antiestrogenic treatments (antiestrogens associated or not associated with progestational agents).
2. The more precise indication for such therapy offered by measurement of hormone receptors.

If systematic assay of estrogen receptors and, especially, progesterone receptors already appears an essential element for an optimal classification of the disease prior to treatment, a rational use of the measurement of these receptors and the development of more informative and sensitive assay techniques would in all likelihood make it possible to resolve a number of important problems concerning hormone-dependent tumors and thus improve our knowledge of therapeutic indications.

These are the channels of therapeutic research that attempt to specify the present article.

References

1. Anonymous (1982) Compilation of experimental cancer therapy protocol summaries, 6th ed. US Department of Health and Human Services, Washington, DC
2. Baulieu EE (1975) Some aspects of the mechanism of action of steroid hormone. Mol Cell Biochem 7: 157−175
3. Bonadonna G, Valagussa P, Rossi A et al. (1979) CMF adjuvant chemotherapy in operable breast cancer. In: Jones SE, Salmon S (eds) Adjuvant therapy of cancer II. Grune and Stratton, New York, pp 215−226
4. Buzdar A, Smith T, Blumenshein G, Hortobagyi G, Hersh E, Gehan E (1981) Adjuvant chemotherapy with fluorouracil, doxorubicin and cyclophosphamide (FAC) for stage II or III breast cancer: 5 year results. In: Salmon E, Jones SE (eds) Adjuvant therapy of cancer III. Grune and Stratton, New York, pp 419−426
5. Cooke T, George D, Shields R, Maynard P, Griffith K (1979) Estrogen receptor and prognosis in early breast cancer. Lancet 1: 1995−1997
6. Fisher B, Redmond C, participating NSABP investigators (1979) Breast cancer studies on the rational surgical adjuvant breast and colon project (NSABP). In: Jones SE, Salmon S (eds) Adjuvant therapy of cancer II. Grune and Stratton, New York, pp 215−226
7. Horwitz KB, McGuire WL (1978) Estrogen control of progesterone receptor in human breast cancer. J Biol Chem 253: 2223−2228
8. Jensen EV, Polluy TZ, Smith S, Block EG, Ferguson DJ, Desombre ER (1975) Prediction of hormone dependence in human breast cancer. In: McGuire WL (ed) Estrogen receptors in human breast cancer. Raven, New York, pp 37−56
9. Kiang DT, Frenning DH, Goldman AI, Ascensao VF, Kennedy BJ (1978) Estrogen receptors and response to chemotherapy and hormonal therapy in advanced breast cancer. N Engl J Med 299: 1330−1335
10. Legha SS, Buzdar AV, Smith TL, Swenerton KD, Hortobagyi GN, Blumenschein GR (1980) Response to hormonal therapy as a prognostic factor for metastatic breast cancer treated with combination chemotherapy. Cancer 46: 438−445
11. Lippman ME, Cassidy J, Wesley M, Young RC (1982) A randomized attempt to increase the efficacy of cytotoxic chemotherapy in metastatic breast cancer by hormonal synchronization. In: ASCO Conf, Abstract 79, C-305
12. Magdelénat H, Pouillart P, Jouve M et al. (1982) Progesterone receptor as a more reliable prognostic parameter than estrogen receptor in patients with advanced breast cancer. Breast Cancer Res Treat 2, 195−196
13. Magdelénat H, Toubeau M, Picco C, Bidron C (1980) Détermination des récepteurs d'oestrogènes et de progestérone sur foragebiopsies des tumeurs mammaires. In: Martin PM (ed) Récepteurs hormonaux et pathologie mammaire. MEDSI, Paris, pp 107−119
14. Magdelénat H (1979) Simultaneous determination of estrogen and progestin receptors on small amounts of breast tumor cytosols. Cancer Treat Rep 63: 1146
15. Martin PM, Rolland PH, Jacquemier J, Rolland AM, Toga M (1978) Tumeurs mammaires humaines: corrélation entre les récepteurs hormonaux stéroidiens et l'anatomie pathologie. Bull Cancer (Paris) 65: 383−388
16. Martin PM, Benyahia B, Magdelénat H (1982) A new approach for the visualization of estrogen receptors in target tissues: use of autofluorescent ligands and image intensifier. 6th International congress on hormonal steroids, Jerusalem

17. McGuire WL, Horwitz KB, Pearson OH, Segaloff A (1977) Current status of estrogen and progesterone receptors in breast cancer. Cancer 39: 2934–2947

18. McGuire WL, Horwitz KB (1978) Progesterone receptors in breast cancer. In: McGuire WL (ed) Hormones, receptors and breast cancer. Raven, New York, pp 31–42

19. Mauriac L, Wafflart J, Durand M et al. (1981) Apport de la drill-biopsie dans le bilan préthérapeutique des adénocarcinomes mammaires. Bull Cancer (Paris) 68: 417–421

20. Meyer JS, Rao BR, Stevens SC (1977) Low incidence of estrogen receptor in breast carcinomas with rapid rates of cellular replication. Cancer 40: 2290–2298

21. Namer M, Lalanne C, Baulieu EE (1980) Increase of progesterone receptor by tamoxifen as a hormonal challenge test in breast cancer. Cancer Res 40: 1750–1752

22. Pichon MF, Pallud C, Brunet M, Milgrom E (1980) Relationship of presence of progesterone receptors to prognosis in early breast cancer. Cancer Res 40: 3357–3360

23. Pouillart P, Palangie T, Jouve M, Garcia-Giralt E, Asselain B, Magdelénat H (1981) Metastatic breast cancer treated simultaneously by cytotoxic chemotherapy and hormonal therapy. Preliminary results of a randomized trial. Review on Endocrine-Related Cancers (Suppl) Oct: 439–453

24. Pouillart P, Palangie T, Jouve M et al. (1982) Hormonal therapy in advanced breast cancer. Sequential administration of tamoxifen and medroxyprogesterone acetate. Bull Cancer (Paris) 69: 176–177

25. Silfverswärd C, Humla S (1980) Estrogen receptor analysis on needle aspirates from human mammary carcinoma. Acta Cytol (Baltimore) 24: 54–57

26. Silfverswärd C, Skoog L, Humla S, Gustafsson SA, Nordenskjöld B (1980) Intratumoral variation of cytoplasmic and nuclear estrogen receptor concentrations in human mammary carcinoma. Eur J Cancer 16: 59–65

27. Rose C, Mouridsen MT, Palshoff T (1981) Combination of tamoxifen with cytosolic or endocrine therapy. Reviews on Endocrine-Related Cancers (Suppl) Oct: 455–471

28. Tormey DC, Holland JF, Weinberg V, Weiss R, Falkson G, Glidewell O, Leone L, Perloff M (1981) Five drug-vs-3-drug ± MER postoperative chemotherapy for mammary carcinoma. In: Salmon E, Jones SE (eds) Adjuvant therapy of cancer III. Grune and Stratton, New York, pp 377–384

Part V: A Critical Summary

E. Engelsman

Antoni van Leeuwenhoekhuis,
Het Nederlands Kankeninstituut Plesmanlaan 121, 1066 CX
Amsterdam, The Netherlands

Endocrine manipulation in breast cancer patients has been an important tool for palliative treatment since 1896, when Beatson demonstrated that a progressing tumor could be influenced favorably without touching the tumor itself. He also showed that this effect was temporary.

Over the years, more endocrine therapies − both ablative procedures and additive treatments − have been placed at our disposal. Clinical features made it possible to predict response to a moderate degree, and hormone receptors have further improved prediction, thus proving helpful in clinical decision making. Nevertheless, it is important to remember that, whether we can predict a response or not, and whether we use one hormone therapy or another, still only 30% of breast cancers will respond to hormone therapy.

For practical clinical use a cut-off value between receptor-positive and receptor-negative values can often be helpful in the choice between endocrine and cytostatic palliative treatment. The exact quantity of receptor is also important, not least to increase our insight into the mechanisms of action of endocrine treatment. Without interlaboratory quality control, comparison of data has only limited value.

Endocrine Surgery

Badelino and co-workers report on endocrine surgery. Much stress is laid upon the importance of adrenalectomy and hypophysectomy. Adrenalectomy has always been a major operation, with considerable morbidity and significant mortality. Although palliation was obtained for the responders, the nonresponders had a very short survival in those series where these data were provided: considering that patients selected for adrenalectomy had to be in a reasonably good condition, the survival of the nonresponders was probably shortened by the operation. Many centers have never adopted adrenalectomy as a routine procedure for endocrine treatment; instead they have tried to employ oophorectomy and additive therapies to the maximum. Hypophysectomy, especially when performed transsphenoidally, produces less morbidity and mortality than adrenalectomy, but it requires specialised surgeons, and special provisions if yttrium implantation is used. In comparison, oophorectomy is a simple procedure, available in every hospital and imposing a relatively low burden on the nonresponders.

Badelino's remark that adrenalectomy is more effective when it is the first treatment is not untrue, but too specific: all endocrine therapies are more effective when they are the first treatment! I am glad that reference is made to Dargent's ingenious technique of implanting part of an adrenal gland in the spleen, thus using the liver to inactivate the sex steroids and avoiding the need for corticosteroid substitution.

Tamoxifen

Rose and Mouridsen have made an excellent review of what is and what is not known about this widely used antiestrogen. An important and intriguing area seems to be the possible use of tamoxifen in premenopausal patients, and especially in an adjuvant setting. Tamoxifen is supposed to block estrogen receptors, with the possible consequence of elevated estrogen blood levels when the ovaries are still present.
How long should tamoxifen be given, and what are the long-term effects of such treatment? I can imagine premenopausal patients on adjuvant tamoxifen treatment (some of them cured) posing pertinent questions as to the late effects of such treatment.

Medroxyprogesterone Acetate (MPA)

De Lena and co-workers have studied different dose levels of MPA and found equal response rates. Recent publications have stressed high dose levels, without really explaining why the doses should be so high. More studies comparing different dose levels of MPA are underway, but this report gives the first indication that low doses can be as effective as high doses.
Unless MPA is proven to have particular features requiring very high blood levels, one might regard MPA as another mode of changing the endocrine milieu in the patient in such a way that the hormone-sensitive tumor cannot grow in it for a certain period. Although the responses to MPA in this study were all in ER+ tumors, the response rate in such tumors was modest: 33% in patients more than 5 years' postmenopause. So the correlation with ER positivity was present, but "poor". All these patients, however, had been treated already with chemotherapy combinations, and their receptor data were, as a rule, from the primary tumors.

Megestrol Acetate (MA)

Alexieva and co-workers have found MA an effective agent for hormone therapy, responses occurring in 33% of patients. But, just like De Lena for MPA, they did not find the "usual" correlation between ER and response. In fact, they found no correlation between response and estrogen, progesterone and glucocorticoid receptors. Only the duration of response was significantly longer for ER+ tumors.
High levels of androgen receptor were correlated with response; all tumors with high androgen receptor levels were ER+.
Since both MPA and MA are competitors for steroids binding to androgen, progesterone and glucocorticoid receptors, and do not compete with estradiol for ER, it should not be surprising that the correlation between ER and response seems poor.
The clinical concept of hormone sensitivity seems to be developing into a complicated interplay of factors, with increasing nuance. Nevertheless, correlation with estrogen receptors or not, the response rate to progestagens is in the same range as that to other hormone therapies (30%). The question arises whether the 30% of tumors responding to

progestagens are the same 30% which respond to treatments like oophorectomy or antiestrogens.

Aminoglutethimide

Paridaens and co-workers confirm that aminoglutethimide (plus cortisone supplement) is an effective endocrine treatment. They stress again the importance of reaching the dose of 1 g daily gradually, in order to avoid toxicity. They present data on 16 patients for whom the ER content of the tumor was known.

The seven responses in this group were all with tumors containing more than 90 fmol/mg tissue protein (t.p.). Although higher ER values do predict a higher probability of remission, these data might suggest that for breast cancer to respond to medical adrenalectomy, a minimum ER level of 90 fmol/mg t.p. would be required. On the other hand, these 16 patients possibly represent a selected group, because 14 of them (87.5%) had ER levels higher than 10 fmol/mg t.p. Among these 14 patients (usually ER+), the response rate was 50% (the seven responders mentioned above). Thus there is a suggestion that when aminoglutethimide is used, a cut-off level for ER positivity of 10 fmol/mg t.p. is without predictive value. The cut-off level should in this situation be increased to about 100 fmol/mg t.p. If this finding were to be confirmed, the concepts of hormone sensitivity and hormone receptors would need further differentiation.

Palliative Treatment

Adrenalectomy and hypophysectomy are doomed, I am afraid, to become obsolete for palliative endocrine treatment of breast cancer. The range of medical endocrine therapies has been enlarged with antiestrogens, progestagens, and aminoglutethimide. The future of oophorectomy seems questionable. Antiestrogens may become first choice in the treatment of premenopausal patients, possibly with secondary oophorectomy for responders after relapse.

There is also a promise of "medical oophorectomy" by suppression of pituitary gonadotrophins.

Conclusion

Tamoxifen has become an important palliative agent. Questions remain concerning the long-term effects, especially in an adjuvant situation where a proportion of the patients will have normal life expectancy. *MPA* has been shown to be equally effective in low and high doses; the correlation between response and ER seems poor. *Megestrol acetate* responses did not correlate with ER, but with androgen receptor levels. There is no doubt that progestagens can be effective as an endocrine therapy; it seems quite possible that their mechanism of action is different from that of other hormone therapies. Possibly hormone sensitivity is not just equal to estrogen sensitivity. "Medical adrenalectomy" by *aminoglutethimide* is by now an accepted endocrine therapy; there is a suggestion that high ER levels are required to obtain a response.

Summarizing, new medical endocrine therapies will push ablative surgical procedures into the background; our understanding of hormone sensitivity is increasing; and the correlation between ER and response needs reconsideration.

Part VI. Prospects for Future Tests of Hormone Dependence

Peroxidase Activity as a Marker for Estrogen Action in Rat Uteri and Human Mammary Carcinomas*

M. J. Duffy, M. O'Connell, and L. McDonnell

Departments of Nuclear Medicine and Pathology, St. Vincent's Hospital, Dublin 4, Ireland

Introduction

A major effect of estrogen action is regulation of protein synthesis. This is thought to be accomplished by the following sequence of events: binding of estradiol to a cytoplasmic protein termed the cytoplasmic estradiol receptor (CER), translocation of the CER complex into the nucleus, binding of the complex to an acceptor site within the nucleus, increased RNA synthesis including mRNA for specific proteins, and, finally, increased or de novo protein synthesis. For estradiol action it is necessary that this sequence of events be intact. The most widely studied reaction in the above pathway is the binding of estradiol to its cytoplasmic receptor. One of the reasons for the detailed investigation of this step is that the CER level in breast carcinomas and possibly other tumors is of great clinical significance. Its significance relates to the now well-established finding that $50\%-60\%$ of breast cancers containing this protein respond to some form of hormone manipulative therapy while less than 10% respond if tumors are receptor negative. Why the remaining $40\%-50\%$ of CER-positive tumors fail to respond is unknown. However, one hypothesis amenable to biochemical investigation is that although CER is present, it is not biologically active, i.e., does not migrate into the nucleus, bind there, or induce protein synthesis. Receptor defects of these types have previously been reported in mutants of mouse lymphoma cell lines which failed to respond to the killing action of glucocorticoids [19]. On the other hand, the wild type cells possessing the intact glucocorticoid receptor system were killed by the steroid. Also in mice mammary tumors, Shyamala [20] has reported that failure of CER-positive tumors to respond to oophorectomy was due to a defect in translocation of cytoplasmic receptor to the nucleus. Indirect evidence for similar defects in human breast tumors was the finding of CER-positive carcinomas lacking either nuclear ER (NER) [5] or the estrogen inducible protein, progesterone receptor (PgR) [4]. Moreover, tumors with CER and either NER [9] or PgR [4] had an approximately threefold greater chance of responding to hormonal therapy than CER-containing tumors without either of these receptors. Therefore, ideally what should be measured to assess hormone responsiveness is not the first step in estrogen action, but some of the end products of the steroid's action such as inducible proteins. NER and PgR can be regarded

* This work was supported by the Medical Research Council of Ireland and the Irish Cancer Society. We also thank The Endocrinology Department, St. Vincent's Hospital, Dublin for performing the estrogen and progesterone assays and Imelda Duffy for typing this manuscript

as markers for a partially intact or completely intact ER system. However, assay of these receptors is rather difficult, especially for routine hospital laboratories. The enzyme peroxidase is an example of another protein induced by estradiol at least in the immature rat uterus, and in this tissue peroxidase is an excellent marker for estrogen action (for a review see reference [7]). In contrast to either NER or PgR, peroxidase activity is relatively stable and both easy and cheap to assay. In this study we therefore investigated the possibility of using peroxidase as a marker for estrogen action in normal rat tissues and human breast carcinomas.

Materials and Methods

Tumors were stored, homogenized, and assayed for CER, NER, cytosol estrogens, and progesterone as previously described [3]. The cut-off points for CER and NER were 50 and 25 fmol/g wet weight respectively. Peroxidase-positive tumors were defined as those possessing greater than 0.1 U/g wet weight. PgR, androgen receptors (AR), and glucocorticoid receptors (GR) were assayed using single saturating concentrations of 5 nM [^{3}H]ORG-2058, [^{3}H]R-1551 and [^{3}H]-dexamethasone respectively in the presence and absence of 100-fold excess appropriate unlabeled steroid. Binding of R-1551 to PgR was prevented by the addition of a 100-fold excess of unlabeled R-5020. Lymphocyte infiltration was estimated semiquantitatively on a scale of 1 (few or no lymphocytes) to 4 (very dense infiltrate).

Results

Induction of Peroxidase Activity in Rat Tissues

Table 1 shows that administration of 10 µg estradiol to immature rats resulted in greater than 50-fold induction of peroxidase activity in the uterus. In contrast, the steroid had little or no detectable effect on ovarian, pancreatic, or thyroid peroxidase activity. The estradiol stimulation of uterine peroxidase was specific, as testosterone, progesterone, and cortisol (at similar molar concentrations) and prolactin (20 IU/kg body wt.) had no effect on activity.

Table 1. Alteration in peroxidase activity in different tissues of immature female rats 20 h after the administration of 10 µg estradiol subcutaneously. Numbers of animals used shown in parentheses

Tissue	Peroxidase activity (U/tissue)	
	Control	With estradiol
Uterus	< 0.002 (3)	0.1 (3)
Thyroid	< 0.002 (3)	< 0.002 (3)
Pancreas	0.63 (9)	0.52 (9)
Ovary	< 0.002 (3)	< 0.002 (3)

Table 2. Extent of induction of various protein and enzyme activities in uteri from either immature or oophorectomized rats

Protein	Induction (fold)	Authors
Induced protein (IP)	1.83	Iacobelli et al. 1977 [6]
Progesterone receptor	2.5–4	Walters and Clark 1977 [21]
Hexokinase (cytosol)	2.3	Baquer and McLean 1972 [1]
Hexokinase (particulate)	6.1	Baquer and McLean 1972 [1]
Lactate dehydrogenase	2.2	Baquer and McLean 1972 [1]
Prolyl hydroxylase	5.0–25.0	Salvador et al. 1976 [17]
Gluthathione peroxidase	1.75	Soujanen et al. 1980 [18]
γ-Glutamyl transpeptidase	1.82	Soujanen et al. 1980 [18]
Glucose-6-phosphate dehydrogenase	15	Ringler and Hilf 1975 [15]
Alkaline phosphatase	4.52	O'Connell and Duffy (unpubl.)
Plasminogen activator	46	Katz et al. 1976 [8]
Peroxidase	202	Lyttle and DeSombre 1977 [11]
Peroxidase	~ 200	Lucas et al. 1955 [10]

Table 2 compares the magnitude of peroxidase induction with that of other estrogen-inducible proteins in either immature or oophorectomized rats. Whereas the induction of most proteins or enzyme activities is less than 20-fold, the induction of peroxidase can be greater than 200-fold. The conclusion from these data is that peroxidase activity should be one of the best markers for estrogen action in the immature or oophorectomized rat. The term 'induction' used here should be interpreted with caution, as in no case has increased specific mRNA been demonstrated for these uterine proteins. The increased activity of some of the enzymes following estradiol administration could thus be due to direct enzyme activation, removal of an inhibitor, or increased influx of blood cells containing the specific enzyme into the uterus. However, the increase in uterine peroxidase activity following estradiol administration is inhibited by the antiestrogen CI-628 and by actinomycin D and cycloheximide [12]. These findings suggest that estrogen action, at least on peroxidase activity, is receptor mediated and requires DNA and RNA synthesis.

Correlation Between Peroxidase Activity and CER in Human Breast Carcinomas

If peroxidase activity is a specific marker for a functional CER in human breast carcinomas, activity should mostly be confined to receptor-positive tumors with little or no activity in receptor-negative carcinomas. However, as shown in Fig. 1, the median peroxidase activity was similar in tumors with or without CER.

Attempts to Explain Lack of Correlation Between CER and Peroxidase Activity in Breast Carcinomas

1. *False CER-negative tumors due to high concentrations of endogenous estrogens occupying the receptor:* Since the CER assay carried out at 4° C measures mostly free or unoccupied receptor, endogenous estrogens saturating the receptor might cause at least

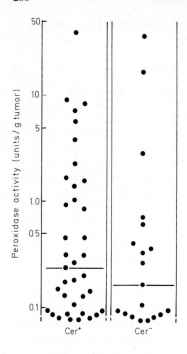

Fig. 1. Distribution of peroxidase activity in CER-positive and CER-negative breast carcinomas. *Bar* represents median activity in each group

some false-negative receptor results. Thus in some tumors without measurable CER but possessing peroxidase activity, receptor negativity could have been due to endogenous estrogens occupying the receptor. If this hypothesis is correct, levels of cytoplasmic estrogens should be higher in the CER negative-peroxidase positive group than in the CER negative-peroxidase negative group. Measurement of endogenous estrogens showed that the former group had a significantly higher median concentration than the latter (1.69 vs 0.75 pmol/g tumor, $P = 0.039$ using a Mann-Whitney U test). However, the median NER concentration was not significantly different in these two groups, suggesting that the peroxidase activity was not induced through the ER mechanism.

2. *Possible antiestrogenic effects of endogenous progesterone:* Progesterone is an estrogen antagonist and high levels of endogenous progesterone might thus inhibit estrogen-inducible peroxidase activity in some tumors. Endogenous progesterone was therefore measured in CER-positive carcinomas with and without peroxidase activity. No significant difference in mean levels of progesterone was found between the two groups, suggesting that endogenous progesterone was unlikely to be inhibiting estrogen-inducible peroxidase activity.

3. *NER in the absence of CER:* Another possible explanation for the lack of correlation between CER and peroxidase could be the presence of NER in the absence of CER. However, NER was found in only six of 17 tumors without CER, and the median peroxidase activity in this group was not significantly different from the tumors without both CER and NER.

4. *Induction of peroxidase by other steroid hormones:* As described above, neither testosterone nor progesterone nor cortisol induced peroxidase activity in the immature rat uterus. However, receptors for all of these steroids have been found in human mammary carcinomas and thus might be involved in peroxidase induction. However, in

the present investigation no correlation was found between peroxidase activity and PgR, AR, or GR in the human tumors. Furthermore, peroxidase did not correlate with cytosol progesterone levels.

5. *Infiltration of lymphocytes:* White blood cells contain high levels of peroxidase activity and infiltrate breast carcinomas to varying extents. Peroxidase activity was therefore correlated against levels of lymphocyte infiltration. A moderate but statistically significant correlation was found between the two parameters ($r = 0.37$, $P = 0.001$, $n = 44$), suggesting that some of the peroxidase measured in breast tumor extracts may be derived from lymphocytes. The varying levels of lymphocyte may explain in part the lack of correlation between ER concentrations and peroxidase activity. Using data from all the tumors, there was a random relationship between NER levels and peroxidase activity ($r = 0.013$, $P = 0.44$, $n = 56$); however, the correlation approached statistical significance when tumors with only level 1 lymphocyte infiltration were compared ($r = 0.19$, $P = 0.065$, $n = 31$).

Discussion

Our results confirm that peroxidase activity is one of the best available markers for estrogen action in the immature rat uterus. Recently also, a fivefold increase in peroxidase activity has been found in R3230AC rat mammary tumors following the administration of estradiol [16], and in dimethylbenz(a)anthracene-induced rat mammary tumors Jellinck et al. [7] found a moderate ($r = 0.45$) correlation between NER and peroxidase activity. In both mice [13] and rat [14] mammary tumors, peroxidase activity was higher in the hormone-dependent group than in the hormone-independent group. However, in this study and in that of Collings and Savage [2] no correlation was found between CER and basal levels of peroxidase activity in human mammary carcinomas, suggesting that the latter is unlikely to be an adjunct to the ER in predicting endocrine-sensitive tumors. One reason for this lack of correlation appears to be the varying levels of lymphocyte infiltration in the human tumors. Infiltration of other types of white cells are also likely to contribute to the measured peroxidase activity.

However, an alternative explanation for the correlation between lymphocyte infiltration and peroxidase activity could be that the former was a host response to peroxidase-rich tumors. Further investigation is necessary to clarify the relationship between these two parameters in breast cancers.

In conclusion, if peroxidase is to be used as a marker for a functional ER in human breast carcinomas, a specific tumor peroxidase must first be shown to be present and then either separated from the white cell peroxidase or assayed by a specific method such as that of radioimmunoassay.

References

1. Baquer NZ, McLean P (1972) The effect of oestradiol on the profile of constant and specific proportion groups of enzymes in rat uterus. Biochem Biophys Res Commun 48: 729−734
2. Collings JR, Savage N (1979) Peroxidase as a marker for oestrogen dependence in human breast cancer. Br J Cancer 40: 500−503
3. Duffy MJ, O'Connell M (1981) Estrogens, estradiol receptors and peroxidase activity in human breast carcinomas. Eur J Cancer 17: 711−714

4. Edwards DP, Chamness GC, McGuire WL (1979) Estrogen and progesterone receptor proteins in breast cancer. Biochim Biophys Acta 560: 457–486

5. Fazekas AG, MacFarlane JK (1980) Studies on cytosol and nuclear binding of estradiol in human breast cancer. J Steroid Biochem 13: 613–622

6. Iacobelli S, King RJB, Vokaer A (1977) Antibody to estrogen induced protein (IP) and quantification of the protein in rat uterus by a radioimmunoassay. Biochem Biophys Res Commun 76: 1230–1237

7. Jellinck PH, Newcombe A, Keeping HS (1979) Peroxidase as a marker enzyme in estrogen-responsive tissues. Adv Enzyme Regul 17: 325–342

8. Katz J, Levitz M (1976) Estrogen-dependent trypsin-like activity in the rat uterus, localization of activity in the 12,000 g pellet and nucleus. Arch Biochem Biophys 173: 347–354

9. Leake RE, Laing L, Calman KC, Macbeth FR, Crawford D, Smith DC (1976) Oestrogen-receptor status and endocrine therapy of breast cancer: response rates and status of stability. Br J Cancer 43: 59–65

10. Lucas FV, Neufeld HA, Utterback JG, Martin AP, Stotz E (1955) The effect of estrogen on the production of a peroxidase in the rat uterus. J Biol Chem 214: 775–780

11. Lyttle CR, DeSombre ER (1977) Generality of oestrogen stimulation of peroxidase activity in growth responsive tissues. Nature 268: 337–339

12. Lyttle CR, DeSombre ER (1977) Uterine peroxidase as a marker for estrogen action. Proc Natl Acad Sci USA 74: 3162–3166

13. Lyttle CR, Thorpe SM, DeSombre ER, Daehnfeldt JL (1979) Peroxidase activity and iodide uptake in hormone-responsive and hormone-independent GR mouse mammary tumors. J Natl Cancer Inst 62: 1031–1034

14. Penney GC, Scott KM, Hawkins RA (1980) Endogenous peroxidase: an alternative to oestrogen receptor in the management of breast cancer. Br J Cancer 41: 648–651

15. Ringler MB, Hilf R (1975) Effect of estrogen on synthesis of glucose-6-phosphate dehydrogenase in R3230AC mammary tumors and uteri. Biochim Biophys Acta 411: 50–62

16. Rorke EA, Katzenellenbogen BS (1980) Comparative effects of estrogen and antiestrogens on enzyme activities in R3230AC rat mammary tumors and uteri of tumor-bearing animals. Cancer Res 40: 3158–3162

17. Salvador RA, Tsai I, Stassen FLH (1976) On the mechanism of the increase in prolyl hydroxylase activity in the uterus of the rat given estradiol-β 17. Biochem Pharmacol 25: 907–912

18. Soujanen JN, Gay RJ, Hilf R (1980) Influence of estrogens on glutathione levels and glutathione-metabolizing enzymes in uteri and R3230AC mammary tumors of rats. Biochim Biophys Acta 630: 485–496

19. Sibley CH, Tomkins GM (1974) Mechanisms of steroid resistance. Cell 2: 221–222

20. Shyamala G (1972) Estradiol receptors in mouse mammary tumors; absence of the transfer of bound estradiol from the cytoplasm to the nucleus. Biochem Biophys Res Commun 46: 1623–1629

21. Walters MR, Clark JH (1977) Cytosol progesterone receptors of the rat uterus: assay of receptor characteristics. J Steroid Biochem 8: 1137–1144

Estrogen-Induced Proteins in Human Breast Cancer Cells*

H. Rochefort, F. Capony, M. Garcia, F. Veith, F. Vignon, and B. Westley

Institut National de la Saute et de la Recherche Medicale,
Unité d'Endocrinologie Cellulaire et Moléculaire, INSERM (U 148),
60 Rue de Navacelles, 34100 Montpellier, France

Introduction

Estrogens regulate both gene expression and cell proliferation in breast cancer. Specific intracellular estrogen receptors (ER) are required to mediate these effects. However, they are not in themselves sufficient since 50% of human breast cancers containing estrogen receptors do not respond to endocrine therapy [1]. In order to evaluate estrogen responsiveness, McGuire et al. [2, 3] have successfully proposed that the progesterone receptor (PgR), which is known to be stimulated by estrogen in the uterus [4], should also be assayed. However, there are many examples of discrepancy between the effect of estrogens on PgR induction and the stimulation of breast cancer growth both in animals [5−8] and in humans. Thus the antiestrogens prevent cell growth while they induce the PgR, as shown in MCF$_7$ cells [3]. Moreover, there are still 20% of PgR− patients who respond to endocrine therapy and 20% of PgR+ patients who do not respond [2]. In an attempt to find a better marker for estrogen-responsive cell growth and proliferation than PgR, we and others have looked to other estrogen-induced proteins in human breast cancer cell lines.

In the present paper we will not discuss further PgR, which is currently assayed in human breast cancer monitoring; rather we will focus on these other estrogen-induced proteins which might improve the reliability of predictive tests of hormone dependency.

Intracellular Proteins

A double-labeling technique with ^{3}H- and ^{14}C-leucine has been successfully used to demonstrate an estrogen-induced protein (ip) in the rat uterus [9]. Using this technique, McGuire et al. [10] found in MCF$_7$ cells previously inhibited by antiestrogens, two estrogen-stimulated proteins of molecular weights 24 and 36 K as well as an increase of

* This study was supported by INSERM, the NCI-INSERM cooperative group on "Hormones and Cancer", the Fondation pour la Recherche Médicale Française, and an INSERM grant (No. 49.77.81). We thank Mrs. D. Derocq, Mrs. S. Ladrech, and Mrs. J. Vanbiervliet for their excellent technical assistance and Miss E. Barrié for the preparation of the manuscript. We are grateful to Drs. M. Lippman, M. Rich, and I. Keydar, and the Mason Research Institute, for their gifts of mammary cell lines

Table 1. Enzymatic activities stimulated by estrogens in MCF$_7$ cells

Enzymes	Cell fraction	Increase	Optimal time of induction
Lactico-dehydrogenase [15]	Cytosol	× 2	10 days
Plasminogen activator [16]	Total cell extract	× 1.9	2 days
DNA polymerase [17]	Cytosol	× 1.5	3 days
Thymidine kinase [18]	Cytosol	× 2	1 day
Ornithine decarboxylase [19]	Total cell extract	× 1.5−3.5	12 h

poly A$^+$ RNA coding for the 24 K and for a 54 K protein [11]. By labeling the proteins of MCF$_7$ cells with ^{35}S-methionine and analyzing them by the two-dimensional gel analysis of O'Farrell, we have demonstrated three cellular proteins, C_1, C_2, and C_3, with molecular weights between 50 and 160 K [12, 13]. Mairesse et al. [14] have also suggested early induction of a 46 K protein in the cytosol of ER+ cell line. Other authors have reported the stimulation of various enzyme activities (Table 1) in MCF$_7$ cells, even though the hormonal specificity of the induction was not always stated.

Other estrogen-induced proteins have been proposed as markers for hormone responsiveness, e.g., the peroxidase which is being studied extensively by De Sombre's group [20] in the uterus. However, this enzyme does not seem to be of any use in human breast cancer and was absent from MCF$_7$ cells (De Sombre, personal communication). Some of these cellular proteins are of potential interest but can only be assayed in tumor collected during surgery. We have therefore tried to find estrogen-induced proteins secreted by cells, which might be liberated in the plasma and which could therefore be used as circulating markers of hormone dependency in breast cancer [21].

"Secretory" Proteins

In MCF$_7$ cells, using the same labeling by ^{35}S-methionine followed by SDS polyacrylamide gel electrophoresis and fluorography, we found that estrogens stimulated two- to threefold the synthesis of proteins which were released into the medium [22]. Some of them were more particularly induced, i.e., a 160 K protein and a major one, representing 20%−40% of the total amount of secretory proteins, with a molecular weight of 52,000 in denaturing conditions[1] [13]. The induction of this protein was specific for physiological concentrations of estrogens. Progesterone and dexamethasone were inactive.

The effects of nonsteroidal antiestrogens on these secreted proteins are particularly interesting since they appear to be closely related to effects of antiestrogens on MCF$_7$ cell growth. Tamoxifen was totally inactive in inducing the 52 K protein but prevented E$_2$ action in a molar ratio of 10^4. The metabolite monohydroxy-tamoxifen was 200-fold more potent than tamoxifen in blocking the cell growth [23] and the estrogen-induced secretion of the 52 K protein [12]. It is worthy of note that monohydroxy-tamoxifen binds to ER with very high affinity and is accumulated in vivo in the nuclei of estrogen target tissues such as rat uterus and chick liver [24].

---

1 The molecular weight was first found to be 46,000 using 15% polyacrylamide gel. It seems to be closer to 52,000 in 10% polyacrylamide gel and by taking the NEN proteins as markers

The 52 K protein was also induced by the estrogen 3 sulfate but not the 17 sulfate cells. This finding was surprising since estrogen sulfates have either no or only a low affinity for ER. However, we found that MCF_7 cells are able to hydrolyze the sulfate ester bond of ^3H-estrone 3 sulfate, thus liberating ^3H-estrone which was recovered, bound to the nuclear ER [25]. Previous results from our laboratory showed that estrogen sulfates in serum are not completely removed by charcoal treatment. Serum treated by charcoal in order to deplete steroids for cell culture experiments in fact contained up to 30 nM estrogen sulfate [25]. These results led us to propose that the culture medium containing charcoal-treated serum contains estrogen sulfate which can be used as biologically active estrogens by the cells. The presence of estrogen sulfate can explain the difficulty in obtaining an effect of estrogen on the growth of MCF_7 cells.

For pharmacological concentrations of DHT ($\simeq 0.5 \mu M$) [21] and physiological concentrations of 5-androstenediol (10 nM) [26], we were also able to show that androgens behave as estrogen agonists as far as their affinity for ER was sufficient to bind to and activate the receptor. This effect of androgens on the induction of the 52 K protein was inhibited by antiestrogen [21]. These observations led to the conclusion that the specificity of induction of this protein was due to the nature of the receptor protein which was activated, rather than to the structure of the steroid which was administered and was present in the nucleus [21].

The 52 K protein is most likely a glycoprotein, as shown by its micro-heterogeneity in two-dimensional gel electrophoresis, its sensibility to neuraminidase and tunicamycin, its labeling by ^3H-fucose, and its selective retention on Con A Sepharose. Its induction is likely at the transcriptional level, as suggested by the effect of actinomycin D and α-amanitin (M. Garcia, unpublished data). The identity and function of this 52 K protein is presently unknown. We can, however, exclude the major milk proteins such as the human casein and α-lactalbumin, which have different molecular weights and do not seem to be present or induced in MCF_7 cells. Its relationship with the MMTV gp52 [27] is under study. An enzymatic activity such as a protease activity is not excluded, since estrogen also stimulates in MCF_7 cells the plasminogen activator [16] and a collagenase [28]. It is tempting to speculate that this protein has an important function in mediating some effect of estrogens on breast cancer, since its regulation has been shown in all ER+ cell lines which have been looked at (MCF_7, ZR_{75-1}, $T_{47}D$) but was not found in two ER− lines (HBL 100 and BT 20) [12]. Whether this protein is acting directly on cancer cells by stimulating cell attachment or cell proliferation or whether it is acting on other cells is unknown but can be experimentally tested. In any case, this protein appears to be an excellent probe for studying the mechanism of action of estrogen and antiestrogen in breast cancer.

Possible Clinical Applications

In addition to their basic interest for understanding the mechanism of hormonal modulation of breast cancer, the induced proteins might also have clinical applications. The evidence that the 52 K protein might be a better marker of estrogen responsiveness than PgR is presently circumstantial:

1. It is present in cells which contain ER and whose growth is stimulated by estrogens.
2. It is not induced in ER− cells but might be present in ER− cells and/or induced in cells resistant to estrogens for growth.

Table 2. Comparison between two markers of estrogen responsiveness in human breast cancer cells

	PgR	52K
Without estrogen	Present	Absent?
With tamoxifen	Induced	Not induced
Hormone-independent tumors	Induced in MTW$_9$, DMBA	Absent in two $R_E < 0$ cell lines
Localisation	Cellular	Secreted
Time lag before induction	3 days	12 h
Assay sensitivity	5×10^7 cells	5×10^4 cells
Relation with cell proliferation	Not always	Yes?
Present in the tumor	Yes	To be confirmed

3. The antiestrogen which prevented cell growth totally inhibited the synthesis of this protein, but not that of the PgR.
4. The 52 K protein being released into the medium could be secreted into the blood and serve as a useful circulating marker of hormone dependency in human breast cancer.

Compared with PgR, the 52 K protein therefore appears to be a potentially interesting marker for estrogen responsiveness of breast cancers (Table 2). To establish this definitely, we would have first to demonstrate clearly its induction in cancer patient and second to develop a radioimmunoassay.

Preliminary evidence indicates that the 52 K protein is indeed induced in breast cancer patients. A radioimmunoassay for this protein not yet being available, we have looked to the effect of antiestrogens (in vivo) and estradiol (in vitro) on the labeling of secretory proteins by ^{35}S-methionine. In patients with cutaneous metastases, biopsies were taken before and after tamoxifen treatment. This work, performed in collaboration with the Centre Paul Lamarque of Montpellier (Profs. Pujol and Pourquier), allowed us to show that in some patients the pattern of secretory proteins was different before and after tamoxifen treatment [29]. In most cases, a major protein located in the 40−60 K region was markedly decreased after antiestrogen. In another series of experiments, we have shown in primary culture of several human metastatic breast cancer a 52 K protein which was similar to that of MCF$_7$ cells and was specifically induced in vitro by estrogens [30]. These results indicate that this protein is not restricted to continuous cell lines but is also present in clinical breast cancer. The next step will be to develop a radioimmunoassay for this protein in order to evaluate its concentration in the tissue and the plasma of several patients and to correlate it with the ER and PgR content and with the clinical evolution of breast cancer. The use of antibodis to the 52 K protein for breast cancer monitoring can also be considered if it happens that this protein is restricted to transformed cells or to metastasing breast cancers [31].

References

1. McGuire WL, Carbone PP, Vollmer EP (1975) Estrogen receptors in human breast cancer. Raven, New York

2. Osborne CK, McGuire WL (1979) The use of steroid hormone receptors in the treatment of human breast cancer: a review. Bull Cancer (Paris) 66: 203–210
3. Horwitz KB, Kosedi Y, McGuire WL (1978) Estrogen control of progesterone receptor in human breast cancer: role of estradiol and antiestrogen. Endocrinology 103: 1742–1751
4. Milgrom E, Atger M, Perrot M, Baulieu EE (1972) Endocrinology 90: 1071–1078
5. Koenders AJM, Geurts-Moespot A, Zolinger SJ, Benraad TJ (1977) Progesterone receptors in normal and neoplastic tissues. Raven, New York, p 71
6. Ip M, Milholland RJ, Rosen F, Kim U (1979) Mammary cancer: selective action of the estrogen receptor complex. Science 203: 361–363
7. Rochefort H, Coezy E, Joly E, Westley B, Vignon F (1981) Hormonal control of breast cancer in cell culture. In: Iacobelli S, King RJ, Lindner HR, Lippman ME (eds) Hormones and cancer. Raven, New York, p 21
8. Vignon F (1979) Etapes initiales du mécanisme d'action des oestrogènes dans les tumeurs mammaires. PhD Thesis, University of Montpellier I
9. Notides A, Gorski J (1966) Estrogen-induced synthesis of a specific uterine protein. Proc Natl Acad Sci 56: 230–235
10. Edwards DP, Adams DJ, Savage N, McGuire WL (1980) Estrogen-induced synthesis of specific proteins in human breast cancer cells. Biochem Biophys Res Commun 93: 804–812
11. Adams DJ, Edwards DP, McGuire WL (1980) Estrogen regulation of specific messenger RNA's in human breast cancer cells. Biochem Biophys Res Commun 97: 1354–1361
12. Westley B, Rochefort H (1980) A secreted glycoprotein induced by estrogen in human breast cancer cell lines. Cell 20: 353–362
13. Westley B, Rochefort H (1979) Estradiol induced proteins in the MCF_7 human breast cancer cell line. Biochem Biophys Res Commun 90: 410–416
14. Mairesse N, Deuleeschonuer N, Leclercq G, Galand P (1980) Estrogen-induced protein in the human breast cancer cell line MCF_7. Biochem Biophys Res Commun 97: 1251–1257
15. Burke RE, Harris SC, McGuire WL (1978) Lactate dehydrogenase in estrogen-responsive human breast cancer cells. Cancer Res 38: 2773–2776
16. Butler WB, Kirkland WL, Jorgensen TL (1979) Induction of plasminogen activator by estrogen in a human breast cancer cell line (MCF_7). Biochem Biophys Res Commun 90: 1328–1334
17. Edwards DP, Murthy SV, McGuire WL (1980) Effects of estrogen and antiestrogen on DNA polymerase in human breast cancer. Cancer Res 40: 1722–1726
18. Dronzert DA, Monaco ME, Pinkus L, Aitken S, Lippman ME (1981) Purification and properties of estrogen-responsive cytoplasmic thymidine kinase from human breast cancer. Cancer Res 41: 604–610
19. Mercier-Bodard C, Baulieu EE (to be published) Innsbruck Conferences, 1981
20. Anderson WA, Kang YH, De Sombre FR (1975) Endogenous peroxidase: specific marker enzyme for tissues displaying growth-dependency on estrogen. J Cell Biol 64: 668
21. Rochefort H, Garcia M, Vignon F, Westley B (1980) Steroid induced uterine proteins. In: Beato M (ed). Elsevier/North-Holland Biomedical, Amsterdam, p 171
22. Garcia M, Westley B, Rochefort H (1981) 5-bromodeoxyuridine specifically inhibits the synthesis of estrogen induced proteins in MCF_7 cells. Eur J Biochem 116: 297–301
23. Coezy E, Borgna JL, Rochefort H (1982) Tamoxifen and metabolites in MCF_7 cells: correlation between binding to estrogen receptor and cell growth inhibition. Cancer Res 42: 317–323
24. Borgna JL, Rochefort H (1981) Hydroxylated metabolites of tamoxifen are formed in vivo and bound to estrogen receptor in target tissues. J Biol Chem 256: 859–868
25. Vignon F, Terqui M, Westley B, Derocq D, Rochefort H (1980) Effects of plasma estrogen sulfates in mammary cancer cells. Endocrinology 106: 1079–1086
26. Adams J, Garcia M, Rochefort H (1981) Estrogenic effects of physiological concentrations of 5-androstene-$3\beta,17\beta$-diol and its metabolism in MCF_7 human breast cancer cells. Cancer Res 41: 4720–4726.
27. Mesa-Tejeda R, Keydar I, Ramanarayanan M, Ohno T, Penoglio C, Spiegelman S (1978) Detection in human breast carcinomas of an antigen immunologically related to a group-specific antigen of mouse mammary tumor virus. Proc Natl Acad Sci USA 75: 1529–1533

28. Paranjpe M, Engel L, Young N, Liotta LA (1980) Activation of human breast carcinoma collagenase through plasminogen activator. Life Sci 26: 1223–1231
29. Veith F, Rochefort H, Saussol J, Bressot N, Pourquier H, Pujol H (1981) Proteins secreted by human breast cancer: effect of tamoxifen. In: Anti-hormones and breast cancer. Reviews on Endocrine-Related Cancer [Suppl] 9: 229–231
30. Veith F, Capony F, Garcia M, Chantelard I, Pujol H, Veith F, Zajdela A, Rochefort H (1983) Release of estrogen-induced glycoprotein with a molecular weight of 52,000 by breast cancer cells in primary culture. Cancer Res 43: 1861–1868
31. Blythman HE, Casellas P, Gros O, Gros P, Jansen FK, Paolucci F, Pau B, Vidal H (1981) Immunotoxins: hybrid molecules of monoclonal antibodies and a toxin subunit specifically kill tumour cells. Nature 290: 145–146

Stimulation by 17β-Estradiol of a Secreted Glycoprotein in MCF-7 Cells and Human Breast Cancer

S. Iacobelli, V. Natoli, and P. Marchetti

Laboratorio di Endocrinologia Molecolare, Università Cattolica del Sacro Cuore, Largo Gemelli 8, 00168 Rome, Italy

Introduction

At present there is no single test which can accurately predict the effectiveness of hormonal therapy in patients with breast cancer. Even patients whose tumors contain both estrogen and progesterone receptors show variations in sensitivity to therapy [5]. Therefore other indicators of hormone action are needed to further rationalize treatment. Westley and Rochefort [7, 8] have recently reported that estrogens induce the synthesis of a 46,000 daltons secreted protein (46 K) in three estrogen receptor-positive human breast cancer cell lines. In this paper we present evidence that a protein similar to the 46 K is present in freshly obtained human breast cancer tissue. This finding may prove to be extremely useful for both diagnostic and therapeutic purposes.

Experimental Procedures

Breast cancer tissue was obtained at mastectomy. A sample was dissected free of adipose and necrotic tissue and very finely sliced (thickness less than 1 mm). Ten to fifteen randomly selected slices were incubated in 2 ml of Gay's Balanced Salt Solution at 37° C for 6−8 h under an atmosphere of 5% CO_2 : 95% O_2. Incubations were done in the presence of 17β-estradiol or its vehicle. Tissues were labeled with 100 μCi/ml ^{35}S-methionine. MCF-7 cells were generously provided by Dr. H. Rochefort (INSERM, Montpellier, France). Cells were grown in Dulbecco's Modified Eagle's Medium supplemented with 100 U/ml penicillin, 100 μg/ml streptomycin, 0.6 μg/ml insulin, 0.025 M Hepes, and 10% fetal calf serum. To test the effects of steroids on protein synthesis, the protocol described by Westley and Rochefort [7] was used with minor modifications. Twenty-four hours before subculturing the cells, the medium was replaced with a medium of the same composition except that it contained serum treated with dextran-coated charcoal [2]. The cells were trypsinized and plated out in microwells (0.6 cm diameter) at the density of 150,000/ml. After 48 h, the medium was replaced and cells were incubated with fresh medium containing 17β-estradiol or its vehicle. After 24−48 h, cells were labeled in 0.05 ml of Eagle's Minimum Essential Medium (minus methionine) containing 200 μCi/ml ^{35}S-methionine for 6 h at 37° C. For SDS-polyacrylamide gel electrophoresis, 30,000−50,000 trichloroacetic acid precipitable cpm were mixed with protein denaturing buffer as described [3]. Samples were

Recent Results in Cancer Research. Vol. 91
© Springer-Verlag Berlin · Heidelberg 1984

boiled for 3 min and analyzed on 15% polyacrylamide gel (containing 0.09% bis-acryl-amide). Two-dimensional electrophoresis was carried out as described by O'Farrel [6]. Gels were processed for fluorography [1] and exposed to Kodak X-Omat S0282 film at −85° C for various periods.

Results

Figure 1 shows a typical SDS-polyacrylamide gel electrophoresis separation of newly labeled proteins found in the medium of MCF-7 cells (lanes a, b) or human breast cancer tissue (lanes c, d). It is evident that in the medium of breast cancer tissue, estrogen has increased the rate of synthesis of a single protein which has the same electrophoretic mobility as that found in the culture medium of MCF-7 cells. The electrophoretic mobility of this protein in our gel conditions corresponded to that of a peptide of approximately 51,000 daltons. However, for practical reasons, we will continue to refer to this protein as the "46 K". Increased rate of synthesis of the 46 K began after 6 h of exposure to 17β-estradiol [4]. No consistent effect of estrogen was observed in the labeling pattern of either MCF-7 cells or breast cancer tissue cytosol proteins (data not shown).

For a more reliable comparison of these estrogen-induced proteins, labeled mediums from MCF-7 cells and breast cancer tissue were additionally analyzed by the sensitive two-dimensional electrophoresis procedure. Figure 2 shows the pattern observed in the absence or presence of 17β-estradiol. About 15 different proteins of which only the 46 K

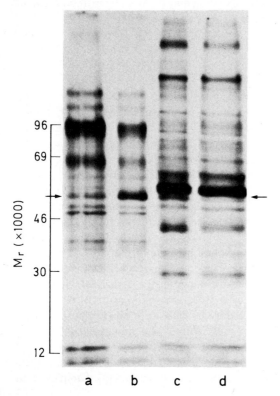

Fig. 1. Demonstration of the presence and estrogen-inducibility of the 46 K protein in human breast cancer and MCF-7 cells. Samples were subjected to SDS-polyacrylamide gel electrophoresis followed by fluorography. The lanes are: medium from *a* control; *b*, 17β-estradiol-treated (48 h, 1×10^{-9} *M*) MCF-7 cells; medium from *c* 17β-estradiol-treated (6 h, 1×10^{-9} *M*); *d*, control breast cancer tissue. The *arrows* indicate the migration position of the 46 K protein

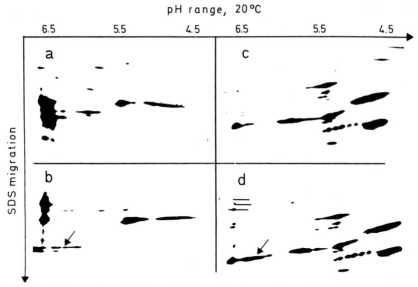

Fig. 2. Two-dimensional electrophoresis of proteins found in the medium of human breast cancer tissue and MCF-7 cells. Samples were isoelectric focused in Nonidet P-40, urea gels containing ampholines [6]; gels were then applied to second dimension SDS-polyacrylamide gel electrophoresis followed by fluorography. Medium from *a* control and *b* 17β-estradiol-treated (48 h, 1×10^{-9} M) MCF-7 cells; medium from *c* control and *d* 17β-estradiol-treated (7 h, 1×10^{-9} M) breast cancer tissue. The *arrows* indicate the position of the 46 K protein

Table 1. Percentage of the 46 K protein in human breast cancer[a]

Sample	% of 46 K protein	
	Control	17β-Estradiol
1	7.2	6.9
2	1.4	2.0
3	3.5	4.0
4	6.0	5.1
5	3.2	7.9
6	12.1	9.9
7	6.5	5.9
8	4.7	8.8
9	2.0	4.4
10	1.9	2.4
11	9.5	9.9
12	2.2	1.8
13	0.9	1.0
14	1.8	3.2
15	2.4	3.1

[a] Explants of human breast cancer were incubated for 6−8 h in the presence of ^{35}S-methionine in either control medium or medium containing 1×10^{-9} M 17β-estradiol. Proteins released in the medium were analyzed by SDS-polyacrylamide gel electrophoresis followed by fluorography. The percentage of radioactivity in the 46 K protein band was evaluated by densitometric scanning of the fluorograms. A stimulatory effect of estradiol on the synthesis (and/or release) of 46 K protein is evident in samples 5, 8, 9, and 14

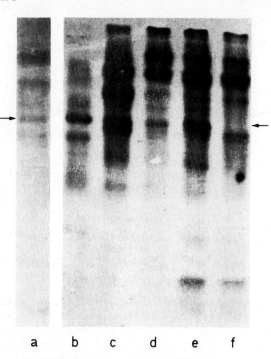

Fig. 3. Protein patterns of mediums from MCF-7 cells separated by DEAE-cellulose chromatography and then subjected to SDS-polyacrylamide gel electrophoresis and fluorography. The lanes are: *a*, proteins not absorbed to the column; proteins eluted by *b* 0.2 *M* NaCl; *c*, 0.25 *M* NaCl; *d*, 0.5 *M* NaCl; medium from *e* 17β-estradiol-treated; *f*, control MCF-7 cells. The *arrows* indicate the migration position of the 46 K protein

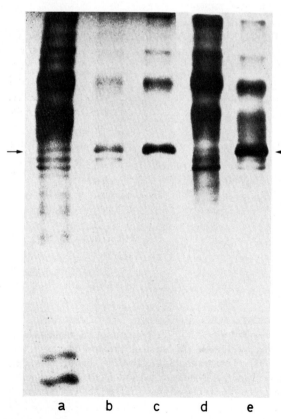

Fig. 4. Protein patterns of mediums from MCF-7 cells separated by concanavalin A-Sepharose chromatography and then subjected to SDS-polyacrylamide gel electrophoresis and fluorography. The lanes are: *a*, proteins not absorbed to the column; *b*, proteins eluted by 0.4 *M* α-methylglucopyranoside; *c*, proteins recovered from the concanavalin A-Sepharose after boiling with SDS and mercaptoethanol; medium from *d* control; *e*, 17β-estradiol-treated MCF-7 cells. The *arrows* indicate the migration position of the 46 K protein

was found to be stimulated by hormone treatment were visualized using this procedure. The isoelectric points of these estrogen-induced proteins ranged between 6.0 and 6.5. Synthesis of the 46 K was detected, although at variable rates, in 15 different breast cancer specimens examined (Table 1). However, a clear effect of estrogen was observed in only four of the samples, independent of tumor histology and menopausal status.

Some of the behavioural characteristics of the 46 K may be relevant to any purification study. First, the protein was found to bind to an anionic exchange cellulose and to elute at an anionic strength of 0.2–0.25 M (Fig. 3). Second, consistent with its glycoprotein nature [4], the 46 K adsorbed to the plant lectin concanavalin A. In Fig. 4, it can be seen that the majority of labeled proteins in the medium did not attach to the specific adsorbent and were washed through by the starting buffer. A very small percentage ($\sim 5\%$) of the 46 K was found in this fraction; approximately 10% was recovered after eluting the column with α-methylglucopyranoside whereas the majority ($\sim 70\%$) remained tightly bound and could only be detached after boiling with a buffer containing SDS and mercaptoethanol. The purity of the 46 K, evaluated in terms of radioactivity, recovered from the concanavalin A chromatography was in the order of 80%. In addition, its concentration, as judged by the intensity of the band after staining with Coomassie Brillant Blue, amounted to approximately 5 µg/l medium. Third, the 46 K had no affinity for Cibacron Blue F3 G-A, which indicates that it is probably not an enzyme requiring adenyl-containing cofactors (including NAD and NADP) (data not shown).

Conclusion

This study has shown that freshly obtained human breast cancer tissue produces a 51,000 dalton protein which, by the criteria utilized, appears to be identical to the so-called "46 K" protein previously described in long-term human breast cancer cell lines. Moreover, estrogen directly stimulates the synthesis of this protein when present for 6 h during incubation. This protein seems to possess several characteristics of practical interest. First, the fact that its synthesis is not a function exclusively restricted to or acquired by cells maintained in tissue culture for a long time, such as MCF-7 or ZR 75-1, but occurs even in primary breast cancer, suggests that this synthesis actually takes place in vivo and calls for the immediate use of this protein as a marker of estrogen dependency in breast cancer. Hopefully, evaluation of the 46 K as an adjunct to other existing prognostic indicators, such as steroid hormone receptors, will provide better insight into the treatment of breast cancer. Second, purification of this molecule may lead to the development of a specific immunologic assay for determining its presence in the circulation. Because the 46 K is released (possibly secreted) into the incubation medium of breast cancer cells, it might also be used as an early indicator of the onset of the disease. Third and finally, as this protein is only produced by malignant cells [4], it is conceivable that the production of a cytotoxic agent-antibody conjugate might be used to selectively destroy breast cancer cells.

References

1. Bonner WM, Laskey RA (1974) A film detection method for tritium-labelled proteins and nucleic acids in polyacrylamide gels. Eur J Biochem 46: 83–88
2. Burke RE, McGuire WL (1978) Nuclear thyroid hormone receptors in a human breast cancer cell line. Cancer Res 38: 3769–3773

3. Iacobelli S, Marchetti P, Bartoccioni E, Natoli V, Scambia G, Kaye AM (1981) Steroid-induced proteins in human endometrium. Mol Cell Endocrinol 23: 321–331
4. Westley B, Rochefort H (1980) A secreted glycoprotein induced by estrogen in human breast cancer cell lines. Cell 20: 353–362
5. McGuire W (1978) Hormones, receptors and breast cancer. Raven, New York
6. O'Farrel PH (1975) High resolution two-dimensional electrophoresis of proteins. J Biol Chem 10: 4007–4021
7. Westley B, Rochefort H (1979) Estradiol induced proteins in the MCF_7 human breast cancer cell line. Biochem Biophys Res Commun 90: 410–416

Estrogen Action on the Synthesis and Secretion of a Broad Spectrum of Proteins in Mammary Tumor Cells

N. Mairesse, P. Galand, G. Leclercq, and N. Devleeschouwer

Biology Unit, Institute of Interdisciplinary Research, School of Medicine, Free University of Bruxelles, Campus Erasme, Route de Lennik 808, 1070 Bruxelles, Belgium

Introduction

About 60% of human breast cancers containing estrogen receptor (ER) respond to endocrine treatment [1]. One may assume that some of these tumors contain altered receptors unable to bind efficiently to the acceptor loci involved in the regulation of cell growth. In any case, it seems likely that measurement of specific estrogen-controlled biochemical products might improve the characterisation of hormone dependency. In this context, the estrogen-induced increase of the progesterone receptor level [2] has been studied. However, this may be a side-effect unrelated to the trophic response. It is therefore interesting to extend the number of estrogen-specific responses to increase the probability of detecting a relevant defect of the ER in a given cell population.

In the rat uterus, an early estrogenic event is the induction of the so-called "induced protein" (IP) first described by Notides and Gorski [3]. The latter has been assumed to play a role in the trophic action of estrogen. This assumption may fit with the recent demonstration [4] that the major component of IP is the BB isozyme of creatine kinase (CK), an enzyme which regulates the intracellular concentration of ATP. Concerning mammary tumors, we reported previously on the in vitro estrogen-stimulated synthesis of IP (or IP-like protein) in most DMBA-induced rat tumors [5] as well as in one out of six human breast cancers [6]. The fact that IP response can be induced in tissue samples incubated for a short time makes IP a potentially useful marker of hormone dependency in clinical investigations.

Human breast cancer cell lines, such as MCF-7 cells, containing ER [7] appeared a good in vitro model for studying the estrogen-dependent events under defined conditions. This prompted us to investigate IP and IP-like responses in cytosolic and secreted proteins from the responsive MCF-7 line. A cell line lacking ER (Evsa-T) was used as unresponsive control.

Cytosolic Proteins

Using electrophoretic fractionation of [^{35}S]methionine-labeled proteins and fluorography, we have shown [8, 9] that in MCF-7 cells, estradiol-17β (E$_2$) triggers the synthesis of a protein very similar in charge and molecular weight to the uterine IP. This protein, referred to as "tumor IP", is also synthesized in the control cell line Evsa-T. However, in this

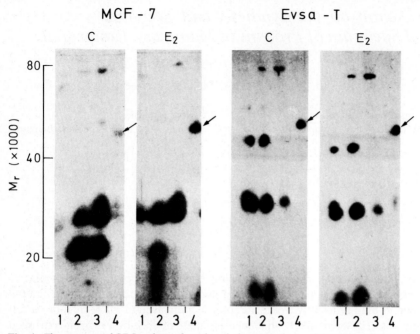

Fig. 1. *Fluorogram of SDS-polyacrylamide gel electrophoresis of the Cellogel-IP region from MCF-7 and Evsa-T cytosol.* Cells were incubated for 3 h with [^{35}S]methionine (100 μCi/ml) in the absence (C) or presence (E$_2$) of 10^{-8} M E$_2$. Samples of cytosol proteins were subjected to Cellogel electrophoresis [17]. The Cellogel region corresponding to IP position for a uterine cytosol (mobilities: 1 to 1.2 relative to BSA run in parallel) was excised and separated into four fractions that were directly applied into the wells of a 8% polyacrylamide gel. Electrophoresis was performed as described by Laemmli [18]. Electrophoretograms were treated for fluorography as described by Bonner and Laskey [19] and exposed on Rx-O-mat films for about 1 week. The *arrows* indicate the 48,000 dalton protein(s)

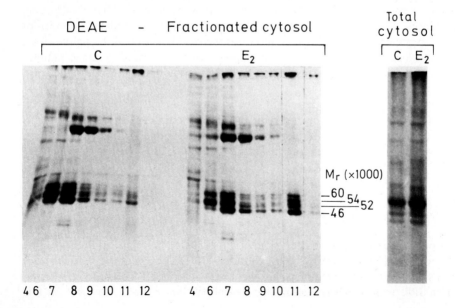

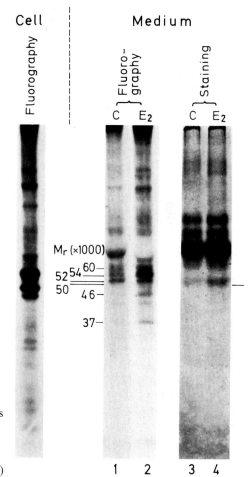

Fig. 3. Analysis of secreted proteins from untreated (C) and E_2-treated MCF-7 cells (E_2) on SDS-polyacrylamide gel. Cells were incubated for 24 h with [^{35}S]methionine (25 μCi/ml), with or without 10^{-8} M E_2; secreted proteins were precipitated and samples corresponding to 30 μl medium were submitted to the modified SDS-PAGE as in Fig. 1. Proteins were revealed by fluorography (lanes 1, 2) or by Coomassie Blue staining (lanes 3, 4)

Fig. 2. *Fluorogram of 7%−20% polyacrylamide gradient gel electrophoresis of samples obtained by fractionation of MCF-7 cytosol on DEAE cellulose.* Cells were incubated for 3 h with [^{35}S]methionine (100 μCi/ml) in the absence (C) or presence (E_2) of 10^{-8} M E_2. Cytosol samples corresponding in each case to 3×10^6 cpm were applied on a DEAE cellulose column and eluted in a linear gradient of 0−250 mM NaCl in 100 mM Tris-HCl buffer pH 5.2 (total volume of 40 ml). The fractions so obtained were precipitated and analyzed on a modified polyacrylamide gel SDS-PAGE according to Reiss and Kaye [4]. This includes a gradient of polyacrylamide concentration (containing a higher proportion of acrylamide and an increase in the molarity of the resolving buffer). Proteins were revealed by fluorography [18]. Lanes 8 and 9 (C and E_2) contain CK activity; lane 11 (C and E_2), the tumor-IP. Note in lane "11-E_2", compared with lane "11-C", the increased labeling intensity in four bands corresponding to proteins of 46,000, 52,000, 54,000, and 60,000 M_r

insensitive line, estradiol does not stimulate the rate of IP synthesis (Fig. 1). A two-step fractionation of the cytosolic proteins according to charge (Cellogel electrophoresis; DEAE cellulose chromatography) and molecular weight (SDS-polyacrylamide gel electrophoresis) reveals that the tumor IP is heterogeneous. Indeed, IP separates into two major bands of 46,000 and 52,000 M_r and two minor ones of 54,000 and 60,000 M_r. All bands are stimulated by E_2 (Fig. 2, lanes 11). On the other hand, the tumor IP is slightly more acidic than the uterine IP (as shown by its later elution from DEAE-cellulose column in a gradient of NaCl) and also lacks the CK activity associated with the latter (legend, Fig. 2). The fact that different proteins are stimulated by E_2 in different target cells may provide some clue as to their role in the full development of the trophic action of estrogens. It would therefore be important to elucidate the function (enzymatic?) of the tumor IP, and also to characterize the "IP-like" protein described previously in most DMBA-induced rat tumors [5] and in one human cancer [6].

Secreted Proteins

Using electrophoretic fractionation and fluorography, about 15 [^{35}S]methionine-labeled proteins are detected in the incubation medium of MCF-7 cells after about 24 h (Fig. 3, lanes 1, 2). The electrophoretic pattern is quite different from that of the cytosol, indicating that the accumulation of proteins in the medium results essentially from secretion rather than from cell lysis. All secreted proteins are detected in the incubation medium of untreated (lane 1) as well of E_2-treated cells (lane 2). However, under E_2 action, the labeling intensity is markedly increased in several bands corresponding to secreted proteins of about 37,000, 46,000, 54,000, and 60,000 M_r. Some of these proteins (46,000, 54,000, and 60,000 M_r) may be identical to the cytosolic induced proteins described in the previous section.

When the secreted proteins are revealed on the gel by Coomassie Brilliant Blue staining (Fig. 3, lanes 3, 4), about six bands are detected, with the most prominent one corresponding to a protein of 65,000 M_r (albumin?). Notably, a protein of about 50,000 M_r is more abundant in the incubation medium of E_2-treated cells (lane 4) than in controls (lane 3). As this protein is not detected by fluorography (lanes 1, 2), it is obvious that its synthesis had essentially occurred before the addition of labeled amino acids. In this case, E_2 stimulates the secretion of (a) preexisting protein(s).

Finally, most of the secreted proteins are common to MCF-7 and Evsa-T cells, but estrogen treatment has no effect on their rate of synthesis and/or secretion in the latter cell line [9].

Conclusions

From this work and similar studies (summarized in Table 1), it is evident that a spectrum of changes is produced by estrogens in the hormone-sensitive MCF-7 cell line. Therefore, it should be stressed that referring to a single protein as a marker of responsiveness to endocrine treatment may be misleading. Indeed, involvement of any of these proteins in the control of growth by the hormone has not yet been demonstrated. Investigation of a spectrum of responses is more likely to reveal eventual correlation between estrogen-induced changes and hormonal sensitivity.

Table 1. Effect of estrogen on the synthesis and secretion of specific proteins in breast cancers

Protein	MCF-7 cells		References
	Intracellular	Extracellular	
PgR	Induction	Not investigated	[10]
LDH	Increased activity	Not detected	[11]
Plasminogen activator	Increased activity	Increased activity	[12]
Collagenase	Not investigated	Increased activity	[13]
160,000 M_r 46,000	Not detected	Increased content[a]	[14]
± 150,000 55,000	Stimulated synthesis	Not investigated	[14]
36,000 24,000	Stimulated synthesis[b]	Not investigated	[15]
60,000[c] 54,000 52,000 46,000	Stimulated synthesis	Increased content[a]	This work
37,000	Not detected	Increased content	This work
50,000	Decreased content	Increased content	This work

[a] The intracellular level of the proteins being low or undetectable in E_2-treated cells, their accumulation in the medium under E_2 action can only be explained by stimulation of synthesis and secretion

[b] Nafoxidine pretreatment

[c] Adams et al. [16] have detected an estrogen-regulated mRNA predicting a protein of 54,000 M_r which, however, was not detected in the cells

Another interesting extension of this study would be the comparison of cellular and secreted proteins from both normal and tumor mammary cells in order to reveal possible specific markers of neoplasia.

References

1. McGuire WL, Carbone PP, Vollmer EP (1975) Estrogen receptors in human breast cancer. Raven, New York, pp 1−7
2. McGuire WL, Horwitz KB (1978) Progesterone receptors in breast cancer. In: McGuire WL (ed) Hormones, receptors and breast cancer. Raven, New York, pp 41−43
3. Notides A, Gorski J (1966) Estrogen-induced synthesis of a specific uterine protein. Proc Natl Acad Sci USA 46: 230−235
4. Reiss N, Kaye AM (1981) Identification of the major component of the estrogen-induced protein of rat uterus as the BB isozyme of creatine kinase. J Biol Chem 256: 5741−5749
5. Mairesse N, Heuson JC, Galand P, Leclercq G (1977) Estrogen-induced protein in rat mammary tumor and uterus. J Endocrinol 75: 331−332

6. Mairesse N, Heuson JC, Galand P, Leclercq G (1977) Estrogen-induced protein in human tumor and rat uterus. 7th Int symposium on the biological characterization of human tumors, Budapest

7. Lippman M, Bolan G, Huff K (1976) The effects of estrogens and antiestrogens on hormone responsive human breast cancer in long-term tissue culture. Cancer Res 36: 4595−4601

8. Mairesse N, Devleeschouwer N, Leclercq G, Galand P (1980) Estrogen-induced protein in the human breast cancer cell line MCF-7. Biochem Biophys Res Commun 97: 1251−1257

9. Mairesse N, Devleeschouwer N, Leclercq G, Galand P (in press) Estrogen-induced synthesis and secretion of proteins in the human breast cancer cell lines MCF-7. J Steroid Biochem

10. Horwitz KB, McGuire WL Estrogen and progesterone: their relationship in hormone dependent breast cancer. In: McGuire WL, Raynaud J-P, Baulieu EE (eds) Progesterone receptors in normal and neoplastic tissues. Raven, New York, pp 103−124

11. Burke RE, Harris SC, McGuire WL (1978) Lactate dehydrogenase in estrogen-responsive human breast cancer cells. Cancer Res 38: 2773−2776

12. Butler B, Kirkland NL, Jorgensen TL (1979) Induction of plasminogen activator in a human breast cancer cell line (MCF-7). Biochem Biophys Res Commun 70: 1328−1334

13. Shafie S, Liotta L (1980) Formation of metastasis by human breast carcinoma cells (MCF-7) in nude mice. Cancer Lett 11: 81−87

14. Westley B, Rochefort H (1980) A secreted glycoprotein induced by estrogen in human breast cancer cell line. Cell 20: 353−362

15. Edwards DP, Adams DJ, Savage N, McGuire WL (1980) Estrogen-induced synthesis of specific proteins in human breast cancer cells. Biochem Biophys Res Commun 93: 804−812

16. Kaye AM, Reiss N, Iacobelli S, Bartoccioni E, Marchetti P (1980) The "estrogen-induced protein" in normal and neoplasic cells. In: Iacobelli et al. (eds) Hormone cancer. Raven, New York

17. Sömjen D, Sömjen G, King RJB, Kaye AM, Lindner HR (1973) Nuclear binding of estradiol-17β and induction of protein synthesis in the rat uterus during postnatal development. Biochem J 136: 25−33

18. Laemmli UK (1971) Cleavage of structural proteins during the assembly of the head of bacteriophorage T_4. Nature 227: 680−685

19. Bonner WH, Laskey PA (1974) A film detection method for tritium-labelled proteins and nucleic acids in polyacrylamide gels. Eur J Biochem 46: 83−88

Part VII.
Laboratories Performing Receptor Assays

Austria

G. Daxenbichler

Universitätsklinik für Frauenheilkunde,
Anichstrasse 35, 6020 Innsbruck, Austria

Steroid receptor determination is limited to four centers. The first receptor laboratory was established at the Dept. of Gynecology, University of Innsbruck in 1976 in collaboration with Dr. J. L. Wittliff, University of Louisville, Kentucky.

In the four centers, about 2,000 mammary carcinoma samples from about 70 hospitals are analyzed each year for ER and PgR. This number represents approximately 55% of all newly detected malign breast tumors per year. The decision to order the receptor assay rests with the surgeon. Unfortunately, some surgeons, particularly those in smaller hospitals, are not sufficiently familiar with the value of the receptor assay to include it in their protocol.

Receptor laboratories are sponsored by the federal and district governments and national health insurance plans. Thus for the majority of patients the costs of the receptor assay are absorbed by the hospitals. Only private patients are charged directly for receptor assay, but they may be refunded by their individual health insurance company.

Quality control for the steroid receptor assays is not coordinated among the laboratories and requires improvement in some cases.

Addresses	Characteristics				
	No. of samples/year	SR assay	Usual technique	Time required for response	Quality control
Graz					
J. Semmelrock Med.-Chem. Labor Univ-Klinik für Chirurgie Auenpruggerplatz 8036 Graz	350	ER PgR	DCC assay Scatchard plot analysis	1–2 weeks	No
P. Pürstner Hormonlabor Univ.-Frauenklinik Auenpruggerplatz 8036 Graz	150	ER PgR	DCC assay Scatchard plot analysis	1 week	ER: commercially available control samples PgR: No
Innsbruck					
G. Daxenbichler Univ-Frauenklinik Anichstrasse 35 6020 Innsbruck	700	ER PgR	DCC assay Scatchard plot analysis	1 week	Internal: Calf uterus External: Italian and EORTC quality control
Wien – Vienna					
J. Spona Hormonlaboratorium I. Univ.-Frauenklinik Spitalgasse 23 1090 Wien	900	ER PgR AR	DCC assay Scatchard plot analysis	1 week	Internal: Rat uterus External: EORTC quality control

Belgium (and Luxembourg)

G. Leclercq

Institut Jules Bordet,
Centre des Tumeurs de l'Université Libre de Bruxelles,
Service de Médicine, Clinique et Laboratoire de Cancérologie Mammaire,
Rue Héger-Bordet 1, 1000 Bruxelles, Belgium

Receptor assays are performed at eight university centers. There is no national quality control but most laboratories participate in foreign controls (EORTC, Italian, or French).
The cost of the receptor assay is refunded by social security.

| Addresses | Characteristics | | | | |
	No. of samples/year	SR assay	Usual technique	Time required for response	Quality control
Antwerpen P. Blockx, D. Becquart Nucleaire Geneeskunde Akademisch Ziekenhuis Antwerpen Wilrijkstraat 10 2520 Edegem 031/29 11 11 (ext. 15 65)	150	ER PgR	Modified DCC[a] Nonlinear regression analysis	± 10 days	EORTC or cytosol from McGuire's lab.
Bruxelles – Brussels G. Leclercq Lab. Cancérologie Mammaire Institut J. Bordet 1, rue Héger-Bordet 1000 Bruxelles 02/5 38 08 58	700	ER PgR	DCC Scatchard plot analysis	1 week	EORTC Italy (Dr. Fumero)
G. Noel Lab. Senobiochemistry Dept. Cancerology U.C.L. – Clin. St Luc P.O. Box U.C.L. 5369 1200 Brussels 02/7 62 34 00 (ext. 53 70)	350	ER PgR AR CR	Modified DCC[a] Nonlinear regression analysis	Max. 5 days	Internal
A. Vokaer Laboratoire de Recherche Fondation FRESERH Service de Gynécologie Hopital Brugmann 4, Pl. Van Gehuchten 1020 Bruxelles 02/4 78 48 70 (ext. 29 89)	130	ER PgR	DCC Scatchard plot analysis	2–7 days	In collaboration with P. M. Martin and H. Magdelenat

Diepenbeek J. Raus Dr. L. Willems-Instituut Universitaire Campus 3610 Diepenbeek 0 11/22 67 21	150	ER PgR	DCC Scatchard plot analysis	Max. 5 days	EORTC
Gent J. de Boever Akademisch Ziekenhuis Vrouwenkliniek/Poli III De Pintenlaan 135 9000 Gent	140	ER PgR	DCC Scatchard plot analysis	Max. 10 days	Calf and rabbit uterine cytosol
Leuven W. de Loecker, J. Janssens Afdeling Biochemie Campus Gasthuisberg Herestraat 49 3000 Leuven 0 16/22 84 21 (ext. 12 84)	700	ER PgR AR CR	DCC Scatchard plot analysis	Max. 7 days	EORTC
Liège J. Duvivier Service de Chimie médicale Tour de pathologie C.H.U. Sart-Tilman (par Liège I) 0 41/56 24 75	60	ER PgR AR	DCC Scatchard plot analysis	Max. 10 days	EORTC
Luxembourg M. Dicato Dept. Hématologie-Cancérologie Centre Hospitalier de Luxembourg 1210 Luxembourg	200	ER CR	Scatchard plot analysis	14 days	In process
J. P. Hoffmann Biochimie Laboratoire National de Santé Luxembourg	100	ER	Scatchard plot analysis	14 days	In process

a G. Noel and H. Maisin Arch Int Physiol Biochim (1981) 89: B 189 – B 190; Rev Endocrine-Related Cancer (1981) Suppl 9: 95–102

Denmark

S. M. Thorpe

The Fibiger Laboratory, Ndr. Frihavnsgade 70,
2100 Copenhagen, Denmark

Steroid hormone recptor determinations are performed in conjunction with the nationwide Danish Breast Cancer Cooperative Group project (DBCG) that registers approximately 2,000 new cases of primary breast cancer annually. Biopsy material is prepared and collected at the pathological departments and transported on dry ice to the receptor laboratories by means of either car or the postal service. Financing of the project is at present primarily through the private organization, The Danish Cancer Society.

The method used for ER and PgR determinations is that recommended by EORTC in 1981 with minor modifications.

Efforts to standardize the ER and PgR analyses have been initiated. A receptor committee has been established under the auspices of the DBCG, and a comparison of the results obtained upon analysis of the standard EORTC lyophilized calf uterine powders has just been completed. It is reported in Part II in this book.

Addresses	Characteristics					
	No. of samples/year	SR assay	Usual technique	Time required for response	Quality control
Ålborg K. O. Pedersen Dept. of Clinical Chemistry Afsnit Syd Box 365 9100 Ålborg 08-1 31 11 11	150	ER PgR	Scatchard plot analysis DCC	1–3 weeks	DBCG
Århus H. Skovgaard Poulsen Kræftforskningsinstitutet Radiumstationen 8000 Århus C 06-12 55 55	350	ER PgR	Scatchard plot analysis DCC	1–3 weeks	DBCG
Copenhagen S. Thorpe Fibiger Laboratory/ Dept. of Clinical Physiology, Finsen Institut Strandboulevarden 49 2100 Copenhagen Ø 01-38 45 90	1,000	ER PgR	Scatchard plot analysis DCC	10 days	EORTC/DBCG

Federal Republic of Germany

W. Jonat

Zentralkrankenhaus, Frauenklinik, St. Jürgen-Strasse, 2800 Bremen, FRG

It was in 1969/70 that steroid hormone receptor analyses were first performed in Hamburg, the slice uptake technique being used. These early studies resulted in the first European publication about clinical correlation of estrogen receptor status and response to endocrine therapy [1]. Later, the agar gel electrophoresis, invented by Wagner [2], was accepted as the most applicable procedure for assaying steroid hormone receptors. Today this method is still widely used in West Germany.

To achieve sufficient methodological standardization, in 1978 a committee of laboratory investigators selected the multiple point dextran-coated charcoal assay analyzed by the method of Scatchard [3] as standard procedure. This committee also established a quality control system (see Part 2).

Although the clinical value of receptor determination is accepted by most clinicians, the refunding of receptor laboratories still remains a problem. In the early 1970s they were paid by the DFG (German Scientific Research Society). Today from a scientific standpoint receptor assay is accepted as a routine method which no longer needs refunding by the DFG. Therefore first attempts have been made by most laboratories to get the analysis paid for by social security companies and the government. The price for the analyses of one tissue sample for ER and PgR is approximately 200 DM.

The list of major laboratories performing SR assays reveals two other important points:

1. Still only four laboratories accept tissue samples from other institutions.
2. Hormone receptor assays are performed in less than 10% of all patients developing breast cancer in West Germany.

The above points stress the need to establish more central laboratories for hormone receptor analyses.

References

1. Maass H, Engel B, Hohmeister H, Lehmann F, Trams G (1972) Estrogen receptors in human breast cancer tissue. Am J Obstet Gynecol 113: 377–382
2. Wagner RK (1972) Characterization and assay of steroid hormone receptors and steroid-binding serum proteins by agar gel electrophoresis at low temperature. Hoppe-Seylers Z Physiol Chem 353: 1235–1245
3. EORTC Breast Cooperative Group (1980) Revision of the standards for the assessment of hormone receptors in human breast cancer. Eur J Cancer 16: 1513–1515

Addresses	Characteristics			Time required for response	Quality control
	No. of samples/year	SR assay	Usual technique		
Berlin M. Schmidt-Gollwitzer Universitätsklinikum Charlottenburg Tel: 0 30/3 20 35 33	200	ER PgR	DCC	Max. 14 days	GCGRS
Bremen W. Jonat Zentralkrankenhaus, Frauenklinik St.-Jürgen-Strasse Tel: 04 21/4 97 34 63	1,500	ER PgR	DCC	Max. 7 days	EORTC, GCGRS
Düsseldorf H. Bojar Abt. für Onkologische Biochemie Physiologische Chemie II Universität Düsseldorf Tel: 02 11/3 11 43 55	1,500	ER PgR	DCC	Max. 7 days	EORTC, GCGRS
Erlangen K. V. Maillot Frauenklinik der Universität Erlangen-Nürnberg Tel: 0 91 31/85 35 53	550	ER PgR AR	DCC	Max. 7 days	GCGRS
Frankfurt R. Th. Michel Universitätsfrauenklinik Frankfurt Tel: 06 11/63 01 52 22					

Addresses	Characteristics				
	No. of samples/year	SR assay	Usual technique	Time required for response	Quality control
Freiburg H. Geyer Universitätsfrauenklinik Freiburg Tel: 07 61/2-70 30	500	ER PgR AR	DCC	Max. 7 days	GCGRS
Göttingen C. Blossey Universitätsklinik Göttingen Tel: 05 51/3 90	500	ER PgR	DCC	Max. 7 days	GCGRS
Hamburg G. Trams Universitätsfrauenklinik Hamburg Tel: 0 40/4 68 26 13	300	ER PgR	Agar-gel electrophoresis	Max. 5 days	GCGRS
Hannover H. O. Hoppen Max-Planck-Institut für experimentelle Endokrinologie Hannover Tel: 05 11/53 21	1,000	ER PgR (estrogen, progesterone concentration in the nucleus)	Agar-gel electrophoresis, DCC	Max. 14 days	EORTC, GCGRS
Heidelberg K. Klinga Universitätsfrauenklinik Heidelberg Tel: 0 62 21/56 50 56	150	ER PgR	DCC	Max. 10 days	GCGRS

Ingelheim B. Heicke Biocientia, Institut für Labormedizin, Ingelheim Tel: 0 61 32/71 71	1,000	ER PgR	DCC	Max. 7 days	EORTC
Köln H. Würtz Universitätsfrauenklinik Köln Tel: 02 21/4 78 49 86	175	ER PgR	Agar-gel electrophoresis	Max. 7 days	GCGRS
Mainz K. Pollow Abt. für experimentelle Endokrinologie Universitätsfrauenklinik Mainz Tel: 0 61 31/19 27 63	1,000	ER PgR	DCC	Max. 7 days	GCGRS, commercial standard by NEN
München C. de Wall I. Universitätsfrauenklinik München Tel: 0 89/5 39 71	100	ER PgR	DCC	Max. 7 days	GCGRS
Würzburg H. Caffier Universitätsfrauenklinik Würzburg Tel: 09 31/2 01 36 21					

France

P. M. Martin

Faculté de Médicine, Laboratoire de Récepteurs Hormonaux,
Boulevard P. Dramard, 13015 Marseille, France

Interlaboratory Quality Control

Receptor assays are performed in almost all regions of the country. A common technical protocol for routine ER and PgR assays on surgical samples has been accepted. In this interlaboratory protocol, each laboratory uses the interassay standard set up in that laboratory and a commercial standard (marketed by Immunotech France, Marseille, since 1983). In 1980–1981 the interlaboratory protocol was utilized in only a few laboratories, while in 1982–1983 quality controls based on the interlaboratory French protocol, organized by the Ligue Contre le Cancer, were used at 24 centers. For 1984–1986 the organization of these controls has been taken over by the Caisse Nationale Assurance Maladie and the Fédération des Centres Anticancéreux, with 29 groups participating. In the interlaboratory quality controls, human breast tumors are the test material. Owing to the small quantity of material in each sample, each tumor sample is divided into only two parts and assayed in two laboratories. Up to four laboratories can exchange samples. Statistical analysis is based on a test of "inter-judge concordance" [1]. Intralaboratory variability is evaluated.

The practical organization for four participating laboratories is as follows: each laboratory sends, frozen, 12 half-tumors to each of the other three laboratories (36 samples) and assays 72 half-tumors (their own 36 and 36 from the other three laboratories). Essential information is collected on a form accompanying each sample.

Reference

1. Ployart F (1981) Contribution à l'étude des données médicales: concordance intra- et inter-juges. Medical dissertation, Paris

Addresses	Characteristics					
	No. of samples/year	SR assay	Usual technique	Time required for response	Quality control
Angers Centre Paul Papin Dr. Davert Laboratoire de Biochimie Hormonale 2, Rue Moll 49036 Angers Tél.: (41) 48 10 66	300	ER PgR	DCC Three concentrations analysis	3 days	Intralaboratory Interlaboratory French protocol
Besancon INSERM U 198 Dr. Dahan Route de Dale Tél.: (81) 52 33 00	200	Er PgR	DCC Single dose assay Scatchard plot analysis	15 days	Intralaboratory Interlaboratory French protocol
Bordeaux Fondation Bergonié Dr. Waffelard Laboratoire des Récepteurs Hormonaux 180, Rue de Saint Genès 33076 Bordeaux Cedex Tel.: (56) 91 34 05	900	ER PgR	DCC Single dose assay	3 days	Intralaboratory quality control
Brest Pr. Floch Laboratoire de Biochemie ERA CNRS 784 C. H. U. Brest Faculté de Médecine Av. Camille Desmoulin 29200 Brest Tél.: (98) 80 01 84	250	ER PgR	DCC Single dose assay	15 days	Intralaboratory

Addresses	Characteristics					
	No. of samples/year	SR assay	Usual technique	Time required for response	Quality control	

Addresses	No. of samples/year	SR assay	Usual technique	Time required for response	Quality control
Caen Centre F. Baclesse Dr. Goussard Route de Lion s/Mer B.P. 5026 14021 Caen Tél.: (31) 94 81 34	400	ER PgR AR	DCC Single dose assay Scatchard plot analysis Microassay	8 days	Intralaboratory Interlaboratory French protocol
Clermont Ferrand Centre Jean Perrin Dr. Gandillon Service Médecine Nucléaire Place H. Dunan BP 392 63011 Clermont Ferrand Tél.: (73) 26 56 56	500	ER PgR	DCC Scatchard plot analysis Microassay	15 days	Intralaboratory Interlaboratory French protocol
Creteil Hopital Henri Mondor Dr. Kouyoumoudjian 94010 Creteil	400	ER PgR	DCC Scatchard plot analysis	15 days	Intralaboratory Interlaboratory French protocol
Dijon Centre G. F. Leclerc Dr. Bordes Laboratoire de Biochimie Hormonale 1, Rue dy Pr Marion 21034 Dijon Tél.: (80) 66 81 36	400	ER PgR	DCC Scatchard plot analysis	2 days	Intralaboratory Interlaboratory French protocol

Location		Receptors	Method	Days	Protocols
Grenoble C. H. U. Dr. Chambaz Laboratoire d'Hormonologie 38700 La Tronche Tél.: (76) 42 81 21	500	ER PgR	DCC Scatchard plot analysis	15 days	Intralaboratory Interlaboratory French protocol
Lille Institut Pasteur Dr. Peyrat Laboratoire d'Endocrinology Expérimentale 20, Bd Louis XIV 59019 Lille Tél.: (20) 52 33 33 poste 289	800	ER PgR	EORTC protocol DCC Scatchard plot analysis	10 days	Intralaboratory Interlaboratory French protocol EORTC
Lyon Centre Léon Bérard Dr. Saez Department de Biochimie Médicale 28, Rue Laennec 69008 Lyon Tél.: (7) 8 74 08 36	1600	ER PgR	DCC Scatchard plot analysis	20 days	Intralaboratory Interlaboratory French protocol
Marseille Faculté de Médecine Nord Dr. Martin Laboratoire des Récepteurs Hormonaux Bd P. Dramard 13015 Marseille Tél.: (91) 51 90 01	2100	ER PgR AR	DCC Scatchard plot analysis Microassay	20 days	Intralaboratory Interlaboratory French protocol EORTC
Montpellier Maternité du CHR Dr. Bressot Laboratoire Hormones Steroides Biochimie A 34000 Montpellier Tél.: (67) 63 53 80	580	ER PgR	DCC Scatchard plot analysis	15 days	Intralaboratory

Addresses	Characteristics				
	No. of samples/year	SR assay	Usual technique	Time required for response	Quality control
Nancy Centre Alexis Vautran Dr. Weber/Marchal Laboratoire de Biochimie Hormonale Av. de Bourgogne R.N. 74 – Bradois 54500 Vandoeuvre les Nancy Tél.: (83) 55 81 06	600	ER PgR AR GR	DCC Single dose assay	15 days	Intralaboratory Interlaboratory French protocol
Nantes Centre René Gauducheau Dr. Riccoleau Laboratoire de Biochimie Hormonale Quai Moscou 44035 Nantes Cedex Tél.: (40) 48 35 55	300	ER PgR	DCC Scatchard plot analysis	7 days	Intralaboratory Interlaboratory French protocol
Nice Centre Lacassagne D' Krebs/Formento Laboratoire d'Endocrinologie 36, Voie Romaine 06054 Nice Tél.: (93) 81 71 33	900	ER PgR AR	DCC Three concentrations analysis Scatchard plot analysis Microassay	7 days	Intralaboratory Interlaboratory French protocol
Paris I C. H. U. Laboratoire de Biochimie Hormonale Dr. Pichon 78, Rue du Général Leclerc 94270 Paris Tél.: (1) 5 21 27 48	600	ER PgR	DCC Single dose assay Scatchard plot analysis	15 days	Intralaboratory Interlaboratory French protocol

Location / Institution	No.	Receptors	Method	Turnaround	Quality control
Paris II Institut Curie Dr. Magdelenat Laboratoire de Radiobiologie 26, Rue d'Ulm 75005 Paris Tél.: (1) 3 29 12 42	1900	ER PgR AR	DCC Scatchard plot analysis Single dose assay Microassay	20 days	Intralaboratory Interlaboratory French protocol
Poitiers C. H. U. Miletrie Dr. Bounaud Service Médecine Nucléaire Hopital Jean Bernard BP 577 86021 Poitiers Cedex Tél.: (49) 46 65 50	300	ER PgR	DCC Single dose assay Scatchard plot analysis	15 days	Intralaboratory Interlaboratory French protocol
Reims Institut Jean Godinot Dr. Gardillier Laboratoire de Biochimie 1, Rue du Général Koenig B.P. 171 51056 Reims Cedex Tél.: (26) 06 05 04	350	ER PgR	DCC Single dose assay	7 days	Intralaboratory
Rennes I Centre Régional de Recherche en Endocrinologie Dr. Jouan Faculté de Médecine et de Pharmacie 2, Av. du Pr. Léon Bernard 35043 Rennes Cedex Tél.: (99) 59 20 20	400	ER Cytosolic + nuclear PgR	DCC Scatcard plot analysis	8 days	Intralaboratory Interlaboratory French protocol
Rennes II Laboratoire de Biochimie Pr. Legal C. H. U. Rennes 35000 Pontchaillou	500	ER PgR	DCC Scatchard plot analysis	8 days	Intralaboratory

Addresses	Characteristics					
	No. of samples/year	SR assay	Usual technique	Time required for response	Quality control	
Rouen Centre Henri Becquerel Dr. Basuyau Laboratoire de Biochimie Rue d'Amiens 76038 Rouen Tél.: (35) 98 20 27	500	ER PgR	EORTC protocol DCC Scatchard plot analysis	8 days	Intralaboratory	
Saint-Cloud Centre René Huguenin Dr. Spyratos Laboratoire de Biochimie Hormonale 35, Rue Dailly 92211 Saint-Cloud Tél.: (1) 7 71 91 91	500	ER PgR	DCC Scatchard plot analysis	15 days	Intralaboratory Interlaboratory French protocol	
Strasbourg I Dr. Hoffner Laboratoire de Boichimie des Pavillons Chirurgicaux A et B Service Pr. Chambon 67005 Strasbourg Cedex Tél.: (88) 36 71 11	200	ER PgR	DCC Single dose assay Scatchard plot analysis	15 days	Intralaboratory Interlaboratory French protocol	
Strasbourg II Dr. Koehl Faculté de Médecine 11, Rue Humann Laboratoire d'Analyses Institut de Chimie Biologique 67085 Strasbourg Tél.: (88) 36 22 31	200	ER PgR	DCC Single dose assay Scatchard plot analysis	15 days	Intralaboratory Interlaboratory French protocol	

Strasbourg III Dr. Abécassis Centre Paul Strauss 3, Rue de la Porte de l'Hopital 67085 Strasbourg Cedex Tél.: (88) 36 20 20	200	ER PgR	DCC Single dose assay Scatchard plot analysis	15 days	Intralaboratory Interlaboratory French protocol
Toulouse I Centre Claudius Regaud Dr. Courriere 20–24 Rue du Pont St. Pierre 31052 Toulouse Cedex	300	ER PgR	DCC Scatchard plot analysis	15 days	Intralaboratory Interlaboratory French protocol
Toulouse II C. H. R. de la Grane Dr. Moatti Laboratoire de Biochimie III Place Lange 31052 Toulouse Cedex Tél.: (61) 42 33 33	300	ER PgR	DCC Scatchard plot analysis	15 days	Intralaboratory Interlaboratory French protocol
Tours C. H. R. Dr. Barnerias Service de Médecine Nucléaire Bd Tonnelé 37044 Tours Cedex	300	ER PgR	DCC Scatchard plot analysis	15 days	Intralaboratory Interlaboratory French protocol
Villejuif Institut Gustave Roussy Dr. Delarue Unité Biochimie Hormonale Rue Camille Desmoulin 94805 Villejuif Cedex Tél.: (1) 5 59 49 09	900	ER PgR	DCC Scatchard plot analysis	15 days	Intralaboratory Interlaboratory French protocol

Great Britain

R. E. Leake

Department of Biochemistry, University of Glasgow,
Glasgow G 12 8QQ, United Kingdom

Entries include only those laboratories which carry out steroid receptor assays on tumour biopsies submitted from different centres and participate in the national quality control programme.

The standard assay for both ER and PgR is a dextran-coated charcoal method (Scatchard plot analysis). Full details are given in Part II.

Each laboratory is funded from its own resources. No national funding, either government or private, has yet been forthcoming.

Recent Results in Cancer Research. Vol. 91
© Springer-Verlag Berlin · Heidelberg 1984

Addresses	Characteristics		Usual technique	Time required for response	Quality control
	No. of samples/year	SR assay			
Birmingham A. Hughes Department of Medicine University of Birmingham Edgbaston Birmingham B15 2TH	400–500	ER PgR	Soluble receptors; DCC with Scatchard plot analysis	5 days	U.K. and EORTC
Cardiff R. I. Nicholson Tenovus Institute for Cancer Research Welsh National School of Medicine The Heath Cardiff CF4 4XXI 02 22 7 55 94 Ext. 25 74	1,500	ER PgR	Cytoplasmic and nuclear ER (nuclear assay by glass bead method)	7 days	U.K.
Edinburgh R. A. Hawkins Dept. of Clinical Surgery The Medical School University of Edinburgh Teviot Place Edinburgh	130–200	ER PgR	Cytosol assay by multiple point DCC adsorption with Scatchard plot analysis	3–7 days	Frozen, minced pool (human uterus); also U.K.
Glasgow R. E. Leake Department of Biochemistry University of Glasgow Glasgow G12 8QQ 041-3 39 88 55 Ext. 72 64	500	ER PgR	Soluble and nuclear receptors; Scatchard plot analysis	7 days	U.K. and EORTC

Addresses	Characteristics		Usual technique	Time required for response	Quality control
	No. of samples/year	SR assay			
London M. Baum Dept. of Surgery King's College Hospital London SE5 8RX 01-2 74 62 22 Ext. 24 41	150	ER PgR	Cytoplasmic receptors; DCC Scatchard plot analysis	1 month	U.K.
Manchester D. M. Barnes Dept. of Clinical Research Christie Hospital Manchester 0 61-4 45 81 23 Ext. 4 37	500	ER PgR	Cytosol and nuclear estrogen receptors and cytosol progesterone receptors by 6-point Scatchard plot analysis	7 days	Internal and U.K.

Ireland

M. J. Duffy

Departments of Nuclear Medicine and Pathology,
St. Vincent's Hospital, Dublin 4, Ireland

Steroid receptor assays are carried out at one centre only, namely in the Nuclear Medicine Laboratory, St. Vincent's Hospital, Dublin. This is a laboratory which specializes in routine clinical biochemical assays utilizing radioisotopes. The ER assay was initially established in 1975 with the help of financial support from the Irish Cancer Society. In 1977 this assay was offered as a routine service not only for patients in St. Vincent's Hospital but for patients with breast cancer all over Ireland. The PgR assay was established in 1978 with continuing support from the Irish Cancer Society. This assay was incorporated into the routine service in 1980. Other receptor determinations established for research purposes include assay of nuclear ER, androgen receptors and glucocorticoids receptors.

Recent Results in Cancer Research. Vol. 91
© Springer-Verlag Berlin · Heidelberg 1984

Addresses	Characteristics				
	No. of samples/year	SR assay	Usual technique	Time required for response	Quality control
Dublin M. J. Duffy Nuclear Medicine Department St. Vincent's Hospital Dublin 4 69 45 33 Ext. 3 78	250	ER	DCC Single saturating concentration	Approx. 4 weeks	None

Italy

A. Piffanelli

Istituto di Radiologia dell' Università,
Corso Giovecca 203, 44100 Ferrara, Italy

Since 1978 an Italian working group for the study of receptrs in neoplastic tissues has been implementing a voluntary external quality assessment scheme to obtain not only a retrospective evaluation of interlaboratory comparability (see results Part II, and Ref. [1]) but also an actual control. All institutions are performing the receptor measurements according to the EORTC recommendations. A few of them are directly involved in the clinical use of receptor measurements, but it seems rather difficult to obtain a large collaborative clinical trial of hormonal therapy.

The cost of assays of ER and PgR are mainly included in the fee of hospitalized patients (National Health Service) and are partially covered by some research programs.

Various practical workshops have been held to train participants from ten new institutions that will join the working group in the near future, in order to create a national network of laboratories involved in the quality control scheme.

The incidence of breast cancer is increasing in Italy [2], and long-term improvements in diagnosis (including receptor assays of all primary tumors) and treatment will be necessary.

References

1. Fumero S, Berruto GP, Pelizolla D et al. (1981) Results of the Italian interlaboratory quality control program for estradiol receptor assay. Tumori 67: 301–306
2. Saracci R, Repetto F (1980) Breast cancer mortality trends in Italy. Br J Cancer 42: 620–623

Addresses	Characteristics				
	No. of samples/year	SR assay	Usual technique	Time required for response	Quality control
Bologna Istituto di Cancerologia Università	70	ER, PgR, AR, CR	DCC	4 days	Italy
Ferrera Istituto di Radiologia Università	250	ER, PgR	DCC	3–4 days	Italy + EORTC
Firenze Laboratorio Centrale Ospedale di Careggi	300	ER, PgR	DCC	7 days	Italy
Ivrea Istituto di Ricerche Biomediche RBM	400	ER, PgR	DCC	2–3 weeks	Italy + EORTC
Lecce Istituto di Istologia Università Ospedale Fazzi		ER	DCC	3–4 weeks	Italy
Milano Istituto per la Cura dei Tumori	1,168	ER, PgR, AR, CR	DCC Sucrose/gradient	7 days	Italy
Napoli Istituto di Zoologia Università Centro Ricerche Ormonali	140	ER, PgR, AR	DCC	7 days	Italy
Istituto Patologia Generale Università (I. Facolt)	50	ER, PgR	DCC Sucrose/gradient	7 days	Italy
Palermo Istituto di Farmacologia Università	60	ER, PgR	DCC	1–2 weeks	Italy

Pavia					
Divisione di Oncologia Università	600	ER, PgR AR: if requested	DCC	7 days	Italy
Parma					
Servizio di Oncologia Ospedali Riun	250	ER, PgR	DCC	7 days	Italy + EORTC
Roma					
Istituto di Anat. Istol. Patol. U.C.S.C.	90	ER, PgR, AR, CR	DCC	1–2 weeks	Italy
Clinica Medica V. Università	900	ER, PgR, AR	DCC	2–3 weeks	Italy
Istituto di Patologia Gen. Sevizio di Oncologia	100	ER, PgR AR, CR: if requested	DCC	7 days	Italy
Torino					
Clinica Medica B. Università	180	ER, PgR, AR, CR	DCC	7 days	Italy
Verona					
Clinica Ostet-Ginecol. Università di Padova	180	ER, PgR	DCC	7 days	Italy

The Netherlands

A. Koenders

Department of Experimental and Chemical Endocrinology,
Medical Faculty, University of Nijmegen,
6500 HB Nijmegen, The Netherlands

Estrogen receptor measurements are presently performed by 16 institutions while 10 laboratories also assay progesterone receptors. Androgen and glucocorticoid receptors are measured by only a very few laboratories. Currently about 6,000 tumor samples, obtained from 150 hospitals, are analyzed for receptor activity per year. Routinely, the time required for response is about 1−3 weeks, while upon request the assay can be performed within 2 days.

All laboratories use a dextran-coated charcoal technique and the cytosolic receptor concentration is most frequently calculated by Scatchard plot analysis. In addition, a few investigators have other techniques available. Arbitrary cut-off levels, ranging between 2 and 10 fmol/mg protein, are most commonly applied to decide whether tumor samples are receptor positive or negative. Three groups establish threshold levels by means of a statistical evaluation of estrogen-binding capacities of benign and malignant breast cancers (probit analysis). The various investigators reported that 60%−75% of the tumors contain ER, while 51%−60% of the samples are classified as PgR positive.

To assess whether the employed method is within control, most laboratories analyze a receptor-positive control preparation together with each series of breast tumor assays. Finally, it should be noted that all laboratories performing receptor assays participate in a national interlaboratory quality control program (see Part 2).

Addresses	Characteristics			
	Receptor assays	Usual technique	Intralaboratory quality control	Interlaboratory quality control
Amersfoort Hospital "de Lichtenberg" Dept. Nuclear Medicine Utrechtseweg 160 3818 ES Amersfoort	ER	DCC-single dose	Receptor-negative preparation	Netherlands
Amsterdam Antoni van Leeuwenhoek Hospital Plesmanlaan 121 1066 CX Amsterdam	ER	DCC-single dose Isoelectric focusing method	Lyophilized calf uterine samples	Netherlands EORTC
Breda Stichting medische laboratoria Bergschot 121 4817 PA Breda	ER	DCC Scatchard plot analysis	None	Netherland
Delft S.S.D.Z. Dept. Pathology Reynier de Graeffweg 7 2600 GA Delft	ER PgR	DCC Scatchard plot analysis Histochemical method	Human uterine cytosol (liq N2)	Netherlands
Eindhoven Catharina Hospital Michel Angelolaan 2 Eindhoven	ER PgR	DCC Scatchard plot analysis	Calf uterus	Netherlands
Enschede Hospital "de Stadsmaten" Ariensplein 1 and Hospital "Ziekenzorg" Haaksbergerstraat 55 Enschede	ER PgR	DCC Scatchard plot analysis	Human uterus	Netherlands

Addresses	Characteristics		Intralaboratory quality control	Interlaboratory quality control
	Receptor assays	Usual technique		
Heerlen de Wever Hospital Henri Dunantstraat 5 6401 CX Heerlen	ER	DCC Scatchard plot analysis	Calf uterus	Netherlands
Leeuwarden Lab. voor de Volksgezondheid in Friesland Jelsumerstraat 6 8917 EN Leeuwarden	ER PgR	DCC Scatchard plot analysis	Rabbit uterine cytosol	Netherlands
Leiden Academic Hospital Dept. Path. Chemistry Rijnsburgerweg 10 2333 AA Leiden	ER (PgR)	DCC-single dose (Agar electrophoresis)	Calf uterus (−80 °C)	Netherlands
Nijmegen Academic Hospital Dept. Exp. and Chem. Endocrinology Geert Grooteplein Zuid 8 6500 HB Nijmegen	ER PgR	DCC Scatchard plot analysis (Gradient method) (H.A.P. adsorption)	Lyophilized reference preparations	Netherlands EORTC
Rotterdam Erasmus University Dept. Urology/Biochemistry II P.O. Box 1738 3000 DR Rotterdam	ER PgR (AR)	DCC Scatchard plot analysis	No	Netherlands

Institution	Receptor	Method	Preparation	Country
Rotterdamsch Radio Therapeutisch Instituut Dr. Daniel den Hoed Kliniek Dept. Biochemistry Groene Hilledijk 301 3075 EA Rotterdam	ER PgR (AR) (CR)	DCC Scatchard plot analysis (Agar electrophoresis) (Gradient method)	Lyophilized calf uterine cytosol	Netherlands EORTC
Tilburg Oncologisch Instituut "Dr. Bernard Verbeeten" Brugsestraat 10 P.O. Box 90120 5000 LA Tilburg	ER PgR	DCC Scatchard plot analysis	Lyophilized calf cytosol	Netherlands
Utrecht Academic Hospital Dept. of Endocrinology Catharijnesingel 101 3500 CG Utrecht	ER PgR	DCC Scatchard plot analysis (Protamine precipitation) (Gradient method) (Agar electrophoresis)	No	Netherlands
Vught Lab. voor Nucleaire Geneeskunde "Voorburg" Boxtelseweg 218 5261 NE Vught	ER PgR	DCC Scatchard plot analysis	Lyophilized calf and bovine uterine preparations	Netherlands
Zwolle Sophia Hospital Klin. Chem. Lab. C. A. Heesweg 2 Zwolle	ER	DCC-single dose	Receptor-positive preparation	Netherlands

Spain

P. Viladiu

Hospital Provincial de Sta. Caterina, Service d'Oncologia,
Girona, Spain

There are eight centers performing steroid receptors assays. Two of them function on a private basis and the remaining six within public hospitals. Social security funds the assays performed in the public institutions.

The methods used are similar in all centers, being based on McGuire's protocol (DCC-Scatchard plot analysis).

There is no national quality control.

Recent Results in Cancer Research. Vol. 91
© Springer-Verlag Berlin · Heidelberg 1984

Addresses	Characteristics				
	No. of samples/year	SR assay	Usual technique	Time required for response	Quality control
Barcelona					
M. A. Navarro C.S.S.S. "Principes de España" Seccion Hormonas Analisis Clínicos Hospitalet de Llob Barcelona	100	ER PgR	DCC Scatchard plot analysis	6–7 days	None
C. Esqué Serv. Bioquímica Hospital S. Pablo Barcelona	200	ER	DCC Scatchard plot analysis	20 days	Female rat uterus homogenates stabilized with DTT and glycerol 60% (stable over 3 months)
J. M. Castellanos Laboratorio Hormonas Residencia "F. Franco" Barcelona	100	ER	DCC Scatchard plot analysis	3 days	None
J. M. Castellanos Unitat Recerca Horm. Huntaner 492 Barcelona	100	ER		3 days	None
F. Rivera Labor. Bioquimi-Hormonal Hospital Clinico y Prov. Barcelona	150	ER PgR	DCC Scatchard plot analysis	15 days	None
D. Pons Centro Tecnico-Isotopos Radioactivos. C/Londres 6 Barcelona	100	ER PgR	DCC Scatchard plot analysis	8–10 days	None

Addresses	Characteristics				
	No. of samples/year	SR assay	Usual technique	Time required for response	Quality control
Madrid P. Gonzalez Gancedo Servicio Bioquimica "La Paz" Madrid	100	ER PgR	DCC Scatchard plot analysis	8 days	None
L. Marcos Servicio Medicina Nuclear Clinica Puerto de Hierro Madrid	160	ER PgR	DCC Scatchard plot analysis	10 days	Blind control

Added in Proofs (Eds.)

Update   Assays are now routinely performed in 3 additional centers
Granada –   V. Pedraza Muriel. Serv. Medicina Nuclear, Hospital Clinico Universitario, Granada
Las Palmas – B.N. Diaz Chico, Dept. Fisiología y Bioquímica, Hospital Universitario de Las Palmas, Aptdo. 550, Las Palmas de Gran Canaria.
Valencia –   J. Muñoz, Dept. Patologia Clinica, Ciudad Sanitaria "La Fe", Valencia.

Sweden (and Norway)

J. F. Sällström, Uppsala

University of Uppsala, Department of Pathology, University Hospital,
Sjukhusvägen 10, 75185 Uppsala, Sweden

Entries include the laboratories participating in the Swedish-Norwegian quality control program (see Part II).

Recent Results in Cancer Research. Vol. 91
© Springer-Verlag Berlin · Heidelberg 1984

Addresses	Characteristics				
	No. of samples/year	SR assay	Usual technique	Time required for response	Quality control
Göteborg J. Waldenström (A. Nilsson) Kliniskt-Kemiska Centrallaboratoriet Sahlgrenska sjukhuset S-413 45 Göteborg	The project started in 1982	ER PgR	DCC Scatchard plot analysis	1 week	Swedish Cancer Society's Coordinating Group for Clinical Steroid Receptor Research
Linköping R. Boll Receptor Laboratory Dept. of Pathology University Hospital S-581 85 Linköping	450	ER PgR	Isoelectric focusing	1–2 weeks	Swedish Cancer Society's Coordinating Group for Clinical Steroid Receptor Research
Lund M. Fernö Dept. of Oncology University Hospital S-221 85 Lund	550	ER PgR	Isoelectric focusing DCC technique with Scatchard plot analysis	Max. 2 weeks	Swedish Cancer Society's Coordinating Group for Clinical Steroid Receptor Research
Malmö R. Ekman Dept. of Nuclear Medicine Malmö General Hospital S-214 01 Malmö	300	ER PgR	Isoelectric focusing Scatchard plot analysis	1–2 weeks	Swedish Cancer Society's Coordinating Group for Clinical Steroid Receptor Research
Oslo O. Børmer Central Laboratory The Norwegian Radium Hospital Montebello N-Oslo 3 Norway	550	ER PgR	5-point DCC with Scatchard plot analysis	7 days	Internal (rat uterine cytosol and intact rat uterine tissue included in each run) plus samples distributed from the Swedish Cancer Society's Coordinating Group for Clinical Steroid Receptor Research

Stockholm L. Skoog Dept. of Tumor Pathology Karolinska Sjukhuset S-104 01 Stockholm	~ 1,000	ER PgR CR	Isoelectric focusing	2–4 days	Swedish Cancer Society's Coordinating Group for Clinical Steroid Receptor Research
Umeå L. Mörtberg Kliniskt-Kemiska Centrallaboratoriet Regionssjukhuset S-901 85 Umeå	100	ER	Isoelectric focusing	Max. 4 weeks	Swedish Cancer Society's Coordinating Group for Clinical Steroid Receptor Research
Uppsala J. F. Sällström Dept. of Pathology Univ. of Uppsala Academic Hospital S-751 85 Uppsala	300	ER PgR CR	Isoelectric focusing	8 days	Swedish Cancer Society's Coordinating Group for Clinical Steroid Receptor Research

Switzerland

G. Martz and D. T. Zava

Kantonsspital Zürich, Department für Innere Medizin, Abteilung Onkologie, Zürich, Switzerland

Estrogen and progesterone receptor assays are performed in six laboratories with a standard dextran-coated method. Receptor concentrations are calculated by Scatchard plot analysis. A quality control study is carried out among these laboratories. The Ludwig Institute for Cancer Research, Inselspital, Bern, is responsible for coordinating the study (Part II).

The cost of the receptor assay is not refunded by social security or by patient insurance.

Addresses	Characteristics				
	No. of samples/year	SR assay	Usual technique	Time required for response	Quality control
Basel U. Eppenberger Univ. Women's Clinic Laboratories 46 Schanzenstrasse 4031 Basel	600	ER PgR	DCC Scatchard plot analysis	Max. 2 weeks	Steroid Receptor Study Group of SAKK (Schweiz. Arbeitsgruppe für klinische Krebsforschung)
Bern D. T. Zava Ludwig Institute for Cancer Research Inselspital 3010 Bern 0 31/25 12 75		ER PgR	DCC Scatchard plot analysis		Steroid Receptor Study Group of SAKK
Genève G. Rosset Centre d'Oncohématologie Hôpital Cantonal 1211 Genève L 0 22/46 92 11	300	ER PgR	DCC Scatchard plot analysis	3 weeks	Steroid Receptor Study Group of SAKK
Lausanne T. Lemarchand-Beraud F. Gomez Division de Biochimie Clinique Département de Médecine C.H.U.V. 1011 Lausanne 0 21/41 54 93	220	ER PgR	DCC Scatchard plot analysis	Ca. 2 weeks	Steroid Receptor Study Group of SAKK

Addresses	Characteristics				
	Receptor assays	Usual technique	Intralaboratory quality control	Interlaboratory quality control
Locarno G. Losa Lab. of Cellular Pathology Istituto Cantonale di Patologia 6604 Locarno 0 93/31 36 60	170	ER PgR	DCC Scatchard plot analysis	4–7 days	Steroid Receptor Study Group of SAKK
Zürich S. Arrenbrecht Laboratorien Onkologie Universitätsspital Häldeliweg 4 8044 Zürich	600	ER PgR	DCC Scatchard plot analysis	2 weeks	Steroid Receptor Study Group of SAKK

Subject Index

Early Detection of Breast Cancer

Editors: **S. Brünner, B. Langfeldt, P. E. Andersen**
1984. 94 figures, 91 tables. XI, 214 pages
(Recent Results in Cancer Research, Volume 90)
ISBN 3-540-12348-2

The contributions presented in this book deal with all aspects of the diagnosis, classification, pathological anatomy, and treatment of breast cancer. Of special interest are reports on the results of screening projects in Sweden and the USA, on progress in early diagnosis using ultrasound and subtraction techniques, and on the current use of irradiation and breast-preserving surgical intervention in place of mastectomy in the USA and Denmark. The book is a synthesis of valuable information from scientists at leading mammographic centers, and will be useful to diagnosticians, radiotherapists, and surgeons as well as to medical students.

Contents: Hypothetical Breast Cancer Risk from Mammography. – Benefits and Risks of Mammography. – Multicentric Breast Carcinoma. – Breast Cancer in the Younger Patient: A Preliminary Report. – Bilateral Breast Carcinoma. – The Radiographic Appearance of Normal and Metastatic Axillary Lymph Nodes. – Evaluation of New Imaging Procedures for Breast Cancer. – Microfocal Spot Magnification Mammography. – Special Techniques in Mammography. – Magnification Mammography. – Enhanced-Image Mammography. – Breast Sonography and the Detection of Cancer. – Breast Cancer Screening: Expected and Observed Incidence and Stages of Female Breast Cancer in Gävleborg County, Sweden, and Implications for Mortality. – Five-Year Experience with Single-View Mammography Randomized Controlled Screening in Sweden. – Breast Cancer Screening in Malmö. – Experience from Randomized Controlled Breast Screening with Mammography in Östergötland County, Sweden: A Preliminary Report. – Breast Cancer Screening: Significance of Minimal Breast Cancers. – Localization and Significance of Clinically Occult Breast Lesions: Experience with 469 Needle-Guided Biopsies. – The Selective Treatment of "Early" Carcinoma of the Breast by Lumpectomy, Level I Axillary Dissection, and Radiation Therapy. – Breast Conserving Treatment in Breast Cancer: Clinical and Psychological Aspects. – Prognostic Pathologic Factors Among Breast Cancers Detected on Screening by Mammography. – What Can We Learn from Interval Carcinomas? – Detection Bias in Mammographic Screening for Breast Carcinoma. – Prognosis of Breast Cancer Related to Intramammary Lymph Nodes. – The Value of Mammography in Estimating the Prognosis for Patients with Breast Cancer. – Screening for Breast Cancer in Europe: Achievements, Problems, and Future. – The First Three Years of the Guildford Breast Screening Project. – Detection of Endocrine Responsiveness by Flow Cytometric DNA Analysis in Experimental Human Breast Cancer. – The Reliability of Frozen-Section Diagnosis in Various Breast Lesions: A Study Based on 3451 Biopsies.

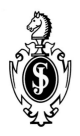

Springer-Verlag
Berlin
Heidelberg
New York
Tokyo

Recent Results in Cancer Research

Managing Editors:
Ch. Herfarth, H. J. Senn

A Selection

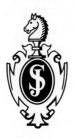

Springer-Verlag
Berlin
Heidelberg
New York
Tokyo

Volume 73
Thyroid Cancer
Editor: **W. Duncan**
1980. 58 figures, 30 tables. X, 142 pages
ISBN 3-540-09328-1

Volume 78
Prostate Cancer
Editor: **W. Duncan**
1981. 68 figures, 67 tables. X, 190 pages
ISBN 3-540-10676-6

Volume 84
Modified Nucleosides and Cancer
Editor: **G. Nass**
1983. 217 figures, 89 tables. XII, 432 pages
ISBN 3-540-12024-6

Volume 85
Urologic Cancer: Chemotherapeutic Principles and Management
Editor: **F. M. Torti**
1983. IX, 151 pages
ISBN 3-540-12163-3

Volume 86
Vascular Perfusion in Cancer Therapy
Editor: **K. Schwemmle, K. Aigner**
1983. 136 figures, 79 tables. XII, 295 pages
ISBN 3-540-12346-6

Volume 87
F. F. Holmes
Aging and Cancer
1983. 58 figures. VII, 75 pages
ISBN 3-540-12656-2

Volume 88
Paediatric Oncology
Editor: **W. Duncan**
1983. 28 figures, 38 tables. X, 116 pages
ISBN 3-540-12349-0

Volume 89
Pain in the Cancer Patient
Pathogenesis, Diagnosis and Therapy
Editors: **M. Zimmermann, P. Drings, G. Wagner**
1984. 67 figures, 57 tables. IX, 238 pages
ISBN 3-540-12347-4